PROFESSIONAL
QUICK REFERENCE

Cardiovascular drug therapy

Springhouse Corporation
Springhouse, Pennsylvania

Staff

Senior Publisher
Matthew Cahill

Clinical Manager
Cindy Tryniszewski, RN, MSN

Art Director
John Hubbard

Senior Editor
Stephen Daly

Clinical Project Manager
Judith E. Meissner, RN, MSN

Editors
Kathleen Beans, Neal Fandek, Ann Lenkiewicz, Jean Wallace

Clinical Editors
George J. Blake, RPh, MS; Marlene Ciranowicz, RN, MSN, CDE; Kathleen McGovern, RN, BSN, CCRN

Designers
Stephanie Peters (associate art director), Donald G. Knauss, Darcy Feralio

Copy Editors
Cynthia C. Breuninger (manager), Priscilla DeWitt, Lynette High, Jennifer George Mintzer, Doris Weinstock

Typography
Diane Paluba (manager), Elizabeth Bergman, Joyce Rossi Biletz, Phyllis Marron, Robin Mayer, Valerie Rosenberger

Manufacturing
Deborah C. Meiris (director), Pat Dorshaw (manager), Anna Brindisi, T.A. Landis

Editorial Project Coordinator
Patricia McCloskey

Editorial Assistants
Beverly Lane, Mary Madden

Indexer
Barbara Hodgson

Ⓡ A member of the Reed Elsevier plc group

Library of Congress Cataloging-in-Publication Data

Cardiovascular drug therapy
    p. cm. — (Professional quick reference)
    Includes index
    1. Cardiovascular agents—Handbooks, manuals, etc.
    2. Cardiovascular system—Diseases—Handbooks, manuals, etc. I. Springhouse Corporation. II. Title: Cardiovascular disorders. III. Series.
    [DNLM: 1. Cardiovascular Diseases—drug therapy—professional instruction. 2. Cardiovascular Diseases—drug therapy—handbooks. 3. Cardiovascular Agents—therapeutic use—professional instruction. 4. Cardiovascular Agents—therapeutic use—handbooks. WG 39 M423 1994]
RM345.M374 1994
616.1'061—dc20
DNLM/DLC   94-3076
ISBN 0-87434-714-9   CIP

Contents

Clinical consultants

Sandra Bixler, RN, MSN
Clinical Nurse Specialist
Berk Cardiologists, Ltd.
Reading, Pa.

Nancy R. Cirone, RN, MSN
Director, Educational Department
Medical College Hospitals
Bucks County Campus
Warminster, Pa.

Jalal K. Ghali, MD
Associate Professor of Medicine,
Cardiology
Louisiana State University Medical
Center
Shreveport

Henry G. Hanley, MD
Professor of Medicine, Chief of
Cardiology
Louisiana State University Medical
Center
Shreveport

Steven B. Meisel, PharmD
Assistant Director of Pharmacy
Fairview Southdale Hospital
Edina, Minn.

Kristine Ann Scordo, RN, PhD
Clinical Director, Clinical Nurse
Specialist
Cardiology Center of Cincinnati

Foreword

In recent years, your role in cardiovascular drug therapy has changed dramatically. And this sweeping trend is likely to continue through the end of this century. Not only do you have greater decision-making responsibilities than ever before, but you see ever-increasing numbers of severely ill patients who require complex drug therapies. What's more, all of this comes at a time when more medications are available than ever before.

So how do you stay current with state-of-the-art cardiovascular drug therapy, particularly when dealing with patients who have complicated cardiovascular disorders? The answer is *Professional Quick Reference: Cardiovascular Drug Therapy*, the first drug book that places medications in their therapeutic context. This handy volume tells you not only *which* drugs are currently being used for cardiovascular disorders, but also *when* and *how* they're used.

Cardiovascular Drug Therapy was conceived, written, and designed for use anywhere: in the hospital, clinic, or office or at the patient's bedside at home. The book contains two parts. The first, *Cardiovascular disorders and treatments*, is alphabetically arranged. It covers the most common and important cardiovascular disorders as well as their treatments, including drug therapy. Each disorder is succinctly defined and described, and the treatments are prioritized, highlighting the role of drug therapy within the course of each treatment plan.

Each cardiovascular drug used for a specific disorder appears with a page reference that refers you to the second part of the book, where you'll find complete drug information.

The second part of the book, *Cardiovascular drugs*, contains detailed information on nearly 100 drugs — also presented in alphabetical order — used to treat cardiovascular disorders. Each entry follows the same easy-to-follow format. A brief introduction describes the drug (detailing selected trade names), its therapeutic classification, and the different forms in which the drug is available. This is followed by *Pharmacokinetics*, where you'll review how the drug is absorbed, distributed, metabolized, and excreted.

The next section, *Indications, dosage, and action*, details the drug's cardiovascular uses and dosages (both adult and pediatric) as well as its action — how the drug works within the body. Next comes *Contraindications and cautions*, which identifies when the drug must be avoided or used cautiously. Also identified are the potential results if the drug is given in these circumstances, along with each drug's pregnancy risk category.

The pregnancy risk category refers to the five categories (A, B, C, D, or X) established by the Food and Drug Administration to indicate a drug's potential for causing birth defects. The categories are:
• A: Adequate studies in pregnant women have failed to show a risk to the fetus in the first trimester of

pregnancy, and there is no evidence of risk in later trimesters.

• B: Animal studies haven't shown an adverse effect on the fetus, but no adequate studies in pregnant women exist.

• C: Animal studies have shown an adverse effect on the fetus, but there are no adequate studies in humans. Or, there are no adequate studies in animals or humans and pregnancy risk is unknown.

• D: Evidence of risk to the human fetus exists, but the potential benefits in pregnant women may be acceptable.

• X: Studies in animals or humans show fetal abnormalities, or adverse reaction reports indicate evidence of fetal risk. The risks clearly outweigh potential benefits.

The next section, *Adverse reactions*, is conveniently divided into three categories: life-threatening, common, and infrequent. Incidence statistics appear for common reactions, when available. The following section, *Interactions*, identifies important drug combinations that can cause potentially hazardous or varying therapeutic responses. Next, *Interventions* tells how to prepare and administer the drug as well as how to monitor the patient receiving it.

Throughout the second part of the book, you'll come upon graphic devices called logos that direct you to essential information. For example, *Interactions alert* warns of the potentially life-threatening hazards of administering multiple drugs to the same patient, while *Incompatibility warning* alerts you to drugs that can't be mixed. *Administration guidelines* provides concise directions on preparing and giving certain drugs, while *Compliance build-er* gives helpful advice on how to get patients to cooperate with their drug therapy regimen. *Patient-teaching checklist* presents a handy rundown of important topics you need to teach the patient.

You'll also find logos, such as *Treatment of choice* in the first part of the book and *Safety tips* in the second part, that call your attention to important considerations when caring for patients taking certain drugs. Finally, after each drug entry, you'll find a *MedTest* — questions that can be used to assess your level of knowledge and to serve as a quick review. The answers to the MedTests appear in the back of the book, where you'll also find helpful appendices that compare cardiovascular drugs within certain classes.

With the development of new and improved drugs, advances in understanding the pathophysiology of cardiovascular disorders, and innovations in diagnostics and treatments, it's little wonder how difficult it is to stay abreast of drug therapies. But I know you'll find *Cardiovascular Drug Therapy* a unique and indispensable resource. It's not only thorough and current, but easy to use — a first-of-its-kind book that will provide exactly the cardiovascular drug information you need to know now.

Patricia E. Casey, RN, MSN
Education Coordinator,
Cardiovascular Nursing
Department of Nursing Education
and Research
Fairfax Hospital,
Falls Church, Va.

Introduction

Recent advances in cardiovascular drug therapy are unparalleled in medical history. As a result of our increased understanding of the pathophysiology and molecular biology of cardiovascular diseases, newer, more effective cardiovascular drugs have been introduced. And their success in preventing and treating cardiovascular diseases is well documented.

These advances, however, make it imperative that health care professionals keep up-to-date with the latest developments in cardiovascular drug therapy so that they can skillfully manage patients with cardiovascular disorders and initiate preventive strategies for those people not yet affected by symptomatic cardiovascular disease.

In recent years, cardiovascular drug therapy has improved in many areas, but progress has been particularly exciting in the treatment of hyperlipidemia, myocardial ischemia and infarction, arrhythmias, and heart failure.

Coronary artery disease (CAD) is still the leading cause of death in the United States. But recognizing the pivotal role that hyperlipidemia — particularly hypercholesterolemia — plays in CAD has helped reduce mortality and morbidity substantially. Cholesterol-lowering drugs have not only reduced atherosclerosis but also helped prevent progression of the disease in patients who are asymptomatic.

Drugs such as lovastatin, pravastatin, and simvastatin have lowered cholesterol levels with few adverse effects and have helped control hypercholesterolemia in patients who are unresponsive to dietary changes alone. Still, identifying and treating more and more of these patients requires waging a continuing campaign to alert the public and educate the health care professionals who care for them. But with an estimated 60 million Americans affected by hypercholesterolemia, the potential benefits are enormous.

Treatment of stable angina pectoris improved markedly when calcium channel blockers were first introduced, and the continuing refinement of these drugs has led to more selective second-generation calcium channel blockers, such as amlodipine, which have proved even more successful.

Thrombolytic agents, such as tissue plasminogen activator, streptokinase, and urokinase, have been shown to reduce mortality in acute myocardial infarction (MI) when used early in treatment. But again, to be effective, thrombolytic therapy requires early diagnosis and intervention, which in turn requires educating the public to seek treatment as soon as possible after the onset of symptoms. And it increases the need for developing newer techniques to diagnose acute MI as early and accurately as possible.

Treatment of ventricular arrhythmias has undergone dramatic change, particularly in patients who have suffered MI. Beta-adrenergic blocking agents have helped reduce mortality in the early and late stages of MI. And one particular beta blocker, sotalol, has shown promise in preventing sudden cardiac death. There is also mounting evidence that another antiarrhythmic agent, amiodarone, improves a patient's chances for survival after MI.

As our population has aged, the lives of patients with ischemic heart disease have been prolonged; however, the prevalence of heart failure also continues to rise. Yet the survival rate of these patients has improved substantially with the use of angiotensin-converting enzyme (ACE) inhibitors, such as captopril, lisinopril, and ramipril. Several studies have shown an increase in survival rate and a corresponding decrease in hospitalization rate when one ACE inhibitor, enalapril, was used in patients with heart failure and impaired left ventricular systolic function. In addition, the use of enalapril in patients with impaired left ventricular systolic function, but with no other symptoms of heart failure, has been shown to prevent or delay the onset of heart failure.

Despite these improvements, however, the full impact of ACE inhibitors on patients with heart failure has yet to be realized. There is still an alarmingly slow response among health care professionals in prescribing these drugs for them. In fact, a recent survey of cardiologists, internists, and family physicians showed that ACE inhibitors were used as first-line drugs in treating heart failure in only 30% of their patients. But there is no question that better education of health care professionals would ensure greater use of such drugs in clinical practice.

Taken as a whole, these advances in cardiovascular pharmacology show great promise in preventing and treating cardiovascular disorders. But before patients can have early access to the newest, most effective cardiovascular drugs, all health care professionals need to have an understanding of cardiovascular pharmacology and its appropriate applications. That's what makes *Cardiovascular Drug Therapy* such a useful and forward-thinking book, one that all health care professionals will find both practical and enlightening.

Henry G. Hanley, MD
Professor of Medicine,
Chief of Cardiology
Louisiana State University
Medical Center
Shreveport, La.

Jalal K. Ghali, MD
Associate Professor of Medicine,
Cardiology
Louisiana State University
Medical Center
Shreveport, La.

Guide to abbreviations

ABG	arterial blood gas	I.M.	intramuscular
a.c.	before meals	IU	International Units
ACE	angiotensin-converting enzyme	lb	pound
		LD	lactate dehydrogenase
ACLS	advanced cardiac life support	MAO	monoamine oxidase
		MI	myocardial infarction
ALP	alkaline phosphatase	0.9% NaCl	0.9% sodium chloride
ALT	alanine aminotransferase	NSAID	nonsteroidal anti-inflammatory drug
APTT	activated partial thromboplastin time		
		OTC	over-the-counter
AST	aspartate aminotransferase	PAC	premature atrial contraction
AV	atrioventricular	$PaCO_2$	partial pressure of arterial carbon dioxide
b.i.d.	twice daily		
BUN	blood urea nitrogen	PaO_2	partial pressure of arterial oxygen
CABG	coronary artery bypass grafting		
		PAP	pulmonary artery pressure
CAD	coronary artery disease	PAT	paroxysmal atrial tachycardia
CBC	complete blood count		
CHF	congestive heart failure	PAWP	pulmonary artery wedge pressure
CK	creatine kinase		
CNS	central nervous system	p.c.	after meals
CO_2	carbon dioxide	PJC	premature junctional contraction
COPD	chronic obstructive pulmonary disease		
		P.O.	by mouth
CPR	cardiopulmonary resuscitation	PVC	premature ventricular contraction
CSF	cerebrospinal fluid	PSVT	paroxysmal supraventricular tachycardia
CV	cardiovascular		
CVA	cerebrovascular accident	PT	prothrombin time
CVP	central venous pressure	PTCA	percutaneous transluminal coronary angioplasty
D_5W	dextrose 5% in water		
ECG	electrocardiogram	PTT	partial thromboplastin time
FDA	Food and Drug Administration	q	every
		q.i.d.	four times a day
GI	gastrointestinal	SA	sinoatrial
GU	genitourinary	S.C.	subcutaneous
HCl	hydrochloride	SSS	sick sinus syndrome
HDL	high-density lipoprotein	TIA	transient ischemic attack
HNKS	hyperosmolar nonketotic syndrome	VLDL	very low-density lipoprotein
		VT	ventricular tachycardia (tachyarrhythmia)
h.s.	at bedtime		
IABP	intra-aortic balloon pump	WBC	white blood cell
ICP	intracranial pressure	WPW	Wolff-Parkinson-White

Cardiovascular disorders and treatments

Abdominal aortic aneurysm

An abnormal dilation in the arterial wall, abdominal aneurysm typically occurs in the aorta between the renal arteries and the aortic bifurcation. A focal weakness in the muscular layer of the aorta (tunica media) stretches the inner layer (tunica intima) and outer layer (tunica adventitia) outward. As the aorta widens, tension in the wall of the aorta weakens the vessel walls and enlarges the aneurysm.

Abdominal aneurysms occur most commonly in hypertensive white males ages 50 to 80. Arteriosclerosis and atherosclerosis account for nearly 95% of abdominal aortic aneurysms; cystic medial necrosis, trauma, syphilis, and other infections cause the rest.

More than 50% of all patients with untreated abdominal aneurysms die of hemorrhage and shock within 2 years of diagnosis; more than 85%, within 5 years. Half of all aneurysms larger than 2½" (6 cm) in diameter rupture within 1 year, compared with less than 20% of smaller aneurysms. However, the prognosis is good with surgical repair.

Treatment

Treatment of choice. Resection of the aneurysm should accompany Dacron graft replacement of the aortic section. If the aneurysm is small and the patient is asymptomatic, surgery may be delayed, with regular physical examinations and ultrasonography used to monitor the aneurysm. However, large aneurysms that cause symptoms risk rupture and require immediate repair.

• In acute dissection, emergency treatment includes fluid replacement therapy and transfusion, I.V. *esmolol* (p. 150) or *propranolol* (p. 280) to reduce myocardial contractility (I.V. esmolol is easier to titrate than propranolol), I.V. *nitroglycerin* (p. 233) and I.V. *nitroprusside* (p. 240) to reduce systolic pressure and maintain it at 100 to 120 mm Hg, and analgesics, such as *morphine sulfate* (p. 233) or meperidine, to relieve pain. An arterial line, an indwelling urinary catheter, and a pulmonary artery catheter are then inserted to monitor the patient's condition and hemodynamic balance.

Aberrant ventricular conduction

A supraventricular impulse, aberrant ventricular conduction refers to a delay in conduction before the ventricles are activated. The QRS complex is prolonged (but usually less than 0.14 second) and reflects the type of intraventricular block, most commonly right bundle-branch block with secondary T-wave changes.

Possible causes of aberrant ventricular conduction include a changing heart rate caused by a sudden shortening in cycle length; metabolic and electrolyte abnormalities; toxic effects of drugs that affect ventricular repolarization time, such as procainamide and quinidine; preexcitation syndromes; and other electrophysiologic changes.

Treatment

• Interventions are usually unnecessary. However, aberrant ventricular conduction may signal an underlying problem that may require treatment, such as an electrolyte imbalance or hypoxia.

• If drug toxicity causes the aberrant ventricular conduction, discontinue the drug. Avoid using other drugs unless the patient is symptomatic or hemodynamically compromised.

Accelerated idioventricular rhythm

A benign escape rhythm, accelerated idioventricular rhythm results from slowed conduction through the SA node, producing AV dissociation. Its onset and termination are typically gradual, occurring with fusion beats because the usual rate of the accelerated idioventricular rhythm commonly approximates that of the normal sinus rhythm. An accelerated idioventricular rhythm may be mistaken for VT if the ventricular rate isn't carefully counted. But it's usually transient and intermittent and doesn't affect the patient's underlying condition or his prognosis.

On an ECG, the atrial rate matches the ventricular rate if retrograde conduction occurs. The ventricular rate ranges from 55 to 120 beats/minute. An inverted P wave may follow the QRS complex, which is usually wide, exceeding 0.12 second. The T wave usually deflects opposite the QRS complex. Abnormal ventricular repolarization occurs when depolarization is abnormal, and the QT interval is usually prolonged.

Accelerated idioventricular rhythm may be caused by MI, slowed sinus rate, or premature beats that cause a long pause in the cardiac cycle. It may be seen as a reperfusion arrhythmia in acute MI patients receiving thrombolytic therapy.

Treatment

• Treatment is needed only if signs of hemodynamic impairment appear.

• With hemodynamic impairment, treatment includes *atropine* (p. 83) or *isoproterenol* (p. 181) and, if needed, atrial pacing to suppress the rhythm.

• Don't give lidocaine because this drug stops ventricular function and may cause asystole in patients with accelerated idioventricular rhythm.

• Treat the underlying condition, such as an electrolyte imbalance or MI, to prevent a recurrence.

Accelerated junctional rhythm

An ectopic rhythm, accelerated junctional rhythm originates in the junctional tissue or bundle of His. The impulses control the ventricular rate at 60 to 100 beats/minute, which exceeds the rate of the junctional pacemaker. Most patients with an accelerated junctional rhythm don't have symptoms because they have adequate cardiac output.

Distinguishing ECG characteristics include a P wave that's usually inverted and that may precede or follow the QRS complex. However, the

P wave may be absent or buried in the QRS complex. If the P wave precedes the QRS complex, the PR interval is less than 0.12 second.

Possible causes are conditions that may produce long pauses in the cardiac cycle, such as SA node ischemia, SSS, increased vagal tone, and digitalis toxicity.

Treatment

• Treatment generally isn't necessary because the ventricular rate is usually normal. If a patient does develop symptoms, however, *atropine* (p. 83) may be administered to increase the sinus rate and enhance conduction through the SA node.
• Alternative treatment may include a temporary pacemaker to enhance the patient's atrial rate and control his ventricular rate. This is used only if the patient has symptoms of decreased cardiac output.

Aortic insufficiency

A chronic disorder, aortic insufficiency (also known as aortic regurgitation) is the backflow of blood through the aortic valve into the left ventricle during diastole. The ventricle gradually becomes overloaded and dilated, and it eventually hypertrophies. The excess blood volume also overloads the left atrium and, eventually, the pulmonary system, potentially causing angina, heart failure, myocardial ischemia, and fatal pulmonary edema.

Aortic insufficiency is most common in men. When associated with mitral valve disease, however, it's more common in women. It's also as-sociated with Marfan syndrome, ankylosing spondylitis, syphilis, and essential hypertension.

Aortic insufficiency most commonly results from rheumatic fever, although it may also stem from endocarditis or trauma.

Following diagnosis, approximately 75% of patients survive for 5 years and 50% for 10 years. Without surgery, death usually occurs within 4 years after development of angina and within 2 years after the onset of heart failure.

Treatment

Treatment of choice. Valve replacement should be performed before significant left ventricular dysfunction occurs.
• Treatment of left ventricular failure may include ACE inhibitors such as *captopril* (p. 99) or *enalapril* (p. 143), digitalis glycosides such as *digoxin* (p. 118), diuretics such as *furosemide* (p. 162), vasodilators such as *nitroglycerin* (p. 233), and a low-sodium diet.
• Long-term administration of arteriolar smooth-muscle relaxers such as *hydralazine* (p. 174) and of calcium channel blockers, such as *diltiazem* (p. 127), *nicardipine* (p. 228), or *nifedipine* (p. 230), may improve systolic function.
• Patients with mild or moderate aortic insufficiency who are asymptomatic and have a normal or slightly enlarged heart require only antibiotic prophylaxis.
• Supplemental oxygen may be necessary in acute episodes.

Aortic stenosis

In this disorder, the opening of the aortic valve becomes narrowed and the left ventricle must exert increased pressure to expel blood through the opening. The added workload causes the left ventricle to hypertrophy, increasing the demand for oxygen and reducing coronary artery perfusion, which causes ischemia of the left ventricle and, eventually, heart failure.

Aortic stenosis is the most significant valvular lesion in elderly men (only 20% of patients are women) and proves fatal in up to two-thirds of patients. Its incidence increases with age. Signs and symptoms may not appear until the patient reaches age 70 or older, even when the lesion has been present since childhood. Sudden death, possibly caused by an arrhythmia, occurs in up to 20% of patients, usually around age 60.

Aortic stenosis may result from congenital aortic bicuspid valve defects (associated with coarctation of the aorta), congenital stenosis of pulmonic valve cusps, rheumatic fever, or atherosclerosis.

Treatment

• Digitalis glycosides such as *digoxin* (p. 118), diuretics such as *furosemide* (p. 162), a low-sodium diet and, in acute cases, oxygen are used to treat heart failure. *Nitroglycerin* (p. 233) may help relieve angina.
• Simple commissurotomy is usually effective in children with normal valves. Adults with calcified valves will need valve replacement surgery once they become symptomatic or are at risk for developing left ventricular failure.
• Percutaneous balloon aortic valvuloplasty may improve left ventricular function in children and young adults who have congenital aortic stenosis and in elderly patients with severe calcification. These patients can then tolerate valve replacement surgery.

Arterial occlusive disease

An obstruction or narrowing of the aorta's lumen and major branches, arterial occlusive disease interrupts blood flow, usually to the legs and feet. This disorder may affect the carotid, vertebral, innominate, subclavian, mesenteric, and celiac arteries.

Arterial occlusive disease occurs more commonly in men than in women. The prognosis depends on the location of the occlusion, the development of collateral circulation to counteract reduced blood flow and, in acute disease, the amount of time between the formation of the occlusion and its removal. Occlusions, which may be acute or chronic, commonly cause severe ischemia, skin ulceration, and gangrene.

The most common cause of an acute arterial occlusion is obstruction of a major artery by a clot. The occlusive mechanism may be endogenous, resulting from formation of emboli, thrombi, or plaques, or it may be exogenous, resulting from trauma or fracture. Chronic arterial occlusive disease is a common complication of atherosclerosis. Predisposing factors include smoking; aging; conditions such as hypertension, hyperlipidemia, and diabetes mellitus; and a family history of vascular disorders, MI, or CVA.

Treatment

• In mild, chronic arterial occlusive disease, treatment usually consists of supportive measures, such as abstention from smoking, control of hypertension, walking for exercise, and appropriate foot and leg care.

• Antiplatelet therapy with aspirin or, for patients unable to tolerate aspirin, ticlopidine may be instituted in carotid artery occlusion. *Heparin* (p. 169) is used for acute TIAs.

• *Pentoxifylline* (p. 246) may improve blood flow through the capillaries for patients with intermittent claudication caused by chronic arterial occlusive disease. This drug is particularly useful for patients who are poor surgical candidates.

• Heparin prevents formation of emboli (from thrombotic occlusion) and usually precedes long-term *warfarin* (p. 321) therapy.

• Thrombolytics, such as *alteplase* (p. 65), *streptokinase* (p. 301), and urokinase, can dissolve clots and relieve the obstruction caused by a thrombus. Intra-arterial thrombolytics are increasingly used in acute arterial occlusive disease.

• The following surgical procedures may also be required:

Embolectomy. A balloon-tipped Fogarty catheter is used to remove thrombotic material from the artery. Embolectomy is used mainly for mesenteric, femoral, or popliteal artery occlusion. Following an embolectomy, patients usually receive long-term warfarin.

Thromboendarterectomy. In this procedure, the artery is opened, and the obstructing thrombus and medial layer of the arterial wall are removed. Plaque deposits remain intact. Thromboendarterectomy is usually performed after angiography and is often used with autogenous vein or Dacron graft bypass surgery (femoropopliteal or aortofemoral).

Percutaneous transluminal angioplasty (PTA). Using fluoroscopy and a special balloon catheter, the doctor dilates the stenotic or occluded artery to a predetermined diameter, taking care not to overdistend it.

Laser surgery. An excimer or a hot-tip laser obliterates the clot and plaque by vaporizing it.

Patch grafting. The thrombotic arterial segment is removed and replaced with an autogenous vein or a Dacron graft.

Bypass graft. Blood flow is diverted through an anastomosed autogenous vein or a woven Dacron graft to bypass the thrombotic arterial segment.

Lumbar sympathectomy. Depending on the condition of the sympathetic nervous system, the sympathetic lumbar nerve may be severed as an adjunct to reconstructive surgery.

• Amputation may be necessary if arterial reconstructive surgery fails or if gangrene, uncontrollable infection, or intractable pain develops.

• Bowel resection with restoration of blood flow is required for mesenteric artery occlusion.

Asystole

A life-threatening arrhythmia, asystole is the total absence of ventricular electrical activity. Some atrial activity may occur, but atrial impulses aren't conducted to the ventricles. Without ventricular electrical activity, ventricular contraction and cardiac output and perfusion don't occur.

Asystole may mimic fine ventricular fibrillation. If all ECG leads aren't placed properly, the resulting waveform may also resemble asystole.

On an ECG, the waveform is an almost flat line. Atrial rhythm and rate are usually indiscernible, and ventricular rhythm and rate are absent.

Possible causes of asystole include severe metabolic deficits, acute respiratory failure, or extensive myocardial damage, possibly from myocardial ischemia, MI, or a ruptured or ventricular aneurysm. Asystole is fatal without successful therapy.

Treatment

- Perform CPR immediately to restore respiration and circulation.
- Carry out ACLS measures, including adjunctive breathing and circulation techniques, cardiac monitoring, I.V. infusions, drug therapy, ABG analysis, and cardiac pacing.
- Drug therapy includes *atropine* (p. 83) and *epinephrine* (p. 146) to restore cardiac rhythm and sodium bicarbonate to treat developing metabolic acidosis.
- Assist with external pacing or temporary transvenous pacemaker insertion, if performed.

- Once the cardiac rhythm is restored, treat the cause of asystole, such as hypoxia or MI.

Atrial fibrillation

Extremely rapid, incomplete contractions of the atria, atrial fibrillation results from impulses in multiple circus reentry pathways in the atria. The impulses usually fire at a rate of 400 to 600 per minute, causing the atria to quiver instead of contract regularly. The ventricles respond only to impulses that pass through the AV node.

Atrial fibrillation eliminates the atrial contraction or kick, which accounts for 10% to 20% of normal end-diastolic volume. If the ventricular rate is fast and diastolic filling time is diminished, cardiac output will decline.

If atrial fibrillation is not treated, a further decline in cardiac output, CHF, hypotension, cardiogenic shock, or myocardial ischemia may follow. Mural thrombi may also develop in the atria, posing the risk of systemic or pulmonary emboli and cerebral vascular occlusion.

Both atrial and ventricular rhythms are grossly irregular. The atrial rate, almost indiscernible, usually exceeds 400 beats/minute. The ventricular rate usually ranges from 100 to 150 beats/minute but can fall below 100 beats/minute.

On an ECG, erratic baseline f (fibrillary) waves appear instead of P waves, representing multiple wavelets of atrial depolarization. When these chaotic f waves are pronounced, the arrhythmia is called *coarse atrial fibrillation*. When they aren't pronounced, the arrhythmia is called *fine atrial fibrillation*. The duration and configuration of the QRS complex are usually normal. If ventricular conduction is aberrant, the QRS complex may be wide and abnormally shaped. Atrial fib-flutter, a rhythm that frequently varies between a fibrillary line and flutter waves, may appear.

Possible causes include rheumatic heart disease, valvular disorders (especially mitral stenosis), hypertension, MI, CAD, CHF, cardiomyopathy, and pericarditis. Noncardiac causes include alcoholism, thyrotoxicosis, and COPD. Digitalis glycosides and, occasionally, increased sympathetic activity from exercise may also cause this arrhythmia. Atrial fibrillation may also be idiopathic.

Treatment

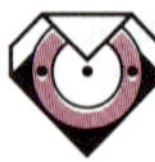 **Treatment of choice.** Drug therapy is the preferred treatment. Give such drugs as *digoxin* (p. 118), *diltiazem* (p. 127), *propranolol* (p. 280), and *verapamil* (p. 316) to block AV nodal conduction and decrease the ventricular response. This gives the SA node a chance to reestablish its role as the heart's pacemaker.

• Following AV blockade, *procainamide* (p. 272) or *quinidine* (p. 284) may be given to prolong the atrial refractory period. However, if these drugs are given without first blocking the AV node, they can worsen the condition by increasing conduction through the AV node.

• Perform synchronized cardioversion immediately if the patient has hypotension, syncope, or worsening angina pectoris. If the patient can't maintain a normal sinus rhythm after repeated cardioversion, such medications as a digitalis glycoside, propranolol, or verapamil are used to control the ventricular rate or response.

• Perform Valsalva's maneuver, carotid sinus massage, or gag reflex stimulation if atrial fibrillation is acute and the patient is hemodynamically stable.

• Institute anticoagulant therapy with *heparin* (p. 169) or *warfarin* (p. 321) as prescribed, especially before cardioversion or in patients with a history of valvular disorders.

• Discover and treat the underlying cause of atrial fibrillation to help prevent a recurrence.

Atrial flutter

Characterized by a rapid atrial rate, atrial flutter results from circus reentry and possibly from increased automaticity. The significance of atrial flutter depends on the extent to which the ventricular rate is accelerated. But even a small rise in the rate can cause angina, syncope, hypotension, CHF, or pulmonary edema, especially in a compromised heart.

On an ECG, ventricular rhythm depends on the AV conduction pattern; it's often regular, although cycles may alternate. The atrial rate is 250 to 400 beats/ minute. The ventricular rate depends on the degree of AV block; usually, it's 60 to 100 beats/ minute, but it may accelerate to 125 to 150 beats/minute. Saw-toothed waves, called flutter (or F) waves, appear. The patient may develop an atrial rhythm that varies between a fibrillary line and flutter waves, called atrial fib-flutter; the ventricular response is irregular.

Possible causes of atrial flutter include acute or chronic cardiac disorders, mitral or tricuspid valve disorders, cor pulmonale, and cardiac infections such as pericarditis. Atrial flutter may also occur as a transient complication of inferior wall MI, digitalis toxicity, hyperthyroidism, or alcoholism. The prognosis depends on the underlying cause.

Treatment
• Immediately perform synchronized cardioversion or give drugs that rapidly prolong AV conduction time, such as *digoxin* (p. 118), *propranolol* (p. 280), *or verapamil* (p. 316), if the patient has a rapid ventricular rate, reduced cardiac output, and signs and symptoms of CHF or myocardial ischemia. However, don't give digoxin if the arrhythmia is caused by digitalis toxicity.
• *Procainamide* (p. 272) or *quinidine* (p. 284) may be given to convert atrial flutter to atrial fibrillation, which is easier to control. However, atrial flutter that is resistant to pharmacologic conversion may require electroconversion. When digoxin and quinidine are used concurrently, digitalization must be achieved before quinidine can be given. This is because quinidine may lower the atrial rate, allowing the AV node to conduct impulses on a 1:1 ratio, which results in an extremely rapid heart rate.

• Use carotid sinus massage, if prescribed, to help identify atrial flutter. This procedure temporarily slows the ventricular rate, allowing flutter waves to be seen more clearly on the ECG. Always have an I.V. line in place and *atropine* (p. 83) available when performing carotid sinus massage.
• Consider atrial flutter controlled if the ventricular rate falls below 100 beats/minute.

Atrial septal defect
An opening between the left and right atria, an atrial septal defect allows blood to shunt between the chambers. Because atrial pressure is normally slightly higher in the left atrium than in the right, blood typically shunts from left to right. The left-to-right shunt results in right ventricular volume overload, which affects the right atrium, right ventricle, and pulmonary arteries. Eventually, the right atrium enlarges and the right ventricle dilates to accommodate the increased blood volume.

The degree of the left-to-right shunt through the defect depends on the size of the defect, the compliance of the ventricles, and pulmonary and systemic vascular resistance. The pressure difference may force large amounts of blood through the defect during late systole and early diastole. If the hole is more than 1 cm in diameter, the atria may act as a single chamber.

Atrial septal defect is found in about 10% of children with congenital heart disease who have survived past their first birthday. The disorder is almost twice as common in girls as in boys and has a strong familial tendency. Delayed development of signs, symptoms, and complications makes this one of the most common congenital heart defects diagnosed in adolescence and adulthood. The cause of this disorder is unknown.

Children with atrial septal defect may be easily fatigued, physically underdeveloped, and prone to respiratory infections. Adults may experience cyanosis, right and left ventricular hypertrophy, atrial arrhythmias, heart failure, and emboli, but children seldom have these complications. The prognosis is excellent in asymptomatic patients, but poor in those with cyanosis.

Treatment

Treatment of choice. Surgical repair of the defect is the primary treatment. No specific drug therapy exists. Because this defect rarely produces complications in infants and toddlers, surgery may be delayed until they reach preschool (ages 2 to 4) or early-school age. A large defect may need immediate surgical closure with sutures or a patch graft.

Atrial tachycardia

Characterized by three or more consecutive ectopic atrial beats occurring at a rate between 160 and 250 beats/minute, atrial tachycardia is benign when it occurs in a healthy person. But this arrhythmia may be dangerous when it occurs in a patient with an existing cardiac disorder.

On an ECG, the P wave is usually positive but may be aberrant. If visible, it precedes each QRS complex.

Digitalis toxicity is the most common cause of atrial tachycardia. This disorder can also be caused by primary cardiac disorders, such as MI, congenital heart disease, cardiomyopathy, pericarditis, valvular disease, or WPW syndrome, or by secondary cardiac problems, such as hyperthyroidism, cor pulmonale, or systemic hypertension. It may also occur in patients with COPD. In otherwise healthy patients, atrial tachycardia can result from physical or psychological stress, hypoxia, hypokalemia, or excessive use of caffeine, other stimulants, or marijuana.

Treatment

• The doctor may prescribe carotid sinus massage, gag reflex stimulation, Valsalva's maneuver, or synchronized cardioversion if signs and symptoms are severe. These measures slow impulses from the SA and AV nodes and trigger atrial standstill, enabling the SA node to function as the main pacemaker again.

• Drug therapy may include *adenosine* (p. 64), *digoxin* (p. 118) (unless digitalis toxicity is the cause of the arrhythmia), *diltiazem* (p. 127), *propranolol* (p. 280), or *verapamil* (p. 316). These drugs increase the AV block, thereby decreasing the ventricular response. After the block occurs, *procainamide* (p. 272) or *quinidine* (p. 284) can be given to establish a normal sinus rhythm.

• When conventional treatments fail, pacing may be used to override the atrial rate.

Atrial tachycardia, multifocal

This form of atrial tachycardia is caused by extremely rapid firing of multifocal ectopic beats. Benign when it occurs in healthy persons, this arrhythmia is usually found in acutely ill patients with pulmonary disease or elevated atrial pressures. Both atrial and ventricular rhythms are irregular, and atrial and ventricular rates range from 100 to 250 beats/minute.

The ECG usually reveals at least three unique P waves, but the configuration may vary. The PR interval also varies. The QRS complex is usually normal but may become aberrant if the arrhythmia persists.

Atrial distention from elevated pulmonary pressure, usually seen in patients with COPD, is a possible cause.

Treatment

• Immediate therapy, if required, is the same as that for atrial tachycardia.
• Antiarrhythmic drugs should not be given until the underlying cause of the arrhythmia is identified and treated.
• Drug therapy may include *digoxin* (p. 118), edrophonium, *esmolol* (p. 150), *propranolol* (p. 280), or *verapamil* (p. 316) to decrease the ventricular response.
• Pacing may be used to override the atrial rate and terminate the arrhythmia when conventional treatments fail.

Atrial tachycardia, paroxysmal

A type of PSVT, PAT arises suddenly. Typically, it follows frequent PACs, one of which precipitates the tachycardia. This arrhythmia is benign when it occurs in a healthy person, unless the PAT is sustained. Both atrial and ventricular rhythms may be regular or may start and stop abruptly. Atrial and ventricular rates range from 160 to 250 beats/minute.

On an ECG, the P wave may be inverted or retrograde and may be indistinguishable from the preceding T wave. Consequently, the PR interval may be unmeasurable. The QRS complex may become aberrant if the arrhythmia persists, and the QT interval is usually shorter because of the rapid rate.

A frequent cause is digitalis toxicity, commonly indicated by an atrial rate that's exactly twice the ventricular rate. Other causes are the same as those for atrial tachycardia.

Treatment

• Immediate therapy is the same as that for atrial tachycardia.
• The drug of choice is *adenosine* (p. 64) or *verapamil* (p. 316), both of which terminate most PATs or slow ventricular conduction to facilitate diagnosis. Verapamil is almost as effective as adenosine but is considerably less expensive.
• Other drug treatments are the same as those for atrial tachycardia.

Atrial tachycardia with block

In this arrhythmia, the atrial rate accelerates and AV conduction is impaired, leading to AV block. Ventricular rhythm is regular if the block is constant, but irregular if it's variable. The atrial rate ranges from 160 to 250 beats/minute and will be a multiple of the ventricular rate, which varies.

On an ECG, the P wave configuration is slightly abnormal. More than one P wave appears for each QRS complex.

Possible causes include increased automaticity and digitalis toxicity.

Treatment
- Immediate therapy is the same as that for atrial tachycardia.
- Drug therapy is the same as that for multifocal atrial tachycardia.
- Pacing may be used to override the atrial rate and terminate the arrhythmia when conventional treatments fail.

Atrioventricular block, first-degree

A heart block in which impulses are normal through the SA node, but delayed at the AV node, is classified as a first-degree AV block. The block may be slight, moderate, or severe, depending on the duration of the PR interval. First-degree AV block is seen in approximately 8% of healthy adults and is usually considered clinically insignificant; however, in some cases, it may progress to complete AV block.

On an ECG, the PR interval is prolonged but constant, exceeding 0.2 second but rarely more than 0.35 second. The QRS complex is usually normal if the conduction delay occurs in the AV node. If the duration of the QRS complex exceeds 0.12 second, the conduction delay may be in the His-Purkinje fibers.

A possible cause of first-degree AV block is drug toxicity caused by digitalis glycosides, quinidine, procainamide, or propranolol. Cardiac causes include chronic degenerative disease of the conduction system or inferior wall MI. Extracardiac causes include hypokalemia or hyperkalemia, hypothermia, and hypothyroidism.

Treatment
- Treatment aims to correct the underlying cause, such as digitalis toxicity or an electrolyte imbalance.
- Monitor carefully for worsening heart block, especially if severe myocardial damage has occurred or if the patient is receiving a new drug, such as a digitalis glycoside, *procainamide* (p. 272), or *quinidine* (p. 284).
- Give 0.5 to 1 mg of *atropine* (p. 83) I.V. for symptomatic bradycardia.

Atrioventricular block, second-degree (Type I)

In Type I (Wenckebach or Mobitz I) second-degree AV block, delayed conduction through the AV node increases with each impulse until one impulse is blocked.

After several beats, an impulse arrives during the absolute refractory period, when the tissue can't conduct it. The next impulse arrives during the relative refractory period and is conducted normally. The cycle is then repeated.

Type I second-degree AV block occurs in approximately 6% of healthy young adults and 9% of athletes. If it's associated with an inferior wall MI but produces no signs or symptoms, this type of AV block may be transient, with a good prognosis. But if the block becomes chronic, especially in patients with organic heart disease, the prognosis is usually poor.

On an ECG, this block can usually be distinguished by grouped beats, referred to as the "footprints of Wenckebach." The atrial rhythm is regular, but the ventricular rhythm is irregular. The atrial rate exceeds the ventricular rate, but both usually remain within normal limits. The R-R interval shortens progressively, and the PR interval lengthens progressively until a P wave appears without a QRS complex. The cycle is then repeated.

Possible causes include inferior wall MI, cardiac surgery, electrolyte imbalance, vagal stimulation, and sinus tachycardia. Type I AV block may also be caused by digitalis toxicity or use of procainamide, quinidine, or propranolol.

Treatment

- For most patients, treatment addresses the underlying cause, usually MI, thereby correcting the heart block.
- Check the ECG frequently for development of more severe types of AV block.

- If the patient develops symptomatic bradycardia, the doctor may prescribe *atropine* (p. 83) or insert a temporary pacemaker.

Atrioventricular block, second-degree (Type II)

Produced by a conduction disturbance in the His-Purkinje fibers, Type II (Mobitz II) second-degree AV block causes an intermittent conduction delay or block. On the ECG, you won't see any warning before a nonconducted beat, as you would with Type I second-degree AV block. In Type II second-degree AV block, the PR and R-R intervals are constant. The block commonly progresses to third-degree, or complete, heart block.

The atrial rhythm is regular, but the ventricular rhythm may be irregular. Some P waves aren't followed by a QRS complex. The PR interval is normal or prolonged, but always constant for the conducted beats. The duration of the QRS complex is within normal limits if the block occurs at the bundle of His; the duration is prolonged if the block occurs below the bundle of His.

Causes include such organic heart diseases as acute anterior wall MI, severe CAD, acute myocarditis, or calcification of the conduction system. The prognosis depends on the underlying cause.

Treatment

- No immediate treatment is needed if the patient is asymptomatic. However, patients may require *atropine* (p. 83) for symptomatic bradycardia

and a temporary external, transvenous, or permanent pacemaker.
• If the patient is hypotensive, treatment aims to increase his heart rate, thereby increasing cardiac output. *Isoproterenol* (p. 181) is used to increase SA impulses and accelerate conduction through the AV node and the His-Purkinje system.

Atrioventricular block, third-degree

When all supraventricular impulses are prevented from reaching the ventricles and a secondary pacemaker develops that stimulates the ventricles or AV junction, the patient has third-degree AV block, also known as complete heart block. This disorder's significance depends on the patient's response to any decrease in the ventricular rate and on the stability of the subsidiary pacemaker. Junctional escape rhythms are typically stable and may resolve without intervention. Ventricular escape rhythms, however, are slower and less stable and pose the risk of intermittent or permanent ventricular standstill. The prognosis depends on the nature and severity of the underlying heart disease.

On an ECG, the atrial rate exceeds the ventricular rate. The slow ventricular rate ranges from 25 to 40 beats/minute, depending on the block's location and the origin of the subsidiary impulse. Blocks proximal to the bundle of His generally produce a normal QRS complex; those distal to the bundle of His, a wide QRS complex. The T wave is normal with a narrow QRS complex or abnormal with a wide or bizarre QRS complex.

Acute blocks may be caused by severe digitalis toxicity, beta blockers or calcium channel blockers, anterior or inferior wall MI, cardiac catheterization, or myocarditis due to Lyme disease.

Chronic blocks may be caused by widespread changes in the His-Purkinje fibers (leading to bilateral bundle-branch block), congenital abnormalities, rheumatic fever, hypoxia, Lev's disease, Lenegre's disease, and complications of surgery to repair mitral valve prolapse, atrial septal defect, ventricular septal defect, or other congenital heart defects.

Treatment

• If the patient has adequate cardiac output, no treatment is generally needed.
• If cardiac output isn't adequate or the patient's condition seems to be deteriorating, therapy focuses on improving the ventricular rhythm. Initially, this may include *atropine* (p. 83) or *isoproterenol* (p. 181) and insertion of a temporary pacemaker. A permanent pacemaker may be required later.

Atrioventricular dissociation

In this arrhythmia, the atria and ventricles beat independently but usually at about the same rate. Since AV dissociation is never a primary disturbance but a symptom of some underlying disorder, its significance depends on the underlying cause.

On an ECG, the QRS complex configuration varies according to the origin of the ventricular beat. A high AV junctional pacemaker produces a narrow QRS complex; a pacemaker in the bundle of His, a wide QRS complex. The T wave is altered or inverted, depending on the underlying cause.

Causes of AV dissociation include conditions that result in slowed or impaired sinus impulse formation or SA conduction, such as sinus bradycardia, sinus arrest, or SA block. It may also be caused by accelerated impulse formation in the AV junction or ventricular pacemaker, such as junctional tachycardia or VT, or by an AV conduction disturbance, such as third-degree AV block. Drug toxicity from a digitalis glycoside, verapamil, or disopyramide may also cause this condition.

Treatment

- If drug toxicity is the cause, the drug must be discontinued.
- No treatment is necessary if the rhythm disturbance caused by AV dissociation is clinically insignificant.
- If the rhythm disturbance reduces cardiac output, treatment aims to resolve the arrhythmia and manage the underlying cardiac disorder. Specific measures include therapy with *atropine* (p. 83) or *isoproterenol* (p. 181), cardioversion, and pacemaker insertion.

Buerger's disease

An inflammatory, nonatheromatous occlusive condition, Buerger's disease causes segmental lesions and subsequent thrombus formation in the small and medium-sized arteries (and sometimes the veins), resulting in decreased blood flow to the hands, legs, and feet. Also called thromboangiitis obliterans, the disease affects the legs more commonly than the arms. Cerebral, visceral, and coronary vessels may also be affected. Incidence is highest among 20- to 40-year-old men of Asian and Jewish ancestry who smoke heavily.

The cause of Buerger's disease is unknown, but a definite link exists between smoking and an increased incidence of human leukocyte antigens B5 and A9, suggesting a hypersensitivity reaction to nicotine.

Impaired tissue perfusion, a complication of Buerger's disease, can cause ulcerations, poor wound healing and, ultimately, gangrene and systemic infection requiring amputation.

Treatment

- Abstention from smoking is the first and most important treatment.
- An aerobic exercise program that uses gravity to fill and drain the blood vessels may also help in mild to moderate disease.
- Calcium channel blockers such as *nifedipine* (p. 230) may dilate arterioles.
- Severe Buerger's disease may require a lumbar sympathectomy or arterial bypass grafting to increase blood supply to the skin.
- Parenteral or oral antibiotics may be used to treat secondary infections.
- As a last resort, amputation may be necessary for intractable ulcers and associated pain or gangrene.

Cardiac tamponade

A rapid rise in intrapericardial pressure that impairs diastolic filling time, cardiac tamponade usually results from the accumulation of blood or fluid in the pericardial sac. If the fluid accumulates rapidly, as little as 200 ml can create an emergency. Slow accumulation, as in pericardial effusion associated with cancer, may not produce immediate symptoms because the gradual stretching of the pericardial sac's fibrous wall can accommodate as much as 2 liters of fluid.

Cardiac tamponade may be idiopathic (Dressler's syndrome) or result from effusion (cancer, bacterial infections, tuberculosis and, rarely, acute rheumatic fever), hemorrhage, viral or idiopathic pericarditis or pericarditis following radiation therapy, acute MI, chronic renal failure during dialysis, a drug reaction (to procainamide, hydralazine, minoxidil, isoniazid, penicillin, methysergide, or daunorubicin), or connective tissue disorders.

Treatment

• Pericardiocentesis or surgical creation of an opening in the pericardial sac dramatically improves systemic arterial pressure and cardiac output with aspiration of as little as 25 ml of fluid.
• A drain may also be inserted in the pericardial sac to syphon off the fluid. The drain may be left in place until the effusion stops or a pericardial window is created.

• If infection develops, antibiotics can be instilled through the drain or administered systemically.
• Dilute *heparin* (p. 169) or, in some cases, antineoplastic agents may be instilled to prevent clotting.
• In hypotensive patients, trial volume loading with I.V. 0.9% NaCl solution with albumin and an inotropic drug such as *dopamine* (p. 139) is necessary to maintain cardiac output.
• Additional treatment varies, depending on the cause of cardiac tamponade. In traumatic injury, a blood transfusion or a thoracotomy may be necessary to drain reaccumulating fluid or repair bleeding sites. In heparin-induced tamponade, the heparin antagonist protamine sulfate may reverse the adverse effects of heparin. In warfarin-induced tamponade, vitamin K may be administered.

Cardiogenic shock

Sometimes called pump failure, cardiogenic shock is a state of diminished cardiac output that severely impairs tissue perfusion. Cardiogenic shock occurs as a serious complication in nearly 15% of all patients hospitalized with acute MI. It typically affects patients whose infarction involves 40% or more of left ventricular muscle mass; in such patients, mortality may exceed 85%. Most patients with cardiogenic shock die within 24 hours of onset.

Cardiogenic shock can result from any condition that causes significant left ventricular dysfunction with reduced cardiac output, such as MI (most common), myocardial ischemia, papillary muscle dysfunction, and end-stage cardiomyopathy. Other causes include myocarditis and decreased myocardial contractility after cardiac arrest or prolonged cardiac surgery. Mechanical abnormalities of the ventricle, such as acute mitral or aortic insufficiency or ventricular aneurysm, may also result in cardiogenic shock.

Regardless of the cause, left ventricular dysfunction triggers a series of compensatory mechanisms to increase heart rate, left ventricular filling pressure, and peripheral resistance to flow in order to enhance venous return to the heart. These responses initially stabilize the patient but later cause deterioration as rising oxygen requirements place even greater demands on the already compromised myocardium. This cycle of low cardiac output, sympathetic compensation, myocardial ischemia, and then even lower cardiac output usually ends in death.

Treatment

• CV drugs may include *dopamine* (p. 139), a vasopressor that increases cardiac output, blood pressure, and renal blood flow; *amrinone* (p. 78) or *dobutamine* (p. 136), which increases myocardial contractility; and *norepinephrine* (p. 243) when a more potent vasoconstrictor is necessary. *Morphine sulfate* (p. 223) may be given for pain.
• *Nitroprusside* (p. 240), a vasodilator, may be used with an inotropic agent to further improve cardiac output by decreasing peripheral vascular resistance (afterload) and reducing left ventricular end-diastolic pressure (preload). However, the patient's blood pressure must be adequate to support nitroprusside therapy and must be monitored closely.
• Treatment may also include the IABP, an inflatable pump inserted through the femoral artery into the descending thoracic aorta. The balloon inflates during diastole to increase coronary artery and renal perfusion pressures and deflates before systole (before the aortic valve opens) to reduce resistance to ejection (afterload) and therefore lessen cardiac workload.
• When drug therapy and IABP insertion fail, a ventricular assist device may be used, or the patient may undergo rescue PTCA or emergency CABG.
• Thrombolytics such as *streptokinase* (p. 301) may be used to lyse a clot, reperfuse the myocardium, and improve cardiac pump function.

Chronic venous insufficiency

A chronic failure of the vein valves to function properly, chronic venous insufficiency interferes with venous return to the heart. This condition results from venous occlusion or valve incompetence, usually in the iliac and femoral veins and occasionally in the saphenous veins.

When veins are unable to drain properly, pressure in the venules and capillary beds behind them increases, resulting in edema and, possibly, severe stasis ulcers.

Chronic venous insufficiency may occur secondary to atherosclerosis, arteriosclerosis, CHF, CAD, cardiomyopathy, pulmonary disease, hypertension, diabetes mellitus, or renal insufficiency. Other risk factors include pregnancy, obesity, and occupations that require prolonged standing. Postmenopausal women are at greatest risk for this disorder.

Treatment
• Appropriate treatment for small ulcers is bed rest, elevation of the legs, warm soaks, and antimicrobial therapy for infection.
• Large ulcers unresponsive to conservative treatment may require excision and skin grafting. Care includes daily inspection to assess healing and measures similar to those for varicose veins.
• Treatment to counteract increased venous pressure may include compression dressings such as Unna's boot, beginning after massive swelling subsides.

Coarctation of the aorta

This disorder involves a narrowing, or coarctation, of the aorta, usually just below the left subclavian artery and near the site where the ligamentum arteriosum joins the pulmonary artery to the aorta. The ligamentum arteriosum is a remnant of the fetal blood vessel called the ductus arteriosus.

By restricting blood flow, the constriction increases pressure on the left ventricle so much that it may fail, causing increased end-diastolic and pulmonary capillary pressures, pulmonary edema, a low-output state and, possibly, sudden circulatory collapse. This restricted flow also dilates the proximal aorta and causes left ventricular hypertrophy.

Coarctation may be associated with mitral or aortic valve lesions (usually the bicuspid aortic valve) and with severe cases of hypoplasia of the aortic arch, patent ductus arteriosus, or a ventricular septal defect.

This disorder accounts for about 8% of all congenital heart defects in children and is more common in boys than in girls. When it occurs in girls, it's commonly associated with Turner's syndrome, a chromosomal disorder that causes ovarian dysgenesis.

The prognosis depends on the severity of associated cardiac anomalies; it's good if the condition can be surgically corrected before it induces severe systemic hypertension or degenerative changes in the aorta.

Treatment
• For an infant with left ventricular failure caused by coarctation of the aorta, treatment consists of prostaglandins, inotropic agents such as *digoxin* (p. 118), and diuretics such as *furosemide* (p. 162).
• Most patients require surgery. The procedure may involve end-to-end anastomosis or subclavian flap angioplasty. If the narrowed segment is long, the doctor may use a tubular graft, patch, or bypass conduit.

Coronary artery disease

The largest single cause of death in North America, CAD is an umbrella term for various diseases that diminish or halt blood flow in the coronary arteries, reducing myocardial oxygen and nutrient supplies. CAD strikes more whites than blacks or Asians and more men than women; it usually occurs in middle age. Men are eight times more susceptible than premenopausal women, and more than 50% of men age 60 or older show signs of CAD on autopsy.

Atherosclerosis, the most common cause of CAD, has been linked to many risk factors. Some, such as age, sex, and race, can't be controlled; others, such as blood pressure, diabetes mellitus, smoking, obesity, a sedentary lifestyle, and stress, may be controlled with medical treatment and lifestyle changes.

Uncommon causes of reduced coronary artery blood flow include dissecting aneurysms, infectious vasculitis, syphilis, congenital defects in the coronary vascular system, and coronary artery spasm.

The classic symptom of CAD is angina, the direct result of inadequate flow of oxygen to the myocardium.

Treatment

• In angina, treatment aims to reduce myocardial oxygen demand or increase the oxygen supply, thus relieving ischemia and reducing pain. Performing activities slowly rather than eliminating them and using stress-reduction techniques help prevent pain.
• Drug therapy consists primarily of nitrates, such as *isosorbide dinitrate* (p. 185), *isosorbide mononitrate* (p. 185), or *nitroglycerin* (p. 233), to relieve angina; beta blockers, such as *atenolol* (p. 80), *metoprolol* (p. 213), or *propranolol* (p. 280), to decrease myocardial oxygen demand; and cal-

cium channel blockers, such as *diltiazem* (p. 127), *nicardipine* (p. 228), or *nifedipine* (p. 230), to decrease myocardial contractility.
• Obstructive lesions may necessitate atherectomy or CABG, using autogenous vein grafts. PTCA may be performed during cardiac catheterization to compress fatty deposits and correct the occlusion.
• Laser angioplasty corrects occlusion by vaporizing fatty deposits with an excimer or hot-tip laser device.
• Rotational ablation (or rotational atherectomy) removes atheromatous plaque with a high-speed, rotating burr covered with diamond crystals.
• Prevention is critical because CAD is so widespread. Dietary restrictions to reduce intake of calories, salt, fats, and cholesterol may minimize the risk, especially when supplemented with regular exercise. Stress reduction and abstention from smoking are also essential.
• Other preventive actions include control of hypertension with diuretics, such as *hydrochlorothiazide* (p. 177); beta blockers, such as atenolol, metoprolol, or propranolol; or calcium channel blockers, such as diltiazem, nicardipine, or nifedipine.
• Elevated serum cholesterol or triglyceride levels may be controlled with antilipemics such as *lovastatin* (p. 199). Platelet aggregation and the danger of blood clots may be defused with aspirin.

Dilated cardiomyopathy

Formerly known as congestive cardiomyopathy, this disorder results from extensively damaged myocardial muscle fibers. Dilated cardiomyopathy interferes with myocardial metabolism and grossly dilates the ventricles without proportional compensatory hypertrophy. This causes the heart to assume a globular shape and contract poorly, thus ejecting blood less efficiently than normal. A large volume of blood remains in the left ventricle after systole, causing signs of heart failure.

Dilated cardiomyopathy most commonly affects middle-aged men but can occur in any age-group. Because the disease isn't usually diagnosed until the advanced stages, the prognosis is generally poor. About 75% of patients die within 5 years of the onset of symptoms.

The cause of most cardiomyopathies is unknown. Dilated cardiomyopathy can result from myocardial destruction by toxic, infectious, and metabolic agents; endocrine and electrolyte disorders; and nutritional disorders. Other causes include muscle disorders, infiltrative disorders, and sarcoidosis. Cardiomyopathy is also a possible complication of alcoholism.

Treatment

- The goal of treatment is to correct the underlying cause and improve the heart's pumping ability with *digoxin* (p. 118), diuretics such as *furosemide* (p. 162), oxygen, and a low-sodium diet supplemented with vitamin therapy. If alcoholism is the suspected cause, alcohol ingestion must stop.
- Antiarrhythmics, such as *amiodarone* (p. 72), *procainamide* (p. 272), *quinidine* (p. 284), or *sotalol* (p. 294), may be used to treat symptomatic arrhythmias.
- Therapy may also include selective use of corticosteroids, particularly when myocardial inflammation is present.
- Vasodilators such as *nitroglycerin* (p. 233) reduce preload and afterload, thereby decreasing congestion and increasing cardiac output. ACE inhibitors, such as *captopril* (p. 99) or *enalapril* (p. 143), may also be used to reduce afterload.
- Beta blockers such as *propranolol* (p. 280) may be prescribed to decrease myocardial oxygen demand, reduce damage due to catecholamines, and improve diastolic relaxation.
- Acute heart failure may require vasodilation with I.V. nitroglycerin or *nitroprusside* (p. 240). *Amrinone* (p. 78), *dobutamine* (p. 136), or *dopamine* (p. 139) may increase cardiac output in the acute stage. Long-term treatment may include *hydralazine* (p. 174), *isosorbide dinitrate* (p. 185), or *prazosin* (p. 265); ACE inhibitors, such as captopril or enalapril; and calcium channel blockers, such as *amlodipine* (p. 75) or *nifedipine* (p. 230).
- If the patient is on prolonged bed rest, anticoagulants such as *warfarin* (p. 321) may be prescribed.
- In appropriate patients, heart transplantation may be performed.

Endocarditis

An infection of the endocardium, the heart valves, or a prosthetic valve, endocarditis is caused by bacterial or fungal invasion. In endocarditis, fibrin and platelets cluster on endothelial and valve tissue, forming sterile vegetations. Infective endocarditis occurs when bacteria or fungi are engulfed in or deposited on these vegetations, causing deformities and destruction of valve tissue. It may also rupture the chordae tendineae, leading to valve insufficiency.

Vegetation may also form on normal surfaces and on the endocardium, usually in areas scarred by rheumatic, congenital, or syphilitic heart disease.

Endocarditis can be classified as native valve endocarditis, prosthetic valve endocarditis, endocarditis of I.V. drug users, or according to the infecting organism. It can be acute or subacute. Untreated, endocarditis is usually fatal; with prompt treatment, about 70% of patients recover. The prognosis is worse when endocarditis causes severe valve damage leading to insufficiency and left ventricular failure, or when it strikes a patient with a prosthetic valve.

Preexisting conditions, including rheumatic heart disease, congenital heart disease, mitral prolapse, degenerative heart disease, calcific aortic stenosis (in elderly people), asymmetrical septal hypertrophy, Marfan syndrome, syphilitic aortic valve, I.V. drug abuse, and long-term hemodialysis with an arteriovenous shunt or fistula, can predispose a patient to endocarditis. However, up to 40% of patients have no underlying heart disease.

Treatment

• The goal of treatment is to eradicate all infectious organisms from the vegetation, usually with I.V. antibiotic therapy lasting 4 weeks. Gentamycin is used to treat penicillinase-producing staphylococcal infection, and amphotericin B is used to treat fungal infections.

• Supportive treatment includes bed rest, aspirin or acetaminophen for fever and aches, and sufficient fluid intake. Severe valve damage, especially aortic insufficiency or infection of a prosthetic valve, may require corrective surgery if refractory heart failure develops or if an infected prosthetic valve must be replaced.

Heart failure

When the myocardium can't pump effectively enough to meet the body's metabolic needs, heart failure occurs. Heart failure is classified as high- or low-output, acute or chronic, left ventricular or right ventricular, forward or backward, systolic or diastolic, and congestive.

Heart failure commonly results from a primary abnormality of the heart muscle (such as an infarction) that impairs ventricular function to the point that the heart can no longer pump sufficient blood. Heart failure can also result from underlying structural abnormalities — congenital or acquired — that lead to an increased hemodynamic burden, valvular disorders, or coronary insufficiency. Heart failure with pulmonary congestion can lead to life-threatening pulmonary edema. This can result in decreased perfusion to major organs, such as the brain and kidneys, causing them to fail, and may lead to MI.

Other precipitating factors include:
— arrhythmias, such as tachyarrhythmias, which can reduce ventricular filling time; bradycardia, which can reduce cardiac output; and arrhythmias that disrupt the normal atrial and ventricular filling synchrony, such as atrial fibrillation
— pregnancy, thyrotoxicosis, and anemia, which can increase the demand for cardiac output
— pulmonary embolism, which elevates PAPs and can cause right ventricular failure
— infections, which may increase metabolic demands and further burden the heart
— increased physical activity, emotional stress, increased sodium or water intake, or failure to comply with the prescribed treatment regimen.

Treatment

• The aim of therapy is to preserve and improve pump function by reducing the heart's workload and limiting sodium and water retention, usually with drugs, thus reversing the damaging compensatory mechanisms.
• Heart failure can usually be controlled quickly by diuretics, such as *bumetanide* (p. 96), *ethacrynic acid* (p. 153), *furosemide* (p. 162), *hydrochlorothiazide* (p. 177), *spironolactone* (p. 298), or *triamterene* (p. 313), to reduce total blood volume and circulatory congestion; inotropic drugs such as *digoxin* (p. 118) to strengthen myocardial contractility; sympathomimetics, such as *dobutamine* (p. 136) and *dopamine* (p. 139), in acute situations; or *amrinone* (p. 78) or *milrinone* (p. 218) to increase contractility and cause arterial vasodilation.
• Venous and arterial vasodilators, such as *hydralazine* (p. 174), *isosorbide dinitrate* (p. 185), *nitroprusside* (p. 240), or *prazosin* (p. 265), can decrease preload and afterload. ACE inhibitors, such as *captopril* (p. 99) or *enalapril* (p. 143), or calcium channel blockers, such as *amlodipine* (p. 75) or *nifedipine* (p. 230), may decrease afterload.
• Heart failure may also be brought under control by restricting physical activity; administering oxygen, when necessary, to increase oxygen delivery to the myocardium and other vital organ tissues; and having the patient wear antiembolism stockings to prevent venostasis and possible thromboembolus formation.
• In chronic CHF, the patient usually must continue taking digoxin, diuretics, potassium supplements, and sometimes low-dose beta blockers such as *metoprolol* (p. 213), and he must remain under medical supervision.
• If the patient with valve dysfunction has recurrent acute heart failure, surgical valve replacement may be necessary.

Hyperlipidemia

An elevated blood lipid level, hyperlipidemia contributes to CAD and MI. High plasma levels of cholesterol and triglycerides, the two major lipids, enhance atherogenesis. Lowering lipid levels reduces the progression of CAD.

High concentrations of LDL and VLDL, which transport cholesterol and triglycerides, also contribute to the formation of atheromatous plaques within coronary arteries. Low levels of HDLs, which increase absorption of cholesterol for excretion, may diminish clearance of cholesterol, causing increased cholesterol deposits in the coronary arteries. Reduced HDL levels can be caused by cigarette smoking, a sedentary lifestyle, and certain drugs, including progestins, corticosteroids (such as prednisone), and beta blockers (such as propranolol).

Factors that contribute to hyperlipidemia may include a diet high in saturated fats and cholesterol; such conditions as hypothyroidism, nephrotic syndrome, liver disease, and diabetes mellitus; a family history of hyperlipidemia; and decreased estrogen levels in menopausal women.

Treatment

• Administer antilipemic agents specific to the lipid abnormality, such as *cholestyramine* (p. 102), *gemfibrozil* (p. 166), *lovastatin* (p. 199), niacin, *pravastatin* (p. 262), *probucol* (p. 269), and *simvastatin* (p. 291).
• Modify the patient's diet to include foods low in cholesterol and saturated fats; total cholesterol intake should not exceed 300 mg/day, and dietary fat intake should amount to less than 30% of total calories.
• Develop a regular exercise program for the patient to establish ideal body weight, increase HDL levels, and reduce cholesterol levels.
• Eliminate or reduce factors associated with low HDL levels, such as cigarette smoking and a sedentary lifestyle, and those associated with high triglyceride levels such as alcohol intake.
• Discontinue progestins, corticosteroids, or beta blockers such as *propranolol* (p. 280), which may contribute to increased lipid levels.

Hypertension

This disorder is marked by a sustained elevation in diastolic or systolic blood pressure (or both), with a systolic pressure of 140 mm Hg or higher or a diastolic pressure of 90 mm Hg or higher. A systolic pressure of 160 mm Hg or higher along with a normal diastolic pressure qualifies as isolated systolic hypertension.

Two major types of hypertension exist. Essential (also called primary or idiopathic) hypertension accounts for 90% to 95% of the cases; secondary hypertension results from renal disease or another identifiable cause. Malignant hypertension is a severe, fulminant form of hypertension common to both types.

If untreated, even mild hypertension can cause significant complications and result in death. In many cases, however, stepped-care treatment can improve the prognosis. It begins with diet modifications and exercise. Later, single- or multiple-drug regimens are begun and often modified to fit each patient's specific needs.

Hypertension affects more than 60 million adults in North America. Blacks are twice as likely as whites to be affected, and they're four times as likely to die of complications from this disorder. Hypertension is also a major cause of CVA, cardiac disease, and renal failure. Cardiac, neurologic, and renovascular complications, such as CAD, MI, heart failure, cerebral infarctions, hypertensive encephalopathy, and blindness, can occur late in the disease. Complications of hypertension can affect any organ system.

Treatment

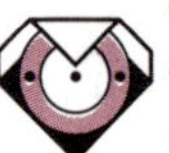 **Treatment of choice.** Although essential hypertension has no cure, lifestyle modifications (exercise, weight loss, reduced alcohol intake, and stress management) are the primary treatments, especially in early, mild cases.
• If needed, further treatment is provided in steps and may include drug therapy.

Step 1: Lifestyle modifications continue, but no drugs are administered.

Step 2: If blood pressure isn't adequately reduced by lifestyle modifications, single-drug treatment may include diuretics, such as *furosemide* (p. 162) or *hydrochlorothiazide* (p. 177), or beta blockers, such as *atenolol* (p. 80), *nadolol* (p. 226), or *propranolol* (p. 280), to decrease oxygen demand. If the patient has other underlying medical problems, alternative drugs may be substituted, including ACE inhibitors, such as *benazepril* (p. 85), *enalapril* (p. 143), or *lisinopril* (p. 196); calcium channel blockers, such as *amlodipine* (p. 75), *diltiazem* (p. 127), *nifedipine* (p. 230), or *verapamil* (p. 316); alpha$_1$-receptor blockers, such as ferazosin or *prazosin* (p. 265);

and combination alpha and beta blockers such as *labetalol* (p. 189).

Step 3: If the patient fails to respond to treatment in 1 to 3 weeks, therapy modification may include increasing drug dose, substituting another drug, or adding a second agent from a different class.

Step 4: If the desired blood pressure still hasn't been achieved, a second or third agent and, if not already prescribed, a diuretic may be given to the patient.
• This stepped-care approach may continue to require modification. For instance, most blacks respond poorly to beta blockers; however, for unclear reasons, they respond well to a combination of a diuretic and an ACE inhibitor. Many elderly patients can be treated with a diuretic alone.
• Treatment of secondary hypertension includes correcting the underlying cause and controlling hypertensive effects.

Hypertensive crisis

A life-threatening emergency, hypertensive crisis occurs when the diastolic blood pressure rises above 130 mm Hg, causing acute and potentially fatal vascular damage. If left untreated, the patient may die quickly from brain damage or more gradually from renal damage.

Most cases of hypertensive crisis occur in patients with preexisting hypertension. Hypertensive crisis can result from untreated or inadequately controlled hypertension, which may be due to noncompliance with the prescribed antihypertensive drug regimen. Other causes include toxemia of pregnancy, renal disease, pituitary tumors, coarctation of the aorta, concurrent use of catecholamine-like drugs (such as pseudoephedrine and MAO inhibitors), adrenocortical hyperfunction, Cushing's syndrome, and polycythemia. Advanced age and the presence of arteriosclerosis can also decrease arterial compliance (elasticity) and contribute to hypertensive crisis.

Hypertensive crisis can lead to vascular changes in the brain, such as vasospasm and ischemia, precipitating a stroke or cerebral hemorrhage; myocardial ischemia and MI if the patient also has CAD; dissection of an aortic aneurysm; and renal failure.

Treatment
• Administer rapidly acting I.V. drugs, such as *diazoxide* (p. 116), *labetalol* (p. 189), *nitroglycerin* (p. 233), or *nitroprusside* (p. 240), to reduce blood pressure by 30% or decrease diastolic pressure to below 105 mm Hg. Sublingual *nifedipine* (p. 230) also rapidly reduces blood pressure.
• Monitor cardiac status to assess for arrhythmias and ischemic changes.
• Administer supplemental oxygen if chest pain, ST-segment ischemic changes, or signs of CHF are present.
• If CHF or pulmonary edema is present, diuretic therapy will include *ethacrynic acid* (p. 153) or *furosemide* (p. 162).
• *Morphine sulfate* (p. 223) reduces peripheral resistance and pulmonary hypertension.
• Treat arrhythmias with antiarrhythmic drugs, such as *atropine* (p. 83),

bretylium (p. 93), *lidocaine* (p. 192), *procainamide* (p. 272), and *verapamil* (p. 316).
• Long-term management of hypertension may include ACE inhibitors such as *enalapril* (p. 143); calcium channel blockers such as nifedipine; beta blockers, such as *atenolol* (p. 80) and *metoprolol* (p. 213); and alpha-adrenergic agents, such as *clonidine* (p. 108) and *prazosin* (p. 265).
• Restrict the patient's intake of simple carbohydrates (such as soft drinks, baked goods, candy, fruit, milk, and ice cream), which increase sympathetic nervous system activity and circulating norepinephrine, altering the effects of antihypertensive drugs. And avoid I.V. 0.9% NaCl solution to limit sodium levels and fluid retention, which can aggravate the hypertensive state.

Hypertrophic cardiomyopathy
Also called idiopathic hypertrophic subaortic stenosis, hypertrophic cardiomyopathy is characterized by left ventricular hypertrophy and a disproportionate, asymmetrical thickening of the interventricular septum, particularly in the anterosuperior part. Abnormal stiffness of the left ventricle and narrowing of the subaortic area, caused by septal hypertrophy in the mitral valve, may obstruct the left ventricular outflow. This may cause pulmonary hypertension and heart failure. The majority of patients with hypertrophic cardiomyopathy are asymptomatic, and sudden

death usually results from VT, PVCs, or atrial fibrillation.

The most common symptoms are dyspnea and angina. These may result from elevated left ventricular end-diastolic pressure and impaired ventricular filling from diastolic malfunction. Angina occurs in 75% of patients. Fatigue and syncope are common, and exertion tends to exacerbate symptoms. About half of all cases are due to an autosomal dominant trait.

Treatment

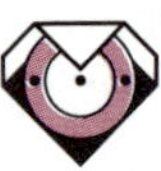 **Treatment of choice.** Drug therapy with a beta-blocking agent such as *propranolol* (p. 280) slows the heart rate and increases ventricular filling, decreasing myocardial oxygen demand and thereby reducing angina, syncope, dyspnea, and arrhythmias.

• Calcium channel blockers, such as *amlodipine* (p. 75), *diltiazem* (p. 127), *nifedipine* (p. 230), or *verapamil* (p. 316), and ACE inhibitors, such as *captopril* (p. 99) or *enalapril* (p. 143), may reduce elevated diastolic pressure and increase exercise tolerance.

• Atrial fibrillation, a medical emergency in hypertrophic cardiomyopathy, requires immediate cardioversion. It also requires administration of anticoagulants, such as *heparin* (p. 169) or *warfarin* (p. 321), prior to cardioversion and until fibrillation subsides because of the high risk of systemic embolism.

• *Amiodarone* (p. 72) may be effective in reducing ventricular and supraventricular arrhythmias and can be used unless an AV block exists.

• Diuretics such as furosemide, vasodilators such as nitroglycerin, sympathetic stimulators such as isoproterenol, and digitalis glycosides should be avoided because they worsen the degree of obstruction.

• Ventricular septal myectomy (resection of the hypertrophied septum) alone or combined with mitral valve replacement may ease outflow tract obstruction and relieve symptoms. Ventricular myectomy may cause complications, such as complete heart block, but new surgical techniques using intraoperative echocardiography have established a mortality rate of less than 5%.

Hypovolemic shock

Potentially life-threatening, hypovolemic shock results from insufficient intravascular blood volume, which leads to decreased cardiac output and inadequate tissue perfusion. This tissue perfusion, in turn, causes a shift in cellular metabolism from aerobic to anaerobic, resulting in an accumulation of lactic acid that produces metabolic acidosis.

Hypovolemic shock most commonly results from acute blood loss (20% of total volume) from GI bleeding, internal or external hemorrhage, or any condition that reduces circulating intravascular volume or other body fluids.

Other causes include intestinal obstruction, peritonitis, acute pancreatitis, ascites, and dehydration from excessive perspiration, severe diarrhea, protracted vomiting, diabetes insipidus, burns, diuresis, or inadequate fluid intake.

Without sufficient blood or fluid replacement, hypovolemic shock can cause rapid and irreversible adult respiratory distress syndrome, acute tubular necrosis and renal failure, cerebral damage, disseminated intravascular coagulation, multisystem organ failure, and death.

Treatment

• Emergency treatment consists of prompt and adequate blood and fluid replacement to restore intravascular volume and to raise diastolic blood pressure and maintain it above 60 mm Hg. Rapid infusion of 0.9% NaCl or lactated Ringer's solution and, possibly, albumin, hetastarch, or other plasma expanders may expand volume adequately until whole blood can be matched and infused.

• Treatment may also include application of a pneumatic antishock garment, administration of oxygen, control of bleeding, administration of *dopamine* (p. 139) or another inotropic drug to increase cardiac output and, possibly, surgery. To be effective, inotropic drugs must be combined with vigorous fluid resuscitation.

Idioventricular rhythm

This slow ventricular arrhythmia results when the cells of the His-Purkinje fibers take over as the heart's pacemaker. When all potential pacemakers above the ventricle fail to discharge or when a block prevents supraventricular impulses from reaching the ventricles, atrial-ventricular synchrony is lost and no atrial kick occurs, resulting in idioventricular rhythm.

The atrial rhythm usually can't be determined. The ventricular rate is 20 to 40 beats/minute. The P wave is absent; consequently, the PR interval can't be measured. The QRS complex is wide and bizarre in configuration; its duration exceeds 0.12 second. The T wave is abnormal, and deflection usually occurs in the direction opposite that of the QRS complex. The QT interval usually is prolonged.

Idioventricular rhythm commonly occurs with third-degree AV block. Other possible causes include MI, metabolic imbalances, digitalis toxicity, beta blockers, calcium antagonists, and tricyclic antidepressants. The prognosis is poor, especially if the condition is accompanied by pulseless electrical activity.

Treatment

• Perform an ECG immediately and assess the patient's condition to help determine the course of treatment.

• Determine the underlying cause and treat accordingly.

• Give drugs such as *atropine* (p. 83) to treat bradycardia.

• External pacing or temporary transvenous pacing may be required.

• *Caution:* Never give lidocaine. It can suppress ventricular activation and cause asystole in a patient with idioventricular rhythm.

Junctional rhythm

This arrhythmia originates in the AV junctional tissue at the rate of the inherent pacemaker (between 40 and 60 beats/minute) and can lead to a reduced heart rate and lowered cardiac output. Its clinical significance and prognosis hinge on the patient's ability to tolerate these conditions and the arrhythmia's underlying cause.

On an ECG, the P wave may be inverted, may occur before or after the QRS complex, may be hidden in it, or may be absent. The PR interval is shortened (less than 0.12 second) if the P wave precedes the QRS complex.

Causes of junctional rhythm include extremely long pauses in the cardiac cycle resulting from SA node ischemia, SSS, digitalis toxicity, and increased vagal tone.

Treatment

• If the patient is asymptomatic, no treatment is needed. However, the underlying cause should be determined and treated.
• If the patient has symptoms, *atropine* (p. 83) may increase the sinus or junctional rate. A pacemaker may also be inserted to enhance the atrial rate and control the ventricular rate.

Junctional tachycardia

In this type of tachycardia, an ectopic impulse originating in the AV node or the bundle of His accelerates the ventricular rate to over 100 beats/minute.

The significance of this arrhythmia depends on the ventricular rate, the underlying cause, and the severity of the accompanying cardiac disease. Patients with junctional tachycardia may suffer the effects of de-

creased cardiac output, such as hypotension and chest pain.

On an ECG, the atrial rate may be difficult to determine if the P wave is absent or hidden in the QRS complex or preceding T wave. The P wave is usually inverted, and the PR interval is shortened (less than 0.12 second) if the P wave precedes the QRS complex. The QT interval is usually normal, but a fast rate may make the T wave indiscernible.

Possible causes of junctional tachycardia include digitalis toxicity, cardiomyopathy, hypoxia, inferior wall MI or myocardial ischemia, myocarditis, open-heart surgery, and electrolyte imbalances.

Treatment

• Treatment aims to correct the underlying cause.
• Maintain adequate cardiac output by using a temporary atrial pacemaker to override the arrhythmia.
• Other measures may include cardioversion, vagotonic maneuvers such as carotid sinus massage, and drug therapy with *digoxin* (p. 118)—if it's not the cause of the arrhythmia—to strengthen myocardial contractility and *propranolol* (p. 280) and *verapamil* (p. 316) to decrease cardiac oxygen demand.
• If junctional tachycardia results from digitalis toxicity, discontinue the drug, or use *digoxin immune FAB* (p. 124), which binds digoxin and digitoxin and blocks their action.
• If the tachycardia is resistant to drug therapy, catheter ablation of the junctional site may be necessary.

Lown-Ganong-Levine syndrome

A preexcitation syndrome, Lown-Ganong-Levine (LGL) syndrome occurs when an atrial bypass tract outside the AV junction connects the atrium to the AV node's lower portion or to the bundle of His. The bypass tract conducts the impulses either by antegrade or retrograde pathways to the atria. With retrograde conduction, circus reentry can arise, resulting in a reentrant tachycardia and symptoms of decreased cardiac output, such as sudden chest pain, shortness of breath, palpitations and, possibly, syncope.

On the ECG, the PR interval is abnormally short (0.1 second or less), but constant.

LGL syndrome is probably congenital, but its exact cause is unknown. The syndrome may lead to abrupt episodes of PAT, atrial fibrillation, and atrial flutter.

The prognosis is good in patients without tachycardia or an associated cardiac anomaly.

Treatment

- No treatment is usually necessary.
- Treat the tachyarrhythmia initially with vagotonic maneuvers to control the heart rate.
- If the tachyarrhythmia is debilitating, catheter-induced electrical or radio-frequency ablation may be necessary to sever the accessory pathway.
- After vagal maneuvers, the initial drug of choice is *adenosine* (p. 64) or antiarrhythmics, such as *pro-cainamide* (p. 272) or *quinidine* (p. 284), to correct the tachyarrhythmia.
- Use *amiodarone* (p. 72), a class III antiarrhythmic, with extreme caution if the patient has received class I drugs. Concomitant use increases the risk of toxicity.
- Cardioversion may be performed if other measures fail.
- *Digoxin* (p. 118) and *verapamil* (p. 316) prolong conduction time in the AV node and should be used with caution or avoided. In the patient with atrial fibrillation, digoxin also shortens refraction in the accessory pathway and may increase the ventricular response. I.V. verapamil may precipitate ventricular fibrillation in a patient with atrial fibrillation.

Mitral insufficiency

Also known as mitral regurgitation, mitral insufficiency occurs when a damaged mitral valve allows the backflow of blood from the left ventricle into the left atrium during systole. As a result, the atrium and the left ventricle dilate to accommodate the backflow and to compensate for diminishing cardiac output. Ventricular hypertrophy and increased end-diastolic pressure result in increased PAP, eventually leading to left and right ventricular failure with pulmonary edema and CV collapse. The larger the ventricular end-diastolic volume, the poorer the prognosis.

Mitral insufficiency tends to be progressive. The mitral valve can be damaged by rheumatic fever, hypertrophic cardiomyopathy, mitral prolapse, MI, severe left ventricular failure, or ruptured chordae tendineae.

Mitral insufficiency is sometimes associated with congenital anomalies, such as transposition of the great arteries. In older patients, mitral insufficiency may occur because the mitral annulus has become calcified.

Treatment

• The nature and severity of associated symptoms determine treatment in heart valve disease. The patient may need to restrict activities to avoid extreme fatigue and dyspnea.

• Heart failure requires *digoxin* (p. 118), diuretics such as *furosemide* (p. 162), a sodium-restricted diet and, in acute cases, oxygen administration.

• Anticoagulant therapy with *heparin* (p. 169) and then *warfarin* (p. 321) to prevent thrombus formation, and ACE inhibitors such as *captopril* (p. 99) may be used when the insufficiency is associated with atrial fibrillation.

• Prophylactic antibiotics are prescribed before and after surgery or dental care.

• If the patient has severe signs and symptoms that can't be managed medically, he may need open-heart surgery with cardiopulmonary bypass for valve replacement.

Mitral prolapse

A leading cause of mitral insufficiency, mitral prolapse occurs when the posterior or both valve leaflets protrude back into the left atrium during ventricular systole. This weakens the outer layer, permitting abnormal degrees of valve prolapse.

Mitral prolapse occurs in up to 5% of the population, with a 2:1 female-to-male ratio in young adults, a more equal distribution between women and men in middle and older age-groups, and peak incidence in patients in their 40s.

Among the factors that may contribute to mitral prolapse are a family history of the disorder; congenital malformations; changes secondary to other cardiac and systemic problems, such as rheumatic heart disease or Marfan syndrome; and autonomic nervous system dysfunction.

Complications of mitral prolapse include arrhythmias, CHF, infective endocarditis, rupture of the chordae tendineae, and cerebral embolism. Approximately 15% of patients develop progressive mitral insufficiency over a 10- to 15-year period and may need mitral valve replacement.

Treatment

• Mitral prolapse is often benign and may require no treatment. A majority of patients remain asymptomatic throughout their lives, but a cardiologist should still see them every 2 to 3 years.

• Since mitral valve repair or replacement is only rarely indicated, treatment usually aims to relieve symptoms.

• Administer anxiolytics to decrease the sympathetic stimulation and anxiety sometimes associated with mitral prolapse.

• Nitrates such as *nitroglycerin* (p. 233) may relieve ischemic chest pain but increase regional ischemia by reducing cardiac size and thus increas-

ing the degree of valve prolapse. Adequate rest is a safer treatment option.
• Treat symptomatic arrhythmias caused by decreased coronary artery blood flow and ischemia with beta blockers such as *propranolol* (p. 280).
• Use diuretics such as *bumetanide* (p. 96) or *furosemide* (p. 162) when CHF is present (caused by mitral insufficiency).
• Provide prophylaxis against infective endocarditis by using antibiotics before dental, respiratory tract, genitourinary, and GI procedures.

Mitral stenosis

In this disorder, valve leaflets become diffusely thickened by fibrosis and calcification. The mitral commissures fuse, the chordae tendineae fuse and shorten, the valve cusps become rigid, and the apex of the valve becomes narrowed, obstructing blood flow from the left atrium to the left ventricle.

As a result, left atrial volume and pressure rise and the atrial chamber dilates. The increased resistance to blood flow causes pulmonary hypertension, right ventricular hypertrophy, a reduction in cardiac output and, eventually, right ventricular failure. What's more, inadequate filling of the left ventricle reduces cardiac output. Two-thirds of all patients are women.

Mitral stenosis most commonly results from rheumatic fever. It may also be associated with congenital anomalies.

Pulmonary hypertension caused by mitral stenosis can rupture pulmonary-bronchial venous connections and cause fibrosis in the alveoli and pulmonary capillaries. This reduces vital capacity, total lung capacity, maximal breathing capacity, and oxygen uptake. Additionally, thrombi may form in the left atrium and, if they embolize, travel to the brain, kidneys, spleen, and extremities. Embolisms occur most commonly in patients with arrhythmias. The prognosis is good with surgery (commissurotomy or valve replacement).

Treatment
• Patients with rheumatic heart disease should receive penicillin for beta-hemolytic streptococcal infections. If the patient is young and asymptomatic, penicillin is an important prophylactic.
• If the patient is symptomatic, treatment may include activity restrictions, diuretics such as *furosemide* (p. 162), a sodium-restricted diet and, in acute cases, oxygen administration. Small doses of beta blockers such as *propranolol* (p. 280) may also be used to slow the ventricular rate when digitalis glycosides such as *digoxin* (p. 118) fail to control atrial fibrillation or flutter.
• Anticoagulant therapy with *heparin* (p. 169) and *warfarin* (p. 321) is used to prevent thrombus formation when the patient is in atrial fibrillation.
• Embolisms require anticoagulants, such as heparin and warfarin, along with treatment of the patient's symptoms.
• If the patient has severe signs and symptoms that can't be managed medically, she may need open-heart

surgery with cardiopulmonary bypass for commissurotomy or valve replacement.
• Percutaneous balloon valvuloplasty may be used in young patients who have no calcification or subvalvular deformity, in symptomatic pregnant women, and in elderly patients with end-stage disease who cannot withstand general anesthesia.

Myocardial infarction

MI results from reduced blood flow through one of the coronary arteries, which causes myocardial ischemia and necrosis. The infarction site depends on the vessels involved. For example, occlusion of the circumflex coronary artery causes a lateral wall infarction; occlusion of the left anterior coronary artery causes an anterior wall infarction. In Q-wave (transmural) MI, tissue damage extends through all myocardial layers; in non–Q-wave (subendocardial) MI, only the innermost layer is usually damaged.

In North America and western Europe, MI is one of the most common causes of death, usually resulting from cardiac damage or other complications. Mortality is about 25%, with more than 50% of sudden deaths occurring within 1 hour after onset of signs and symptoms, often before the patient reaches the hospital.

Men are more susceptible to MI than premenopausal women, although incidence is rising among women who smoke and take oral contraceptives. The incidence in postmenopausal women is similar to that in men.

Treatment

• The goals of treatment are to reduce myocardial ischemia and to preserve myocardial tissue by restoring blood flow, relieving chest pain, stabilizing heart rhythm, and reducing cardiac workload.
• Arrhythmias, the most common problem during the first 48 hours after MI, are treated with anti-arrhythmic drugs, possibly a pacemaker and, rarely, cardioversion.
• Drug therapy includes:
— initial therapy with an intracoronary or systemic thrombolytic, such as *alteplase* (p. 65), *streptokinase* (p. 301), or urokinase, accompanied by aspirin and *heparin* (p. 169). The aspirin is continued long-term. Thrombolytic therapy must be started within 6 hours of the MI. The best response occurs when treatment begins within the first hour after onset of symptoms.
— *lidocaine* (p. 192) for ventricular arrhythmias; if lidocaine is ineffective, *bretylium* (p. 93), *disopyramide* (p. 133), *procainamide* (p. 272), or *quinidine* (p. 284)
— *atropine* (p. 83) I.V. or a temporary pacemaker for heart block or bradycardia
— *isosorbide dinitrate* (p. 185), *nitroglycerin* (p. 233), or calcium channel blockers, such as *diltiazem* (p. 127), *nifedipine* (p. 230), or *verapamil* (p. 316), to relieve pain by redistributing blood to ischemic areas of the myocardium, thus increasing cardiac output and reducing myocardial workload
— *morphine sulfate* (p. 223) I.V. (the drug of choice for pain and sedation), meperidine, or hydromorphone

— inotropic drugs, such as *amrinone* (p. 78), *dobutamine* (p. 136), or *dopamine* (p. 139), to treat reduced myocardial contractility
— beta blockers, such as *metoprolol* (p. 213), *propranolol* (p. 280), or *timolol* (p. 305), during and after acute MI to help reduce infarct size, prevent reinfarction, and decrease mortality
— ACE inhibitors, such as *captopril* (p. 99) or *enalapril* (p. 143)
— magnesium to reduce the risk of arrhythmias.
• Oxygen is usually administered at a modest flow rate for 24 to 48 hours; a lower concentration is necessary if the patient has COPD.
• Pulmonary artery catheterization may be performed on a patient with heart failure or cardiogenic shock to monitor response to treatment or to detect left or right ventricular failure.
• An IABP may be inserted for cardiogenic shock.
• Reperfusion therapy is used if the patient is younger than age 70 and doesn't have a history of CVA, bleeding, GI ulcers, marked hypertension, recent surgery, or chest pain lasting longer than 6 hours.
• PTCA, directional coronary artery atherectomy, and CABG may also be performed.

Myocarditis

A focal or diffuse inflammation of the myocardium, myocarditis is typically uncomplicated and self-limiting and produces no symptoms. It may be acute or chronic and can occur at any age. Myocarditis usually resolves spontaneously and without residual effects.

Occasionally, however, myocarditis may induce myofibril degeneration, right and left ventricular failure with cardiomegaly, arrhythmias, or cardiomyopathy. Myocarditis may also recur or produce chronic valvulitis (when it results from rheumatic fever) or thromboembolism.

This disorder may result from viruses (the most common cause in the United States and western Europe), bacteria, hypersensitivity reactions, radiation therapy, chemical poisoning, parasitic infections, and helminthic infections. The cause of giant cell myocarditis, a rare type of myocarditis, is unknown.

Treatment
• For most patients, treatment includes anti-infectives for the underlying causative infection, modified bed rest to decrease the heart's workload, and careful management of complications.
• Left ventricular failure requires activity restrictions to minimize myocardial oxygen consumption, supplemental oxygen therapy, sodium restriction, diuretics such as *furosemide* (p. 162) to decrease fluid retention, and *digoxin* (p. 118) to increase myocardial contractility. However, digoxin must be administered carefully because some patients with myocarditis may show unusual sensitivity to even small doses of the drug.
• Arrhythmias necessitate prompt but cautious administration of antiarrhythmics, such as *procainamide* (p. 272) or *quinidine* (p. 284).

• Thromboembolism requires antico-agulant therapy with *heparin* (p. 169) or *warfarin* (p. 321).
• Contraindicated during the acute phase (first 2 weeks) because of an increased risk of myocardial damage, NSAIDs such as ibuprofen or aspirin are used in late-phase myocarditis.

Parasystole

A benign arrhythmia, parasystole is the interaction of two foci that inde-pendently initiate cardiac impulses at different rates, one usually in the SA node and the other in the atrium, AV junction, or ventricle. Atrial and junctional parasystole may occur in a healthy heart, but ventricular para-systole is usually associated with heart disease.

On an ECG, atrial and ventricular rhythms are irregular, and atrial and ventricular rates follow the dominant rhythm. The size and configuration of the P wave change in the parasys-tolic beats because the pacemaker is not the SA node. The QRS complex is of normal duration in atrial and junc-tional parasystolic beats but widens in ventricular parasystolic beats; its configuration differs from the QRS complex during a dominant rhythm. The T wave is normal in size and con-figuration in atrial and junctional parasystolic beats but abnormal in ventricular parasystolic beats. The QT interval is of normal duration in atrial and junctional parasystolic beats but may be lengthened in ven-tricular parasystolic beats.

Parasystole may result from MI or may be idiopathic.

Treatment

• Parasystole usually is benign and requires no treatment.
• If the patient is symptomatic or if the arrhythmia is accompanied by myocardial ischemia or hemodyna-mic compromise, administer oxygen or antiarrhythmic drugs.

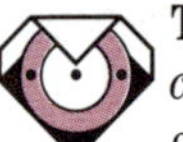 **Treatment of choice.** *Lido-caine* (p. 192) is the drug of choice. If lidocaine is in-effective, however, give *bretylium* (p. 93) or *procainamide* (p. 272).
• If the patient is hypokalemic, give potassium supplements. Also moni-tor magnesium levels and give supple-ments as required.

Patent ductus arteriosus

The ductus arteriosus is a blood ves-sel that connects the pulmonary arte-ry to the descending aorta during fe-tal development. Normally, the duc-tus closes within days or weeks after birth, its closure routing oxygenated blood to the body and unoxygenated blood to the lungs.

In patent ductus arteriosus, how-ever, the lumen of the ductus re-mains open after birth. This abnor-mal opening allows blood to shunt from the aorta to the pulmonary arte-ry, recirculating oxygenated arterial blood through the lungs. The left atri-um and left ventricle must then accommodate increased pulmonary venous return, which raises left ven-tricular filling pressure and workload and may lead to left ventricular fail-ure.

The most common neonatal con-genital heart defect, patent ductus arteriosus typically affects twice as many girls as boys (both sexes equally when accompanied by rubella syndrome). The prognosis is good if the shunt is small or can be surgically repaired.

Patent ductus arteriosus may be familial, or it may have no known cause. It commonly accompanies rubella syndrome and may be associated with other congenital defects, such as coarctation of the aorta, a ventricular septal defect, and pulmonic and aortic stenoses.

Treatment

• Asymptomatic infants require no immediate treatment.
• If signs and symptoms are mild, surgery is usually delayed until the infant is 1 year old. Before surgery, the child requires antibiotics to protect against infective endocarditis.
• Infants with left ventricular failure require fluid restriction and diuretics, such as *digoxin* (p. 118) or *furosemide* (p. 162), to close the ductus until surgery can be performed.
• Other treatments include cardiac catheterization to deposit a plug or umbrella in the ductus or administration of indomethacin I.V. to induce the ductus to spasm and close.

Pericardial effusion

The major complication of pericarditis, pericardial effusion is an accumulation of more than 50 ml of pericardial fluid. (Normally, the pericardial sac contains between 15 and 50 ml of fluid.) This excess fluid, which may be bloody or contain exudates, accumulates and impairs the heart's ability to fill in diastole and contract in systole.

When excess fluid accumulates quickly, the pericardium cannot adjust to the sudden rise of volume and pressure. Pericardial effusion must be treated immediately to avoid cardiac compression, cardiac tamponade, and death. Recurrent pericardial effusion can lead to scarring and thickening of the pericardium.

Pericardial effusion may develop as a response to viral or bacterial pericarditis, idiopathic infections, metastatic disease, trauma, MI, radiation therapy, systemic lupus erythematosus, rheumatoid arthritis, endocarditis, uremia, post-pericardiotomy syndrome, or acquired immunodeficiency syndrome. Drugs such as heparin, warfarin, procainamide, hydralazine, dantrolene, and methysergide may provoke pericardial effusion.

Treatment

• If cardiac compression occurs, pericardiocentesis may be necessary to quickly reduce the amount of pericardial fluid.
• If effusion is not excessive and the patient is not hemodynamically compromised, bed rest, supplemental oxygen, and Fowler's position may ease dyspnea associated with compression of the heart and adjacent lung tissue.
• Give antianxiety agents and provide a quiet, calm environment to decrease anxiety associated with dyspnea. Administer analgesics such as *morphine sulfate* (p. 223) or NSAIDs to relieve pain associated with pericardial effusion (but only if the pa-

tient is not hemodynamically compromised).

• Arrhythmias provoked by excessive pericardial fluid may be treated with antiarrhythmic agents, such as *atropine* (p. 83), *bretylium* (p. 93), *diltiazem* (p. 127), *lidocaine* (p. 192), *procainamide* (p. 272), *propranolol* (p. 280), or *verapamil* (p. 316).

• Hemodynamic monitoring may be required to assess decreased cardiac output, increased left ventricular filling pressures, or a rise in central venous pressure associated with cardiac tamponade.

• CHF may be treated with diuretics, such as *ethacrynic acid* (p. 153) or *furosemide* (p. 162).

• Bacterial or viral pericardial effusion may be treated with antimicrobial agents.

• A pericardiectomy may be indicated for recurrent pericardial effusions or for a thickened pericardium associated with constrictive pericarditis.

• Positive inotropic agents, such as *dobutamine* (p. 136) or *dopamine* (p. 139), may optimize cardiac output.

Pericarditis

An inflammation of the pericardium, the fibroserous sac that envelops, supports, and protects the heart, pericarditis can be acute or chronic. The acute form can be fibrinous or effusive, with serous, purulent, or hemorrhagic exudate. The chronic form, called constrictive pericarditis, is characterized by dense, fibrous pericardial thickening.

Pericardial effusion is the major complication of acute pericarditis. If fluid accumulates rapidly, cardiac tamponade may occur, resulting in shock, CV collapse and, eventually, death. The prognosis depends on the underlying cause but, unless constriction occurs, is typically good even in acute pericarditis.

Common causes of this disorder include bacterial, fungal, or viral infection (infectious pericarditis); neoplasms; high-dose radiation treatments to the chest; uremia; hypersensitivity or autoimmune disorders, such as acute rheumatic fever (the most common cause of pericarditis in children), systemic lupus erythematosus, and rheumatoid arthritis; drugs, such as hydralazine or procainamide; and cardiac injury, such as MI, trauma, or surgery that leaves the pericardium intact but allows blood to leak into the pericardial cavity.

Treatment

• Treatment aims to relieve symptoms, manage underlying systemic disease, and prevent or treat pericardial effusion and cardiac tamponade.

• In idiopathic pericarditis, post-MI pericarditis, and postthoracotomy pericarditis, treatment consists of bed rest as long as fever and pain persist and the administration of NSAIDs, such as aspirin and indomethacin, to relieve pain and reduce inflammation. If symptoms continue, the doctor may prescribe corticosteroids.

• Administer antibiotics when infectious pericarditis results from dis-

ease of the left pleural space, mediastinal abscesses, or septicemia.
• If cardiac tamponade develops, the doctor may perform emergency pericardiocentesis and inject antibiotics directly into the pericardial sac.
• Recurrent pericarditis may require partial pericardiectomy; constrictive pericarditis may require total pericardiectomy to permit the heart to fill and contract adequately.
• Treatment must also include management of the underlying disorder, such as rheumatic fever, uremia, or tuberculosis.

Premature atrial contractions

Originating outside the SA node, PACs usually arise from an irritable focus in the atria that supersedes the SA node as pacemaker for one or more beats. PACs are rarely dangerous in patients free of heart disease. However, they may precipitate a more serious arrhythmia (such as atrial flutter or atrial fibrillation) in patients with heart disease. If PACs occur with an acute MI, they may signal CHF, pericarditis, or an electrolyte imbalance.

On an ECG, atrial and ventricular rhythms are irregular, but the underlying rhythm may be regular. Atrial and ventricular rates vary with the underlying rhythm. The P wave is premature and abnormally shaped and may be lost in the previous T wave. If no QRS complex follows the P wave, a nonconducted PAC may have occurred. This happens when an impulse arrives in the ventricles during their absolute refractory period, so

there's no ventricular response. Don't confuse a nonconducted PAC with either sinus arrest or SA block.

Possible causes of PACs include acute respiratory failure, COPD, or hypoxia; CHF and ischemic, coronary, and heart valve disease; drugs that prolong the SA node's absolute refractory period, such as digoxin, quinidine, and procainamide; excessive use of caffeine, tobacco, or alcohol; and stress, fatigue, or overeating.

Treatment
• Most patients don't require treatment, but once a PAC has been identified, closely monitor the patient's apical pulse rate and rhythm, and assess for increased heart rate, shortness of breath, and chest pain.
• Eliminate known causes of PACs, such as caffeine, tobacco, or alcohol.
• For frequent PACs or those that cause sustained tachycardia, administer drugs that prolong the atrial refractory period, such as *digoxin* (p. 118) (unless it is the cause), *propranolol* (p. 280), or *verapamil* (p. 316).

Premature junctional contractions

An ectopic impulse initiated early by the AV node or bundle of His, a PJC results from enhanced automaticity. PJCs are generally considered harmless, unless they occur frequently (usually defined as more than six per minute). Frequent PJCs indicate junctional irritability and can precipitate a more dangerous arrhythmia, such as paroxysmal junctional tachycardia. In patients taking digitalis glycosides, PJCs are a common early sign of toxicity.

On an ECG, atrial and ventricular rhythms are irregular, but the underlying rhythm may be regular. Atrial and ventricular rates follow the underlying rhythm. The P wave is usually inverted. If the P wave precedes the QRS complex, the PR interval is shortened (less than 0.12 second). A noncompensatory pause reflecting retrograde atrial conduction commonly accompanies PJCs.

Digitalis toxicity is the most common cause of PJCs. Other causes include excessive caffeine or amphetamine ingestion, MI, or myocardial ischemia.

Treatment
• Usually, no treatment is required for this condition.
• If PJCs produce symptoms, treat the underlying cause. For example, if a digitalis glycoside such as digoxin is causing PJCs, withhold the drug. If caffeine is the cause, restrict the patient's caffeine intake.

Premature ventricular contractions

Among the most common arrhythmias, PVCs are ectopic beats that originate low in the ventricles (usually below the bundle of His) and that occur earlier than expected. They may occur singly, in pairs, or in threes and in many cases are followed by a compensatory pause. PVCs may be uniform, arising from the same ectopic focus, or multiform, arising from two different ventricular sites or from one site with abnormal conduction.

PVCs are benign in a healthy asymptomatic patient, but more serious if they occur in a patient with heart disease. In an ischemic or damaged heart, PVCs may develop into ventricular tachycardia, flutter, or fibrillation. Multiform PVCs can be life-threatening and usually indicate severe heart disease or digitalis toxicity.

On an ECG, atrial and ventricular rhythms are irregular; however, the underlying rhythm may be regular. Atrial and ventricular rates follow the underlying rhythm. The QRS complex occurs early, with a duration exceeding 0.12 second and a bizarre configuration. The T wave occurs in the direction opposite that of the QRS complex, and a compensatory pause may follow the T wave.

PVCs may result from caffeine, tobacco, or alcohol ingestion; digitalis toxicity; strenuous or unaccustomed exercise; hypocalcemia; hypokalemia; myocardial irritation by pacemaker electrodes; myocardial scarring secondary to MI; heart valve disease; or sympathomimetic drugs (for example, epinephrine and isoproterenol).

Treatment
• Treatment is required only when PVCs are frequent (six or more a minute) or sustained and the patient is symptomatic (light-headed, experiencing syncope).
• Treatment depends on the underlying cause. For bradycardia, give *atropine* (p. 83) instead of *lidocaine* (p. 192) to elevate the heart rate and

thus override the PVC, because lidocaine may further depress ventricular electrical activity.

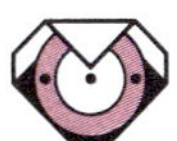 **Treatment of choice.** The drug of choice for acute situations is lidocaine; if it's ineffective, the doctor may prescribe *bretylium* (p. 93) or *procainamide* (p. 272). Administer oxygen concurrently or separately as ordered.

• For patients with chronic PVCs, give *amiodarone* (p. 72), procainamide, or *quinidine* (p. 284), but only if the PVC is life-threatening. Beta blockers, such as *propranolol* (p. 280) or *sotalol* (p. 294), may also be used.

• If the patient is hypokalemic, give potassium supplements. Monitor magnesium levels and provide supplements, if required.

• If the patient has a pacemaker, the electrodes may need to be repositioned; they may be the source of myocardial irritation.

Prolonged QT syndrome

Ventricular depolarization-repolarization, or electrical systole, is represented on the ECG by the QT interval. When the QT interval becomes prolonged, the risk of developing ventricular arrhythmias, syncope, torsades de pointes, and cardiac arrest increases. A prolonged QT interval in myocardial ischemia or MI may herald a life-threatening ventricular arrhythmia.

Causes of prolonged QT syndrome include electrolyte disturbances, such as hypocalcemia, hypomagnesemia, and hypokalemia; antiarrhythmics, such as quinidine, procainamide, disopyramide, flecainide, amiodarone, sotalol, and bepridil; and other drugs, including phenothiazines, probucol, erythromycin, thiazides, and terfenadine.

Other causes of prolonged QT syndrome include myocardial ischemia, subarachnoid hemorrhage, ruptured cerebral aneurysm, streptococcal meningitis, hypothermia, liquid protein diets, and rare congenital syndromes, such as Jervell and Lange-Nielsen syndrome and Romano-Ward syndrome.

Treatment

• The key to treating prolonged QT syndrome is to determine the underlying cause; however, suppressing ventricular arrhythmias is the first priority.

• Electrical cardioversion or defibrillation may disrupt the ventricular arrhythmia.

• Temporary pacing disrupts ventricular tachycardia.

• *Isoproterenol* (p. 181) is used frequently to increase heart rate and shorten the QT interval. But it must be administered with caution in patients with myocardial ischemia.

• Discontinue any contributing drugs.

• Antiarrhythmics, such as *bretylium* (p. 93), *lidocaine* (p. 192), or phenytoin, can shorten repolarization.

• Magnesium sulfate is commonly administered, even to patients with normal serum magnesium levels, to shorten the refractory period.

• The cardiologist may order revascularization by angioplasty to improve or reverse ischemia.

- Congenital prolonged QT syndrome may be treated with beta blockers, such as *metoprolol* (p. 213) or *propranolol* (p. 280), or left stellate ganglionectomy.

Pulmonary edema

A common complication of cardiac disorders, pulmonary edema is marked by an accumulation of fluid in extravascular spaces of the lungs. The disorder may occur as a chronic condition or may develop quickly and rapidly become fatal. Acute pulmonary edema may progress to respiratory and metabolic acidosis, with subsequent cardiac or respiratory arrest.

Pulmonary edema usually results from left ventricular failure caused by arteriosclerotic, cardiomyopathic, hypertensive, or valvular heart disease. The disorder stems from the imbalance of two normally balanced mechanisms: increased pulmonary capillary hydrostatic pressure and decreased colloid osmotic pressure.

Factors that may predispose the patient to pulmonary edema include barbiturate or opiate poisoning, CHF, excessive or overly rapid infusion of I.V. solutions, impaired pulmonary lymphatic drainage, inhalation of irritating gases, mitral stenosis and left atrial myxoma, pneumonia, or pulmonary veno-occlusive disease.

Treatment

- Treatment aims to reduce extravascular fluid, improve gas exchange and myocardial function and, if possible, correct the underlying disease.
- High concentrations of oxygen can be administered by nasal cannula (not mask, which pulmonary edema patients typically cannot tolerate). If the patient's arterial oxygen levels remain too low, mechanical ventilation can improve oxygen delivery to the tissues and usually improves acid-base balance.
- A bronchodilator may decrease bronchospasm and enhance myocardial contractility. Diuretics, such as *bumetanide* (p. 96), *ethacrynic acid* (p. 153), and *furosemide* (p. 162), increase urination, which helps to mobilize extravascular fluid.
- Positive inotropic agents, such as *amrinone* (p. 78) and *digoxin* (p. 118), may enhance contractility in treating myocardial dysfunction.
- Antiarrhythmics, such as *lidocaine* (p. 192) or *procainamide* (p. 272), may also be given, particularly in arrhythmias related to decreased cardiac output. Occasionally, venous and arterial vasodilators, such as I.V. *nitroglycerin* (p. 233) and *nitroprusside* (p. 240), are used to decrease preload, peripheral vascular resistance, and afterload.
- *Morphine sulfate* (p. 223) may reduce anxiety and dyspnea and dilate the systemic venous bed, promoting blood flow from pulmonary circulation to the periphery.
- Other treatments include rotating tourniquets and phlebotomy (to reduce preload). However, phlebotomy will also remove hemoglobin, which may worsen the patient's hypoxemia.
- Albumin may be used to correct causative hypoalbuminemia.

Pulmonary hypertension

In both the rare primary and more common secondary form, pulmonary hypertension is indicated by a resting systolic PAP above 30 mm Hg and a mean PAP above 18 mm Hg.

Primary or idiopathic pulmonary hypertension occurs most commonly in women between ages 20 and 40 and is usually fatal within 3 to 4 years; mortality is highest in pregnant women. Secondary pulmonary hypertension is caused by existing cardiac or pulmonary disease, or both. The prognosis in secondary pulmonary hypertension depends on the severity of the underlying disorder. Both forms may ultimately lead to cor pulmonale, cardiac failure, and cardiac arrest.

The cause of primary pulmonary hypertension remains unknown, but a hereditary defect, collagen disease, and altered immune mechanisms may be responsible. Secondary pulmonary hypertension results from hypoxemia.

Treatment

• Oxygen therapy decreases hypoxemia and resulting pulmonary vascular resistance.
• For patients with right ventricular failure, treatment also includes fluid restriction, *digoxin* (p. 118) to increase cardiac output, and diuretics, such as *bumetanide* (p. 96) or *furosemide* (p. 162), to decrease intravascular volume and extravascular fluid accumulation.
• Drug therapy includes vasodilators, such as I.V. *nitroglycerin* (p. 233) or *nitroprusside* (p. 240), in acute situ-ations, and antihypertensives, such as *hydralazine* (p. 174) or *prazosin* (p. 265), in chronic cases. Calcium channel blockers such as *nifedipine* (p. 230) may also be used to reduce myocardial workload and oxygen consumption. Bronchodilators such as theophylline may also be prescribed.
• For a patient with secondary pulmonary hypertension, treatment must also aim to correct the underlying cause. If that's not possible and the disease progresses, the patient may need a heart-lung transplant.

Pulmonic insufficiency

In this disorder, blood ejected into the pulmonary artery during systole flows back into the right ventricle during diastole, causing fluid overload in the ventricle, ventricular hypertrophy and, eventually, right ventricular failure.

Pulmonic insufficiency may be congenital or result from pulmonary hypertension. Rarely, it may result from prolonged use of a pressure monitoring catheter in the pulmonary artery.

The prognosis depends on the disorder's progression and severity.

Treatment

• Treatment is based on the patient's symptoms. A low-sodium diet and diuretics, such as *bumetanide* (p. 96) or *furosemide* (p. 162), help to reduce hepatic congestion before surgery.
• Valve replacement may be required in severe cases.

Pulmonic stenosis

A narrowing, or stenosis, of the opening of the pulmonary artery from the right ventricle, pulmonic stenosis causes right ventricular hypertrophy as the ventricle attempts to overcome resistance to the narrow valve opening.

Right ventricular failure is the ultimate result of untreated pulmonic stenosis. The prognosis depends on the severity of the obstruction.

Pulmonic stenosis usually results from congenital stenosis of the pulmonic valve cusp. It's also associated with other congenital heart defects, such as tetralogy of Fallot. Occasionally, rheumatic heart disease leads to pulmonic stenosis.

Treatment

• A low-sodium diet and diuretics, such as *bumetanide* (p. 96) or *furosemide* (p. 162), reduce hepatic congestion before surgery.
• Cardiac catheter balloon valvuloplasty is usually effective even with moderate to severe obstruction.
• Use antibiotic prophylaxis to prevent infective endocarditis.
• If the obstruction is not relieved or if the condition is severe, a valvotomy may be performed.

Pulseless electrical activity

An umbrella term for several arrhythmias, pulseless electrical activity is the absence of a detectable pulse or effective myocardial contraction but the presence of some type of electrical activity other than VT or ventricular fibrillation.

Pulseless electrical activity includes the following arrhythmias: electromechanical dissociation, pseudo-electromechanical dissociation, idioventricular rhythms, ventricular escape rhythms, bradyasystolic rhythms, and postdefibrillation idioventricular rhythms. These arrhythmias are frequently associated with conditions, such as hypoxia and hypovolemia, that can be reversed with prompt treatment. If treatment is not successful, however, they're usually fatal.

On an ECG, atrial and ventricular rhythms are the same as the underlying rhythm and become irregular as the rate slows. The atrial and ventricular rates also reflect that of the underlying rhythm but the ventricular rate gradually decreases. The P wave, PR interval, QRS complex, T wave, and QT interval are also the same as in the underlying rhythm but eventually become indiscernible. A flat line tracing indicating asystole usually occurs within several minutes.

Possible causes of pulseless electrical activity include hypovolemia from severe hemorrhage, failure in the calcium transport mechanism, extensive myocardial damage, tension pneumothorax, cardiac tamponade, hypoxemia, acidosis, a massive pulmonary embolus, and advanced left ventricular failure. Other causes include hypothermia, hyperkalemia, and an overdose of a tricyclic antidepressant, digitalis glycoside, beta blocker, or calcium channel blocker.

Treatment

- Pulseless electrical activity is a life-threatening emergency. Start CPR immediately, and administer I.V. fluids and *epinephrine* (p. 146) by I.V. push (repeating epinephrine administration every 3 to 5 minutes as needed). If the heart rate is less than 60 beats/minute, give atropine by I.V. push and repeat every 4 to 5 minutes up to a total of 0.04 mg/kg.
- Identify the cause of the pulseless electrical activity and treat it accordingly. Discontinue the causative drug, if appropriate.
- Provide blood and fluid replacement in severe hemorrhage, hypoxemia, acidosis, and pulmonary embolus.
- In ventricular rupture, the doctor will perform pericardiocentesis and surgically repair the rupture.
- Chest intubation is necessary in tension pneumothorax.
- Use Doppler ultrasound to identify blood flow not detected by arterial palpation. Treat severe hypotension with fluid volume replacement and *dopamine* (p. 139), and initiate transcutaneous pacing.
- Recognize that pacemaker insertion is rarely effective because the myocardial tissue can't respond appropriately to any electrical stimulus.

Raynaud's disease

Also known as vasospastic arterial disease, Raynaud's disease is one of several primary arteriospastic disorders characterized by episodic vasospasm in the small peripheral arteries and arterioles precipitated by exposure to cold or by stress. In rare cases, severe, persistent vasoconstriction may lead to ischemia and gangrene; eventually, amputation may be necessary.

The disease is five times more common in women than in men, particularly between late adolescence and age 40. Although the cause is unknown, several conditions may account for the reduced digital blood flow. These include intrinsic vascular wall hyperactivity in response to cold, ineffective basal heat production, increased vasomotor tone from sympathetic stimulation, stress, and a poorly understood antigen-antibody immune response.

Treatment

- Raynaud's disease is usually benign, requiring no specific treatment and having no serious sequelae.
- Treatment of symptoms consists of avoiding cold, avoiding mechanical or chemical injury, and stopping smoking.
- Because adverse reactions to drugs, especially vasodilators, may be more hazardous than the disease itself, drug therapy with *nifedipine* (p. 230), *phenoxybenzamine* (p. 248), *prazosin* (p. 265), or *reserpine* (p. 288) is reserved for unusually severe signs and symptoms.
- Biofeedback therapy may be useful if signs and symptoms are caused by stress.
- Sympathectomy may be helpful when conservative treatment fails to prevent ischemic ulcers (occurring in fewer than 25% of patients).

Rheumatic fever and rheumatic heart disease

A systemic inflammatory disease of childhood, acute rheumatic fever develops after infection of the upper respiratory tract with group A beta-hemolytic streptococci. Rheumatic fever principally involves the heart, joints, CNS, skin, and subcutaneous tissues.

Worldwide, 15 to 20 million new cases are reported each year. Incidence is highest in children between ages 5 and 15 in lower socioeconomic groups; in the United States, it's most common in the northern states. It commonly recurs.

Rheumatic heart disease, the cardiac sequela of rheumatic fever, develops in up to 50% of patients and may affect the endocardium, myocardium, or pericardium during the early acute phase. It may later affect the heart valves, causing chronic valve disease. The extent of damage to the heart depends on where the disorder strikes.

Rheumatic fever appears to be a hypersensitivity reaction in which antibodies produced to combat streptococci instead react to produce characteristic lesions. The prognosis is good if carditis, the most important manifestation of acute rheumatic fever, doesn't develop. Carditis may permanently scar the heart valves and, in its most severe form, may cause death from acute cardiac failure. Pancarditis, inflammation of all the heart's structures, almost always presents with exudative pericardial lesions, dilation of the heart, and valve lesions.

Treatment

- Effective management eradicates the streptococcal infection, relieves symptoms, and prevents recurrence, thus reducing the chance of permanent cardiac damage.
- During the acute phase, the treatment of choice is a 10-day course of antibiotics. Long-term antibiotic therapy can minimize the risk of recurrence, reducing the risk of permanent cardiac damage and valve deformity.
- Salicylates, such as aspirin, relieve fever and minimize joint swelling and pain in adults. In children, acetaminophen is used for fever and NSAIDs are used for joint pain because of the risk of Reye's syndrome. If the patient has carditis or if salicylates fail to relieve pain and inflammation, the doctor may prescribe corticosteroids.
- Supportive treatment consists of strict bed rest for about 5 weeks during the acute phase, followed by a progressive increase in physical activity. The increase depends on clinical and laboratory findings and the patient's response to treatment.
- After the acute phase subsides, a monthly I.M. injection of 1.2 million units of penicillin G benzathine is most effective. Alternatively, oral sulfadiazine or penicillin G may be given daily to prevent recurrence, although this treatment is less reliable. Such preventive treatment usually continues for at least 5 years or until age 25.
- Heart failure requires continued bed rest and diuretics such as *furosemide* (p. 162).

• Severe mitral or aortic valve dysfunction that causes persistent heart failure will require corrective surgery, such as commissurotomy, valvuloplasty, or valve replacement. Corrective valve surgery is seldom necessary before late adolescence.

Sick sinus syndrome

Also known as tachy-brady syndrome, brady-tachy syndrome, SA syndrome, and Adams-Stokes syndrome, SSS is any combination of sinus arrhythmias. These may include sinus bradycardia, alternating bradycardia and tachycardia, sinus arrest, SA block, atrial standstill, atrial tachycardias, atrial fibrillation, transient asystole and, less frequently, atrial flutter.

SSS may be life-threatening in patients with an underlying heart disease, especially if cardiac output is greatly compromised. Most patients with SSS are elderly, but anyone can develop this arrhythmia.

On an ECG, atrial and ventricular rhythms are irregular because of sinus pauses and abrupt rate changes. Atrial and ventricular rates are fast or slow, or alternate between fast and slow, and are interrupted by a long sinus pause. The P wave varies with the prevailing rhythm.

Possible causes of SSS include cardiomyopathy (especially if caused by amyloidosis and progressive muscular dystrophy), collagen disorders, inflammatory disorders, ischemic heart disease, metastatic disorders, and SA node injury during cardiac surgery. In many patients, however, the cause of SSS is never identified.

Treatment

• If SSS results in symptomatic bradycardia, *atropine* (p. 83) or *isoproterenol* (p. 181) may be given initially, followed by insertion of a pacemaker.

• *Digoxin* (p. 118) or *propranolol* (p. 280) may be prescribed if SSS results in tachycardia. However, these drugs may cause slow sinus discharge and should be used with caution in patients without a pacemaker. Alternatively, a combination of a permanent pacemaker and medication may be used to maintain heart rate and ensure adequate cardiac output.

Sinus arrest and exit block

Sinus arrest and exit block — two separate arrhythmias with different pathophysiologies — are discussed together here because distinguishing between them can be difficult and their clinical significance and treatment are the same.

In sinus arrest, the SA node fails to initiate an impulse. In sinus exit block, the SA node initiates the impulse but it can't be conducted to the atria because of a block in the conduction system.

These arrhythmias may result from increased vagal tone; depressed automaticity and conduction due to certain medications such as digitalis glycosides; or cardiac diseases that impair or destroy the conduction system, such as MI or myocarditis.

On an ECG, sinus arrest is recognizable by a pause in the sinus rhythm. In sinus exit block, the pause is a multiple of the basic P-P interval.

In both of these arrhythmias, the atrial rate may vary but usually is less than 60 beats/minute. The PR interval is usually normal unless another condition, such as first-degree AV block, also exists. If a long pause occurs, escape beats from the AV node or ventricle may appear, in which case the QRS complex will have a longer duration and a wider configuration.

Treatment

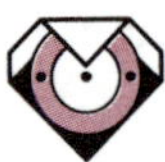

Treatment of choice. If the patient is symptomatic, the drug of choice is *atropine* (p. 83), which prevents the vagus nerve from slowing the heartbeat.

• In patients who experience CHF or symptoms of low cardiac output, a temporary pacemaker may be indicated if atropine does not resolve the sinus arrest or exit block. Until the pacemaker can be inserted, however, a continuous I.V. infusion of *isoproterenol* (p. 181) may be administered.

• If the conduction system is permanently impaired and the pauses exceed 3 seconds, a permanent pacemaker is usually necessary.

Sinus arrhythmia

A normal variation in sinus rhythm related to the respiratory cycle, sinus arrhythmia results from vagal tone inhibition. Unlike sinus bradycardia or sinus tachycardia, the heart rate remains within normal limits.

Sinus arrhythmia may occur normally in athletes and young adults and is usually not significant. However, a marked variation in P-P intervals in an elderly patient may indicate SSS.

On an ECG, the atrial rhythm is irregular, corresponding to the respiratory cycle. Both atrial and ventricular rates are within normal limits but vary with respiration — faster with inspiration, slower with expiration. The P-P and R-R intervals are shorter during inspiration and longer during expiration. The ventricular rhythm is also irregular, corresponding to the respiratory cycle.

Possible causes of sinus arrhythmia include reflex vagal tone inhibition related to the normal respiratory cycle and underlying conditions that increase vagal tone, such as digitalis toxicity, increased ICP, or inferior-wall MI.

Treatment

• No treatment is usually necessary, unless signs and symptoms occur.

• If the patient's heart rate is less than 40 beats/minute and he's symptomatic, he may be given *atropine* (p. 83).

• If sinus arrhythmia is unrelated to the respiratory cycle, it may be due to digitalis toxicity. If so, discontinue digitalis glycoside therapy.

Sinus bradycardia

Characterized by a sinus rate of less than 60 beats/minute, sinus bradycardia is a condition in which all impulses come from the SA node. This arrhythmia is common in athletes, because their well-conditioned hearts can maintain stroke volume with reduced effort, and in patients who have suffered an MI.

Possible causes of sinus bradycardia include hyperkalemia; increased ICP; increased vagal tone that accompanies straining during defecation, vomiting, intubation, mechanical ventilation, SSS, hypothyroidism, eye surgery or intracranial tumors; and adverse reactions to beta blockers, atropine or isoproterenol, digoxin, morphine, or meperidine.

Treatment

• No treatment is necessary unless the patient is hemodynamically compromised.

• If drug toxicity is the cause, normal sinus rates will return when the causative drug is discontinued.

•If the patient is symptomatic, treat the underlying cause and maintain the heart rate with drugs, such as *atropine* (p. 83) or *isoproterenol* (p. 181), or with a pacemaker.

• Give atropine cautiously by rapid I.V. push, particularly in acute MI, because increased oxygen demands caused by a faster heart rate could extend the infarction. If given slowly, it can cause paradoxical slowing of the heart rate.

• Isoproterenol also must be given cautiously if atropine is ineffective because it may increase myocardial irritability and cause ventricular arrhythmias.

Sinus tachycardia

An acceleration of the firing of the SA node beyond its normal discharge rate, sinus tachycardia results in a heart rate of 100 to 180 beats/minute. Rates greater than 180 beats/minute may indicate an ectopic focus.

Sinus tachycardia commonly occurs in healthy patients with no serious adverse effects. However, persistent sinus tachycardia may develop as a normal response to acute MI, leading to further ischemia and myocardial damage by raising the heart's oxygen requirements. In acute MI, it may also be one of the first signs of CHF, cardiogenic shock, pulmonary embolism, or infarct extension.

On an ECG, the QT interval is commonly shortened.

Possible causes of sinus tachycardia include excessive caffeine, nicotine, or alcohol ingestion; digitalis toxicity; hypothyroidism or hyperthyroidism; normal cardiac response to an increased demand for oxygen during anxiety, physical exertion, fever, stress, pain, or dehydration; and treatment with adrenergics, anticholinergics, and some antiarrhythmics.

Treatment

• Treatment aims to correct the underlying cause. Discontinue any causative medications.

• If the patient is symptomatic, beta blockers such as *propranolol* (p. 280) and calcium channel blockers such as *verapamil* (p. 316) may be given to reduce oxygen demand.

• Administer all I.V. fluids cautiously, especially in the hypovolemic patient. Fluid replacement can slow the sinus rate and endanger the patient.

Tetralogy of Fallot

This cardiac defect is really four defects that occur together: a ventricular septal defect, infundibular stenosis (possibly with pulmonic stenosis), right ventricular hypertrophy, and dextroposition of the aorta, which overrides the ventricular septal defect.

The degree of pulmonic stenosis determines the clinical and hemodynamic effects of this complex anomaly. Blood may shunt left to right or right to left, depending on the defect's configuration.

Usually, the ventricular septal defect lies in the outflow tract of the right ventricle and is large enough to equalize right and left ventricular pressures. However, the degree of systemic vascular resistance in relation to the degree of pulmonic stenosis affects how much blood flows across the defect and the direction in which it flows. When blood shunts right to left through the ventricular septal defect, unoxygenated blood mixes with oxygenated blood, which decreases arterial oxygen saturation, leading to cyanosis. Reduced pulmonary blood flow and hypoplasia of all the pulmonary vessels occur. Increased right ventricular pressure related to severely obstructed right ventricular outflow ultimately causes right ventricular hypertrophy.

Tetralogy of Fallot is one of the most common congenital heart defects and occurs equally in men and women. It may coexist with other congenital heart defects, such as patent ductus arteriosus or an atrial septal defect.

Tetralogy of Fallot stems from embryonic hypoplasia of the right ventricle's outflow tract. The cause of the hypoplasia is unknown; however, it has been associated with fetal alcohol syndrome and maternal ingestion of thalidomide during pregnancy.

Treatment

- *Propranolol* (p. 280) may prevent cyanotic episodes. During cyanotic spells, oxygenation will improve if the patient assumes the knee-chest position and receives oxygen and *morphine sulfate* (p. 223).
- Surgery that joins the subclavian artery to the pulmonary artery (Blalock-Taussig operation) may enhance blood flow to the lungs, reducing hypoxia.
- Supportive measures include antibiotics administered before, during, and after dental treatments or surgery. Phlebotomy may also be needed in children with polycythemia.
- Open-heart surgery, usually before age 2, is necessary to relieve pulmonic stenosis and to repair the ventricular septal defect when progressive hypoxia and polycythemia impair the patient's quality of life.

Thoracic aortic aneurysm

An abnormal widening of the ascending, transverse, or descending part of the aorta, a thoracic aortic aneurysm is a potentially life-threatening disorder. The aneurysm may be *dissecting* (a hemorrhagic separation in the aortic wall intima, usually within the medial layer), *saccular* (an outpouching of the arterial wall, involving only a portion of the vessel circumference), or *fusiform* (a spindle-shaped enlargement encompassing the entire aortic circumference).

The ascending aorta is the most common site for the aneurysm, which occurs predominantly in men ages 50 to 70 who have coexisting hypertension. Mortality is high and is directly related to the size of the aneurysm; those that are larger than 2¾″ (7 cm) are more prone to rupture into the pericardium, resulting in cardiac tamponade.

Commonly, an ascending thoracic aortic aneurysm results from atherosclerosis. A descending thoracic aortic aneurysm usually occurs after blunt chest trauma that shears the aorta transversely, as in a motor vehicle accident or penetrating chest injury. A mycotic, or infectious, aneurysm develops from staphylococcal, streptococcal, or salmonella infection, usually at the sight of atherosclerotic plaque. Cystic medial necrosis caused by degeneration of the collagen and elastic fibers in the media of the aorta causes aneurysms during pregnancy and in patients with hypertension and Marfan syndrome. Other causes include congenital disorders, such as coarctation of the aorta, syphilitic infection, and rheumatic vasculitis.

Treatment

• Long-term treatment aims to control hypertension and cardiac output and may include beta blockers such as *propranolol* (p. 280), ACE inhibitors such as *enalapril* (p. 143), calcium channel blockers such as *nifedipine* (p. 230), and other antihypertensive agents, such as *hydralazine* (p. 174) or *prazosin* (p. 265).
• In dissecting ascending aortic aneurysm — an emergency — surgical resection of the aneurysm can restore normal blood flow through a Dacron or Teflon graft replacement.
• With aortic insufficiency, surgery consists of replacing the aortic valve.
• Supportive emergency therapy includes antihypertensives such as *nitroprusside* (p. 240), negative inotropic agents such as *labetalol* (p. 189), analgesics such as *morphine sulfate* (p. 223), oxygen for respiratory distress, and whole blood transfusions.
• Postoperative measures include careful monitoring and continuous assessment in the intensive care unit, antibiotics for routine postsurgical prophylaxis, endotracheal intubation and mechanical ventilation, chest drainage, ECG monitoring, and pulmonary artery catheterization and monitoring.

Thrombophlebitis

An acute condition characterized by inflammation and thrombus formation, thrombophlebitis may occur in deep or superficial veins. It typically occurs at the valve cusps because venous stasis encourages the accumulation and adherence of platelets and fibrin.

Thrombophlebitis usually begins with localized inflammation alone (phlebitis) but rapidly progresses to thrombus formation.

Deep vein thrombophlebitis affects small veins, such as the lesser saphenous vein, or large veins, such as the iliac, femoral, and popliteal veins and the vena cava. It's more serious than superficial vein thrombophlebitis because it adversely affects the veins deep in the leg musculature that carry 90% of the venous outflow from the leg.

Deep vein thrombophlebitis is one of the most serious iatrogenic diseases, affecting up to 35% of hospitalized patients, with the risk increasing dramatically after age 40. The increased use of subclavian vein catheters contributes to this condition.

Three primary factors (Virchow's triad) promote venous thrombosis: hypercoagulability, venous stasis, and intimal damage. Hypercoagulability may be caused by cigarette smoking, estrogen use, systemic infections, and other conditions. Venous stasis may result from acute MI, CHF, dehydration, immobility, or incompetent vein valves. Intimal damage may be caused by infection, infusion of irritating I.V. solutions, trauma, or venipuncture.

The major complications of thrombophlebitis include pulmonary embolism and chronic venous insufficiency.

Treatment

• Superficial vein thrombophlebitis is usually self-limiting and, because these veins have fewer valves than the deep veins, less likely to cause complications.
• Supportive care for severe superficial vein thrombophlebitis may include an NSAID, such as ibuprofen or indomethacin, along with antiembolism stockings, warm compresses, and elevation of the affected limb.
• Treatment for deep vein thrombophlebitis includes bed rest with elevation of the affected limb; application of warm, moist compresses; and anti-inflammatory analgesics, such as ibuprofen, acetaminophen, or aspirin. After the acute episode subsides, the patient may begin to ambulate wearing antiembolism stockings.
• Drug treatment may include anticoagulants—initially *heparin* (p. 169) and later *warfarin* (p. 321)—to prolong clotting time. However, the full anticoagulant dose must be reversed or discontinued prior to most surgical procedures to avoid the risk of hemorrhage.
• After some types of surgery, especially major abdominal or pelvic operations, prophylactic doses of anticoagulants may reduce the risk of deep vein thrombophlebitis.
• For lysis of acute, extensive deep vein thrombophlebitis, treatment may include *streptokinase* (p. 301) or urokinase if the risk of bleeding doesn't outweigh the potential benefits of thrombolytic treatment.
• Rarely, deep vein thrombophlebitis may require venous interruption, performed through simple ligation or clipping, or embolectomy if clots are being mobilized to the pulmonary and systemic vasculature and other treatments fail. Caval interruption with transvenous placement of an umbrella filter can also trap emboli, preventing them from traveling to the pulmonary vasculature.

Torsades de pointes

A potentially life-threatening arrhythmia, torsades de pointes is a form of VT characterized by a prolonged QT interval and a QRS polarity that appears to spiral around the isoelectric line. Any condition that causes a prolonged QT interval can also cause torsades de pointes. Although the sinus rhythm can resume spontaneously, torsades de pointes may degenerate into ventricular fibrillation.

On an ECG, the atrial rhythm and rate can't be determined and the ventricular rate is 150 to 250 beats/minute. The P wave is not identifiable because it's buried in the QRS complex. The QRS complex is wide with a phasic variation in its electrical polarity, shown by complexes that point downward for several beats and then turn upward for several beats, and vice versa. The QT interval is prolonged while the patient is in sinus rhythm. This arrhythmia may be paroxysmal, starting and stopping suddenly.

Possible causes include AV block, drug toxicity, electrolyte imbalance, hereditary prolonged QT syndrome, myocardial ischemia, Prinzmetal's angina, psychotropic drugs, and SA disease.

Treatment

• Treatment differs from standard VT therapy. If misdiagnosed as another arrhythmia, torsades de pointes may not respond to — or may be exacerbated by — such drugs as *procainamide* (p. 272) or *quinidine* (p. 284), which increase the abnormal QT interval and worsen the arrhythmia.
• If the patient is pulseless, immediate CPR and defibrillation are performed, following ACLS guidelines.

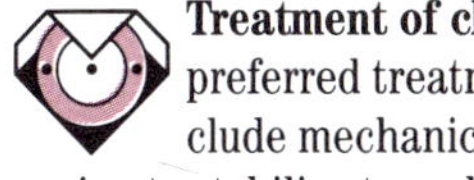
Treatment of choice. The preferred treatments include mechanical overdrive pacing to stabilize torsades de

pointes, I.V. magnesium sulfate replacement to terminate it, and *isoproterenol* (p. 181) and oral *lidocaine* (p. 192) to shorten the refractory period and unify repolarization.
• If torsades de pointes is caused by a specific drug (for example, procainamide or quinidine), discontinue the drug.
• Accompanying electrolyte imbalances are corrected by administering potassium, calcium, or magnesium.
• An implantable cardioverter defibrillator may be considered for refractory torsades de pointes.

Transposition of the great arteries

In this congenital heart defect, the positions of the aorta and the pulmonary artery are reversed. The aorta arises from the right ventricle and the pulmonary artery from the left ventricle. This defect produces two discrete circulatory systems (pulmonary and systemic). Oxygenated blood entering the left side of the heart returns to the lungs by the transposed pulmonary artery, and unoxygenated blood entering the right side of the heart returns to systemic circulation by the transposed aorta.

Transposition accounts for up to 5% of all congenital heart defects and commonly coexists with other congenital heart defects. Transposition is two to three times more common in boys than in girls. The cause is unknown. Serious complications include chronic heart failure, poor oxygenation, arrhythmias, and right ventricular failure.

Treatment
• An infant with transposition of the great arteries may undergo atrial balloon septostomy (Rashkind procedure) during cardiac catheterization. This procedure enlarges the patent foramen ovale, which improves oxygenation by allowing more of the pulmonary and systemic blood to mix. Afterward, *digoxin* (p. 118) and diuretics such as *furosemide* (p. 162) can reduce heart failure until the infant can withstand corrective surgery (usually before age 1).
• One of three surgical procedures can correct transposition. The surgery of choice is the arterial switch, in which the transposed arteries are anastomosed to the correct ventricles. The *Mustard procedure* replaces the atrial septum with a Dacron or pericardial partition or baffle that channels venous blood to the pulmonary artery. The pulmonary artery then carries the blood to the lungs for oxygenation, and oxygenated blood returning to the heart is channeled into the aorta. The *Senning procedure* accomplishes the same result using the atrial septum to create partitions that redirect blood flow.

Tricuspid atresia

The absence of the tricuspid orifice and valve tissue, tricuspid atresia is a rare congenital anomaly found in newborns or infants. It's commonly accompanied by one or more other cardiac deformities, including hypoplasia of the right ventricle, malposition of the pulmonary and aortic arteries, pulmonic valve atresia, pulmonic stenosis, ventricular septal defect, atrial septal defect, coarctation of the aorta, and patent ductus arteriosus.

Absence of a tricuspid valve with a septal defect shunts deoxygenated blood from the right side of the heart to the left atrium or left ventricle. Because of a ventricular septal defect or patent ductus arteriosus, the deoxygenated blood may then be redirected to the right ventricle and pulmonary circulation. It's then injected into the aorta and enters the systemic circulation, causing hypoxia.

With improved surgical procedures, the average life expectancy of an infant with this condition has increased from less than 3 months to 7 to 10 years (depending on associated defects), and to 20 or more years in an infant with no other defect.

Treatment
• The preferred treatment for tricuspid atresia is corrective surgery, which will vary according to associated congenital deformities.
• High concentrations of oxygen are used to treat hypoxia, and *morphine sulfate* (p. 223) is administered to relieve the associated respiratory distress.
• Administer lorazepam or midazolam to reduce anxiety and facilitate mechanical ventilation.
• Elevate the head and chest to 30 degrees or use knee-chest positioning to treat hypoxic episodes. Intubation and mechanical ventilation may be necessary with severe hypoxia.
• Give beta blockers such as *propranolol* (p. 280) to prevent and treat associated arrhythmias.
• Use diuretics, such as *ethacrynic acid* (p. 153) or *furosemide* (p. 162),

or provide inotropic support with drugs such as *dobutamine* (p. 136) or *dopamine* (p. 139) for CHF.
• Administer a vasodilator such as *nitroprusside* (p. 240) in severe CHF.
• Infuse prostaglandin E1 to treat cyanosis. Prostaglandin E1 maintains the patency of ductus arteriosus in the presence of associated pulmonic stenosis.
• *Spironolactone* (p. 298) may be used to supplement diuretic therapy and prevent hypokalemia.
• Oral vasodilator agents, such as *hydralazine* (p. 174) or *prazosin* (p. 265), are used to reduce afterload and preload. *Captopril* (p. 99) is used to reduce afterload and cardiac workload.
• Prophylactic antibiotics reduce the incidence of infective endocarditis and occult infection.
• Adequate hydration prevents increased blood viscosity, reducing the risk of thrombus or embolism.

Tricuspid insufficiency

In this disorder, also known as tricuspid regurgitation, an incompetent tricuspid valve allows blood to flow back into the right atrium during systole, decreasing blood flow to the lungs and the left side of the heart.

Tricuspid insufficiency most commonly is seen in patients with right ventricular hypertension secondary to mitral valve disease, right ventricular infarction, congenital heart disease, and primary pulmonary hypertension. It also may result from congenitally deformed tricuspid valves, AV canal defects, or Ebstein's anomaly of the tricuspid valve. Other causes include infarction of the right ventricular papillary muscles, tricuspid valve prolapse, carcinoid heart disease, endomyocardial fibrosis, infective endocarditis, and trauma.

The prognosis depends on the underlying disorder but is generally good. If pulmonary hypertension is present, however, cardiac output decreases and right ventricular failure develops.

Treatment

• A sodium-restricted diet and diuretics such as *furosemide* (p. 162) help reduce hepatic congestion before surgery.
• In severe insufficiency, the patient may require open-heart surgery for tricuspid annuloplasty or tricuspid valve replacement.

Tricuspid stenosis

A narrowing of the opening of the tricuspid valve, tricuspid stenosis obstructs blood flow from the right atrium to the right ventricle. This causes the right atrium to dilate and hypertrophy, eventually leading to right ventricular failure.

Tricuspid stenosis seldom occurs alone and is most often associated with mitral stenosis. It's most common in women. The prognosis is good with surgical intervention.

Although this disorder is usually caused by rheumatic fever, it may be congenital.

Treatment

• A sodium-restricted diet and diuretics such as *furosemide* (p. 162) can help to reduce hepatic congestion before surgery. Vasodilators such as *ni-*

troglycerin (p. 233) reduce preload and may improve right ventricular performance.
• A patient with moderate to severe stenosis probably will require open-heart surgery for valvulotomy or valve replacement.
• Valvuloplasty may be performed in the cardiac catheterization laboratory on elderly patients with end-stage tricuspid stenosis.

Varicose veins

Dilated, tortuous veins engorged with blood, varicose veins are caused by improper venous valve function. Primary varicose veins originate in the superficial veins — the saphenous veins and their branches — and secondary varicose veins occur in the deep and perforating veins.

Untreated, varicose veins produce venous insufficiency and venous stasis ulcers, particularly around the ankles.

Primary varicose veins tend to be familial, affect both legs, and affect twice as many women as men. Secondary varicose veins usually occur in one leg. Both types are more common in middle adulthood.

Primary varicose veins can result from congenital weakness of the valves or venous wall; conditions that produce prolonged venous stasis, such as pregnancy or wearing tight clothing; or from occupations requiring extended standing.

Secondary varicose veins result from disorders of the venous system, such as deep vein thrombophlebitis, trauma, and occlusion.

Treatment

• Treatment of mild varicose veins involves beginning an exercise program (such as walking), wearing elastic stockings, avoiding tight clothing and prolonged standing, and elevating the legs.
• Treatment of moderate varicose veins consists of wearing antiembolism stockings or elastic bandages.
• Severe varicose veins may require custom-fitted, surgical-weight stockings with graduated pressure.
• Severe varicose veins may require stripping and ligation or, in patients who are poor surgical risks, injection of a sclerosing agent such as sodium tetra decyl sulfate into small segments of affected veins.

Ventricular aneurysm

Characterized by an outpouching of the left ventricle, this potentially life-threatening condition produces ventricular wall dysfunction in about 20% of patients after MI. A ventricular aneurysm may develop days to weeks after MI or be delayed for years. Untreated, a ventricular aneurysm can lead to ventricular arrhythmias, cerebral embolization, heart failure and, ultimately, death.

An MI may destroy a large muscular section of the left ventricle, and the resulting necrosis may reduce the ventricular wall to a thin sheath of fibrous tissue. Under intracardiac pressure, this thin layer stretches and forms a separate noncontractile sac (aneurysm) with abnormal muscle wall movement.

During systolic ejection, these abnormal movements cause the remaining normally functioning myocardial fibers to increase the force of contraction to maintain stroke volume and cardiac output. At the same time, a portion of the stroke volume is lost to passive distention of the noncontractile sac.

Treatment

• Depending on the size of the aneurysm and the degree of complications, treatment may require only routine medical examinations to monitor the patient's condition.
• Emergency treatment of associated ventricular arrhythmias includes *epinephrine* (p. 146), I.V. antiarrhythmics such as *lidocaine* (p. 192), cardioversion, and defibrillation. Preventive treatment continues with oral antiarrhythmics, such as *disopyramide* (p. 133), *procainamide* (p. 272), or *quinidine* (p. 284).
• Emergency treatment for heart failure with pulmonary edema includes oxygen, I.V. *digoxin* (p. 118) and *furosemide* (p. 162), potassium replacement, I.V. *morphine sulfate* (p. 223) and, when necessary, I.V. *nitroprusside* (p. 240) and endotracheal intubation. Maintenance therapy may include oral nitrates such as *hydralazine* (p. 174), *isosorbide dinitrate* (p. 185) or *isosorbide mononitrate* (p. 185), and *prazosin* (p. 265).
• Systemic embolization requires anticoagulation therapy using *heparin* (p. 169) followed by *warfarin* (p. 321) or embolectomy.
• Aneurysmectomy with myocardial revascularization may be indicated in patients with ventricular failure or ventricular arrhythmias.

Ventricular fibrillation

Rapid, tremulous contractions of the ventricles, ventricular fibrillation is a condition in which the ventricles fail to pump blood and cardiac output falls to zero. If fibrillation continues, it leads to ventricular asystole and rapid death.

On an ECG, most components are not measurable and the ventricular rhythm has no pattern or regularity. Coarse fibrillation indicates more electrical activity in the ventricles than does fine fibrillation. The fibrillary waves become finer as acidosis and hypoxemia develop.

Possible causes of ventricular fibrillation include acute MI; digitalis (rarely), epinephrine, or quinidine toxicity; electric shock; electrolyte imbalances; hypothermia; R-on-T phenomenon; and untreated VT.

Treatment

• In accordance with ACLS guidelines, immediate CPR and defibrillation are performed, and epinephrine is administered. Course fibrillation is easier to convert than fine fibrillation. Even when following ACLS guidelines, always consult standing orders and review hospital policy for variations.
• Treat any underlying disorder, such as electrolyte imbalances or drug toxicity.
• For long-term control of this fibrillation, administer antiarrhythmic drugs, such as *bretylium* (p. 93) and *lidocaine* (p. 192).
• If the patient doesn't respond to drug therapy, an internal cardioverter defibrillator may be implanted.

This device recognizes ventricular fibrillation and defibrillates the heart.

Ventricular septal defect

The most common congenital heart disorder, a ventricular septal defect is an abnormal opening in the ventricular septum that allows blood to escape from the left ventricle into the right ventricle. Unoxygenated blood returns to the lungs instead of proceeding into the aortic arch. More than one perforation may exist, or the entire septum may be missing, which creates a single chamber.

Left-to-right shunting and increased pressure in the right ventricle cause hypertrophy, which, in turn, causes the right atrium to enlarge as it works against right ventricular resistance. The patient may ultimately develop heart failure and pulmonary hypertension.

Ventricular septal defect occurs in about 1 in 500 neonates. It may not be apparent immediately because right and left ventricular pressures are nearly equal at birth, so blood may not shunt through the defect. However, 4 to 8 weeks after birth, pulmonary vessels gradually relax and right ventricular pressure decreases. Blood then begins to shunt and symptoms arise.

Up to 30% of smaller defects and 12% of larger ones close without treatment within a year after birth. Untreated defects or defects that have not been surgically corrected can be fatal during the first year after birth, usually because of secondary complications.

Treatment

• Only about 15% of small defects require surgical correction. Infants who don't require surgery may receive an antibiotic to prevent infective endocarditis.
• For an infant with a large defect, treatment focuses on managing heart failure. The infant may receive *digoxin* (p. 118), diuretics such as *furosemide* (p. 162), a sodium-restricted diet, and nutritional supplements. If this regimen is effective, surgery may be delayed to allow the defect to shrink or close spontaneously.
• Surgery for large defects generally requires insertion of a patch graft, usually through the tricuspid valve, or pulmonary artery banding, which normalizes pressures and blood flow distal to the band and prevents pulmonary vascular disease.
• Postoperative treatment usually includes mechanical ventilation, analgesics such as *morphine sulfate* (p. 223), diuretics such as *furosemide* (p. 162) to increase urine output, continuous infusion of *nitroprusside* (p. 240) or adrenergic agents such as *dopamine* (p. 139) to regulate blood pressure and cardiac output and, in rare cases, insertion of a temporary pacemaker.

Ventricular tachycardia

A series of at least three PVCs that occur at a rate of more than 100 per minute, VT originates through reentry of a previous impulse or enhanced automaticity. The rapid ventricular rate reduces effective ventricular filling time, cutting cardiac output sharply and putting the patient at risk for CV collapse and ventricular fibrillation.

Two variations of this arrhythmia are ventricular flutter and torsades de pointes. When the ventricular rate ranges from 150 to 300 beats/minute and the waveform shows a regular up-and-down pattern, the arrhythmia is called ventricular flutter. In torsades de pointes, the ventricular rate ranges from 150 to 250 beats/minute.

On an ECG, the atrial rate and rhythm are not measurable, and the ventricular rhythm is usually regular but rapid (up to 200 beats/minute). The QRS complex has a duration greater than 0.12 second and a bizarre appearance, usually with increased amplitude. The T wave occurs in the opposite direction of the complex.

VT may be caused by coronary or ischemic heart disease, coronary artery spasm, acute MI, cardiomyopathy, drug toxicity, electrolyte imbalance, heart failure, mitral valve prolapse, pulmonary embolism, and rheumatic heart disease.

Treatment

• Treatment depends on the acuteness of the situation. If the patient is alert, expect to administer an antiarrhythmic such as *lidocaine* (p. 192). If lidocaine isn't effective, *bretylium* (p. 93) or *procainamide* (p. 272) may be prescribed.
• Treat underlying conditions. If VT results from drug toxicity, discontinue the causative drug.
• If antiarrhythmic therapy doesn't correct VT, a mechanical method, such as low-energy synchronous cardioversion, may be used.
• If the patient suffers CV collapse and is pulseless, prepare for immediate defibrillation. If the patient's hemodynamic status is stable, an implantable cardioverter defibrillator may be used. Perform CPR until a defibrillator is available.
• Prevent recurrences with antiarrhythmics such as procainamide or *propafenone* (p. 277).

Wandering pacemaker

An atrial arrhythmia in which the site of the impulse shifts, a wandering pacemaker may originate in the SA node, the atrium, or even the AV node. A wandering pacemaker is rarely serious. However, persistence of an AV junctional rhythm may indicate underlying heart disease. This arrhythmia is common in children, athletes, and elderly people.

On an ECG, the atrial rhythm varies slightly, with an irregular P-P interval; the ventricular rhythm also varies slightly, with an irregular R-R interval. The P wave changes in size and configuration because of the changing pacemaker site. When the P wave is present, the PR interval may be shortened.

Possible causes of wandering pacemaker include accelerated atrial or junctional rhythm from digitalis toxicity, increased vagal tone, inflamed or irritated atrial tissue resulting from rheumatic heart disease or other organic heart disease, and pulmonary disease with hypoxemia.

Treatment

- No treatment is indicated if the patient is asymptomatic and hemodynamic deterioration hasn't occurred.
- In the presence of a slow heart rate, encourage the patient to cough. Coughing decreases vagal tone, encouraging the reappearance of a normal sinus rhythm.
- If hemodynamic deterioration occurs, resuscitate the patient with I.V. *atropine* (p. 83).
- If the arrhythmia results from an overdose of a digitalis glycoside, discontinue the drug briefly.

Wolff-Parkinson-White syndrome

The most common preexcitation syndrome, WPW syndrome occurs when an anomalous atrial bypass develops outside the AV junction (probably in the bundle of Kent), connecting the atria and the ventricles. This bypass can conduct impulses either to the ventricles or to the atria. Retrograde conduction may then trigger circus reentry, resulting in a reentrant tachycardia.

Usually, WPW syndrome is considered insignificant if tachycardia doesn't occur or if the patient has no associated cardiac disease. When tachycardia does occur in WPW syndrome, decreased cardiac output, abrupt episodes of premature supraventricular tachycardia, atrial fibrillation, and atrial flutter with rates as fast as 300 beats/minute may develop.

Most likely congenital in origin, WPW syndrome is diagnosed predominantly in young children and in adults ages 20 to 35.

On an ECG, both atrial and ventricular rhythms and rates are normal, except when supraventricular tachycardia occurs. The PR interval is short (less than 0.12 second). The beginning of the QRS complex is slurred because of premature partial ventricular depolarization via the bypass tract. This slurring produces a delta wave, the hallmark of WPW syndrome. Generally, the T wave changes to a direction opposite the major delta and QRS vectors.

Treatment

- This syndrome is generally benign and, unless the patient is symptomatic, requires no specific treatment.
- Accompanying tachyarrhythmias require quick intervention, such as CPR with epinephrine and other vagal maneuvers.

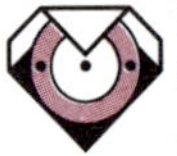 **Treatment of choice.** The drug of choice during tachycardia (after vagal maneuvers) is *adenosine* (p. 64). Antiarrhythmic drugs, such as *procainamide* (p. 272) or *quinidine* (p. 284), may also be used.

- If tachyarrhythmias are debilitating, catheter-induced electrical or radio-frequency ablation may be necessary to sever the bypass tract. Cardioversion may be performed if other measures fail.
- Digoxin and other drugs that prolong conduction time in the AV node, including calcium channel blockers such as verapamil and beta blockers such as propranolol, should be used with extreme caution or avoided.

Cardiovascular drugs

Acebutolol

Also known by the brand names Sectral and Monitan (in Canada), acebutolol is a beta$_1$-adrenergic blocker with intrinsic sympathomimetic activity (ISA). It's therapeutically classified as an antihypertensive and antiarrhythmic. This drug is available in capsules containing 200 and 400 mg. (See *Other ISA beta blockers.*)

Pharmacokinetics
- *Absorption:* First-pass metabolism limits bioavailability. Peak plasma levels occur in about 2½ hours.
- *Distribution:* About 26% protein-bound.
- *Metabolism:* In the liver; peak levels of its major active metabolite, diacetolol, occur in about 3½ hours.
- *Excretion:* 30% to 40% of a dose is excreted in urine; the remainder in feces and bile. The elimination half-life is 3 to 4 hours; the elimination half-life of diacetolol, 8 to 13 hours. Both are excreted in breast milk.

Indications, dosage, and action
Hypertension
- *Adult dosage:* 400 mg P.O. as a single daily dose or divided b.i.d., up to a maximum of 1,200 mg daily.
- *Action:* Acebutolol has cardioselective beta$_1$-adrenergic blocking properties and mild ISA. It decreases heart rate and cardiac output and lowers peripheral vascular resistance.

Ventricular arrhythmias
- *Adult dosage:* 400 mg P.O. daily divided b.i.d., increased as necessary to provide an adequate clinical response. The usual daily dosage is 600 to 1,200 mg.
- *Action:* Acebutolol decreases myocardial contractility, heart rate, cardiac output, and SA and AV node conduction velocity.

Angina
- *Adult dosage:* 200 mg b.i.d. Usual daily dosage is 400 to 800 mg divided b.i.d.
- *Action:* Acebutolol lowers myocardial oxygen demand by decreasing the force of contraction, heart rate, and blood pressure.

Contraindications and cautions
- Don't give acebutolol to patients with persistent severe bradycardia, second- or third-degree AV block, or overt cardiac failure.
- Use cautiously in elderly patients or patients with impaired cardiac, hepatic, or renal function (decrease dosage if creatinine clearance falls below 50 ml/minute).
- Use cautiously in patients with diabetes mellitus or hyperthyroidism because acebutolol may mask tachycardia caused by hypoglycemia or hyperthyroidism.
- Use cautiously in patients with bronchospastic diseases because the drug may cause bronchospasm in such patients.
- Know that acebutolol is excreted in breast milk and is not recommended for breast-feeding women.
- Pregnancy risk category B

Life-threatening adverse reactions
- Hypotension, bradycardia, CHF
- Bronchospasm

Other ISA beta blockers

Acebutolol, carteolol, penbutolol, and pindolol are all beta-adrenergic blocking agents with intrinsic sympathomimetic activity (ISA), a property by which certain beta blockers simultaneously block and stimulate beta-receptors. Beta blockers with ISA produce smaller reductions in resting heart rate and cardiac output than beta blockers without ISA.

Acebutolol is the only one of the four that's $beta_1$-selective and commonly used to treat arrhythmias. The other three drugs block both $beta_1$- and $beta_2$-receptors and are used primarily to treat hypertension.

Carteolol hydrochloride

Also known by the brand name Cartrol, carteolol is available in 2.5-mg and 5-mg tablets. The usual initial adult dosage is 2.5 mg once daily. Gradually increase the dosage as required to 5 mg or 10 mg daily as a single dose. Doses over 10 mg daily may actually be less effective.

Penbutolol sulfate

Also known by the brand name Levatol, penbutolol is available in 20-mg tablets. The usual adult dosage is 20 mg once daily.

Pindolol

Also known by the brand name Visken in the U.S. and Canada, or Novo-Pindol or Syn-Pindolol in Canada, pindolol is available in 5- and 10-mg tablets. In Canada, 15-mg tablets are also available.

Pindolol has the most ISA of any currently available beta blocker. The usual initial adult dosage is 5 mg twice daily. If response is inadequate, dosage is increased in increments of 10 mg per day at 2- to 3-week intervals to a maximum of 45 mg/day (Canada) or 60 mg/day (U.S.).

Common adverse reactions

- Bradycardia
- Pharyngitis
- Fatigue, headache, dizziness, anxiety, hyperesthesia, hypoesthesia, impotence
- Vomiting, abdominal pain
- Conjunctivitis, dry eye, eye pain (with 1,200 mg daily)
- Nausea, constipation, diarrhea, dyspepsia, flatulence
- Impotence, frequent micturition
- Rhinitis
- Abnormal vision, dry eye, eye pain, conjunctivitis
- Rash, pruritus
- Fever, arthralgia, myalgia

Infrequent adverse reactions

- Chest pain, edema
- Dyspnea, wheezing, cough
- Insomnia, depression, abnormal dreams

Interactions

- *Calcium channel blockers:* Increased depressant effect on the myocardium. Monitor closely.

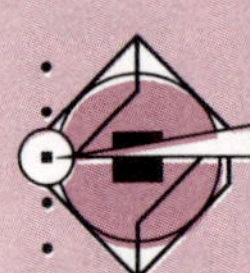

Hazards of multidrug therapy with acebutolol

Interacting drug	Effects
Antihypertensives (such as captopril)	May cause hypotension
Digitalis glycosides (such as digoxin)	May cause excessive bradycardia and increased myocardial depression
Vasodilators (such as nitroglycerin)	May cause hypotension

• *Insulin, oral antidiabetic drugs:* May alter dosage requirements in previously stabilized diabetics.

For dangerous interactions, see *Hazards of multidrug therapy with acebutolol.*

Interventions
Preparation and administration
• Obtain baseline blood pressure and apical pulse rate before therapy and before each dose, especially during initial therapy.

Safety tip. If the patient's apical pulse rate is less than 60 beats/minute, withhold the dose and call the doctor.

• Avoid late-evening doses to minimize insomnia. (See *Taking beta-adrenergic blockers at home.*)

Monitoring and supportive care
• Monitor the effectiveness of acebutolol by frequently checking the patient's cardiac rhythm and assessing for anginal pain.
• Check for adverse reactions, and notify the doctor about severe reactions or those that continue or increasingly disturb the patient. You may need to discontinue the drug or reduce the dosage as ordered.
• Observe diabetic patients closely for indications of hypoglycemia, and monitor blood glucose levels.

Safety tip. Although acebutolol masks tachycardia associated with hypoglycemia, it doesn't mask CNS signs, such as dizziness, headache, restlessness, or changes in mental status.
• Before surgery, notify the anesthesiologist if the patient is receiving this drug.

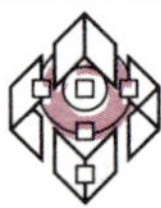

MedTest

1. Acebutolol may mask signs of hypoglycemia, such as:
   - **a.** mental changes.
   - **b.** restlessness.
   - **c.** tachycardia.
   - **d.** headache.

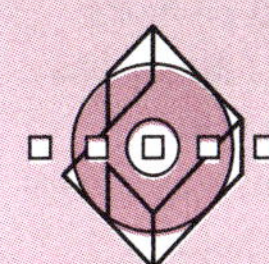

Patient-teaching checklist

Taking beta-adrenergic blockers at home

In addition to explaining the drug's action and dosage, teach the patient who will continue beta-blocker therapy after discharge to follow these important guidelines.

Know when to call your doctor
☐ Measure your pulse rate before each dose and report any rate below 60 beats/minute or any irregularity to the doctor.
☐ Check your blood pressure frequently. Notify your doctor of any significant changes.
☐ If you have diabetes and take medication to control your blood glucose level, you'll need to monitor this level closely because beta blockers may alter your dosage requirements.

Minimize adverse reactions
☐ Remember to change your positions slowly (especially from a supine to an upright position) and dangle your legs over the bedside for a few minutes before standing to minimize dizziness. Lie down immediately if dizziness or faintness occurs.
☐ Take the drug as prescribed even when you're feeling better.

☐ If you have CAD, continue taking the drug even if unpleasant adverse reactions occur because abrupt discontinuation can precipitate MI or exacerbate angina.
☐ Check with your doctor or pharmacist before taking any OTC medications.
☐ Schedule rest periods throughout the day if fatigue occurs. Notify the doctor of any excessive fatigue or dizziness.
☐ Avoid driving, operating machinery, or performing other potentially hazardous activities if you feel tired or lethargic.
☐ Avoid late-evening doses if the drug produces insomnia.

Other instructions
☐ Report to your doctor any weight gain of more than 2 lb (1 kg) per day, difficulty breathing, or swelling of the hands or ankles.

2. Acebutolol is contraindicated in patients with:
  a. first-degree AV block.
  b. PAT.
  c. impaired renal function.
  d. persistent bradycardia.

3. Your patient receiving acebutolol is scheduled for surgery. You should:
  a. discontinue this drug.
  b. remind the doctor to double the dose the morning of surgery.
  c. notify the anesthesiologist that the patient is receiving acebutolol.
  d. remind the doctor to cut the dose in half the morning of surgery.

Adenosine

Also known by the brand name Adenocard, adenosine is a naturally occurring nucleoside that's therapeutically classified as an antiarrhythmic. It's available for injection in 2-ml vials (3 mg/ml).

Pharmacokinetics
- *Absorption:* Rapid I.V. injection.
- *Distribution:* Rapidly taken up by erythrocytes and vascular endothelial cells.
- *Metabolism:* Metabolized within tissues to inosine and adenosine monophosphate.
- *Excretion:* Unknown. Circulating elimination half-life is less than 10 seconds.

Indications, dosage, and action
Conversion of PSVT to sinus rhythm
- *Adult dosage:* 6 mg by I.V. bolus over 1 to 2 seconds. If PSVT isn't corrected in 1 to 2 minutes, 12 mg by rapid I.V. push, and repeat 12-mg dose if necessary. Single doses over 12 mg aren't recommended.
- *Action:* Adenosine acts on the AV node to slow conduction and inhibit reentry pathways. The drug also treats PSVT associated with WPW syndrome.

Contraindications and cautions
- Know that adenosine is not recommended for patients with atrial flutter, atrial fibrillation, or VT because the drug is ineffective in treating these arrhythmias. However, it may be used as a diagnostic tool for these irregular rhythms because fibrillation or flutter waves can be more readily identified if the patient has a slowed ventricular response.
- Because adenosine decreases conduction through the AV node, it may produce a transient first-, second-, or third-degree AV block. For this reason, it's contraindicated in patients with second- or third-degree AV block or SSS unless the patient has a pacemaker. Because the drug has a short half-life, these effects are usually transient; however, patients who develop a significant block after a dose shouldn't receive additional doses.
- More than half of the patients in clinical trials developed new arrhythmias when adenosine was used to convert PSVT to normal sinus rhythm. Such arrhythmias, which are usually transient, may include sinus bradycardia or tachycardia, various degrees of AV block, premature atrial and ventricular contractions, and skipped beats.
- Use with caution in asthma because inhaled adenosine may cause bronchoconstriction. Asthma attacks haven't been reported, however.
- Pregnancy risk category C

Life-threatening adverse reactions
- Asystole, VT, ventricular fibrillation
- Bronchospasm

Common adverse reactions
- Hypotension (with doses greater than 12 mg), PVCs, PACs, sinus bradycardia, sinus tachycardia, skipped beats, various degrees of AV block

(55% of patients), facial flushing (18%)
• Dyspnea, shortness of breath, chest pressure

Infrequent adverse reactions
• Chest pain, headache, hypotension, palpitations, diaphoresis
• Hyperventilation
• Apprehension, neck and back pain, blurred vision, burning sensation, dizziness, heaviness in arms, light-headedness, numbness, tingling in arms
• Metallic taste, nausea
• Tightness in throat, groin pressure

Interactions
• *Carbamazepine, dipyridamole:* May potentiate adenosine's effects.
• *Methylxanthines:* Antagonize effects of adenosine. Patients who take theophylline or drink beverages with caffeine may require higher doses or may not respond to adenosine.

Interventions
Preparation and administration
• Administer directly into a vein or, if using an I.V. line, use the most proximal port and follow with a rapid flush of 0.9% NaCl solution to ensure that the drug reaches the systemic circulation rapidly.
• Check the solution for crystals, which may occur if the solution is cold. If they're present, slowly warm the solution to room temperature.
• Discard any unused drug because it contains no preservatives.

Monitoring and supportive care
• Warn the patient that facial flushing may occur.

• For marked bradycardia, have the patient cough, which usually restores his normal rhythm.

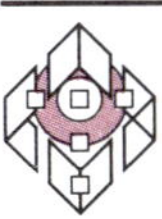 **MedTest**

1. Adenosine is especially useful in treating:
   a. WPW syndrome.
   b. atrial flutter or fibrillation.
   c. VT.
   d. second- or third-degree AV block.

2. When preparing adenosine for injection, you note the presence of crystals in the solution. You should immediately:
   a. discard the drug.
   b. place the drug vial on ice to cool it.
   c. notify the pharmacist.
   d. slowly warm the solution to room temperature.

3. Adenosine may produce a transient first-, second-, or third-degree AV block; therefore, it's contraindicated in:
   a. angina.
   b. tachycardia.
   c. SSS.
   d. left ventricular failure.

Alteplase
Known by the brand name Activase, alteplase is a thrombolytic enzyme that's supplied in 20-mg (11.6 million IU), 50-mg (29 million IU), and

100-mg vials for injection. The drug is classified as a tissue plasminogen activator.

Pharmacokinetics
• *Absorption:* Must be given I.V.
• *Distribution:* 80% of dose is cleared from the plasma by the liver within 10 minutes after infusion is discontinued.
• *Metabolism:* Primarily hepatic.
• *Excretion:* Over 85% of drug is excreted in the urine; about 5%, in the feces. Elimination half-life is less than 10 minutes.

Indications, dosage, and action
Dissolution of coronary artery thrombi in acute MI
• *Adult dosage:* For patients weighing over 143 lb (65 kg), 60 mg in the first hour, with a 6- to 10-mg I.V. bolus over the first 1 to 2 minutes; then 20 mg/hour for an additional 2 hours. Total dose is 100 mg.

For patients weighing 143 lb or less, 1.25 mg/kg; 60% of the dose is administered in the first hour, with 10% of that dose given within the first 1 to 2 minutes.

Alternate dosage: 15-mg bolus, followed by 0.75 mg/kg over 30 minutes, and then 0.5 mg/kg over 60 minutes. Maximum dosage is 100 mg.
• *Action:* Alteplase catalyzes the conversion of tissue plasminogen to plasmin in the presence of fibrin. This fibrin specificity produces local fibrinolysis in the area of recent clot formation, with limited systemic proteolysis. In patients with acute MI, this allows for reperfusion of ischemic cardiac muscle and improved left ventricular function with a decreased incidence of CHF after MI.

Pulmonary embolism
• *Adult dosage:* 100 mg by I.V. infusion over 2 hours. Follow with heparin therapy when the PTT or thrombin time returns to twice normal or less.
• *Action:* Binds to fibrin in a thrombus and locally converts plasminogen to plasmin, which initiates local fibrinolysis.

Contraindications and cautions
• Because of the potential for uncontrolled bleeding, don't give alteplase to patients with active internal bleeding, bleeding diathesis, aneurysm, arteriovenous malformation, history of CVA, recent intraspinal or intracranial surgery or trauma, brain tumor, or severe uncontrolled hypertension.
• Use with extreme caution in patients with acute pericarditis, cerebrovascular disease, diabetic hemorrhagic retinopathy, significant hepatic disease, marked hypertension, subacute infective endocarditis, or septic thrombophlebitis and in patients at risk for thrombi in the left side of the heart (as in mitral stenosis with atrial fibrillation) because of the risk of bleeding.
• Consider risk versus benefit in patients who've had major surgery recently (within 10 days), in pregnancy and the first 10 days postpartum, in organ biopsy, in trauma (including CPR), in GI or GU bleeding, in patients receiving anticoagulants, and in patients ages 75 and older.
• Pregnancy risk category C

Life-threatening adverse reactions

• Arrhythmias (associated with reperfusion of ischemic myocardium)
• Severe, spontaneous cerebral, retroperitoneal, GU, or GI bleeding
• Anaphylactic reaction

Common adverse reactions

• GI bleeding

Infrequent adverse reactions

• Hypotension
• Nausea, vomiting
• Hematuria
• Excessive fibrinolysis leading to bleeding from punctures or recent wounds
• Epistaxis, gingival bleeding
• Urticaria
• Fever

Interactions

• *Aspirin, dipyridamole, and heparin:* Concomitant use of alteplase with these agents increases the risk of bleeding. However, these drugs are commonly used after the alteplase infusion is administered.

Interventions

Preparation and administration

• Expect to begin alteplase infusion within 6 hours after onset of MI symptoms.
• Discontinue the infusion immediately if signs of major bleeding occur.
Safety tip. Avoid I.M. injections, venipuncture, and arterial puncture during therapy because of the risk of bleeding. Also, use pressure dressings or ice packs on recent puncture sites to prevent bleeding. If

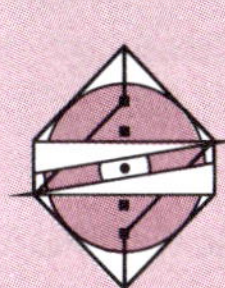

Alteplase combinations to avoid

Don't mix alteplase with bacteriostatic water for injection. The preservatives in bacteriostatic water may react with alteplase, resulting in precipitation of the drug and diminished drug effectiveness.

arterial puncture is necessary, select a site on the arm and apply pressure for 30 minutes afterward.
• Don't mix other drugs with alteplase. (See *Alteplase combinations to avoid,* above, and *Reconstituting alteplase,* page 68.)

Monitoring and supportive care

• Monitor the ECG for transient arrhythmias associated with reperfusion after coronary thrombolysis.
• Have antiarrhythmic drugs and emergency equipment, including a defibrillator, available in case of life-threatening arrhythmias.
• Teach the patient the signs of internal bleeding, and tell him to report these immediately.
• Maintain bed rest during alteplase administration.
• Expect altered results in coagulation and fibrinolytic tests. Adding 150 to 200 units/ml of aprotinin to the blood sample may minimize this interference.

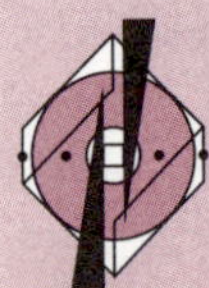

Administration guidelines

Reconstituting alteplase

Use the following guidelines to reconstitute alteplase.

Use sterile water
Using an 18G needle, reconstitute the drug powder in the vial to 1 mg/ml by adding 20 to 100 ml of preservative-free, sterile water for injection. Never use bacteriostatic water, and don't use the contents of the vial if it isn't vacuum sealed.

Gently roll and tilt
Slowly direct the stream of sterile water at the lyophilized cake in the vial. Gently roll and tilt the vial to reconstitute it; *never shake the vial* because this drug requires careful preparation to prevent undue foaming and increased flocculation. The solution should be clear or pale yellow. Let the vial stand for several minutes if slight foaming has occurred.

Use bottle or bag for further dilution
If further dilution is necessary, dilute the drug to 0.5 mg/ml. For a 20-ml vial, add 20 ml of 0.9% NaCl solution or D_5W; for a 50-ml vial, add 50 ml of either solution. Again, avoid undue agitation.

Reconstitute immediately
Reconstitute the alteplase solution immediately before use and use the total reconstituted amount within 8 hours. Discard the unused amount after 8 hours because it contains no preservatives. The drug may be temporarily stored at room temperature or refrigerated during those 8 hours, however.

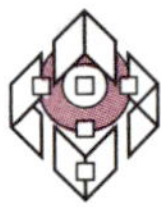

MedTest

1. After the onset of MI symptoms, alteplase should be given within:
   a. 30 minutes.
   b. 1 hour.
   c. 6 hours.
   d. 24 hours.

2. Prepare the alteplase solution using:
   a. bacteriostatic water for injection.
   b. sterile water for injection.
   c. 0.9% NaCl solution.
   d. D_5W.

3. Because of the high risk of bleeding from alteplase infusion, you should:
   a. tell the patient not to brush his teeth for 48 hours.
   b. apply pressure for 10 minutes to arterial puncture sites.
   c. avoid I.M. injections and venipunctures.
   d. avoid fiber in the patient's diet.

Amiloride hydrochloride

Also known by the brand name Midamor, amiloride is a potassium-sparing diuretic that's available in 5-mg tablets. It's therapeutically classified as a diuretic and an antihypertensive.

Pharmacokinetics

• *Absorption:* About 50% of dose is absorbed from the GI tract. Food decreases absorption. Diuresis usually begins in 2 hours and peaks in 6 to 10 hours.
• *Distribution:* Wide extravascular distribution.
• *Metabolism:* Insignificant.
• *Excretion:* Most of dose is excreted in urine; elimination half-life is 6 to 9 hours in patients with normal renal function.

Indications, dosage, and action
Hypertension and CHF-related edema
• *Adult dosage:* 5 mg P.O. daily. Dosage may be increased to 10 mg daily, if necessary, but don't exceed 20 mg daily.
• *Diuretic action:* Acts directly on the distal renal tubules to inhibit sodium and water reabsorption and potassium excretion, thereby reducing potassium loss.
• *Antihypertensive action:* Amiloride is a weak antihypertensive; it probably lowers blood pressure by reducing plasma volume.

Contraindications and cautions
• Don't give amiloride to patients whose serum potassium levels exceed 5.5 mEq/liter or who are receiving ACE inhibitors or other potassium-sparing diuretics or supplements.
• Also don't give the drug to patients with renal insufficiency because of the risk of hyperkalemia.
• Use amiloride cautiously in patients with severe hepatic insufficiency, because electrolyte imbalance may precipitate hepatic encephalopathy, and in patients with diabetes, who are at increased risk for hyperkalemia.
• Closely observe elderly and debilitated patients because they're more susceptible to drug-induced diuresis and hyperkalemia. Reduced dosages may be indicated.
• Pregnancy risk category B

Life-threatening adverse reactions
None noted

Common adverse reactions
• Headache
• Nausea, anorexia, diarrhea, vomiting
• Hyperkalemia (10% occurrence if used without a potassium-depleting diuretic; greater than 10% occurrence in patients with renal impairment or diabetes mellitus and in elderly patients)

Infrequent adverse reactions
• Orthostatic hypotension
• Cough, dypsnea
• Encephalopathy, weakness, dizziness, fatigue

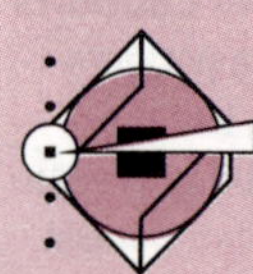

Interactions alert

Hazards of multidrug therapy with amiloride

Interacting drug	Effect
ACE inhibitors (such as captopril and enalapril)	Increase risk of hyperkalemia
Potassium-sparing diuretics (such as spironolactone)	Increase risk of hyperkalemia
Potassium supplements (such as potassium chloride)	Increase risk of hyperkalemia
Salt substitutes containing potassium	Increase risk of hyperkalemia

- Gas pain, appetite changes, abdominal pain, constipation
- Impotence
- Hyperkalemia (when used with a thiazide diuretic and in the absence of renal disease or diabetes)
- Muscle cramps
- Photosensitivity

Interactions

- *Antihypertensive drugs:* Possible risk of hypotension.
- *Lithium:* Possible reduced renal clearance of lithium leading to elevated lithium blood levels.
- *NSAIDs, such as indomethacin or ibuprofen:* May alter renal function and decrease amiloride effectiveness.

   For dangerous interactions, see *Hazards of multidrug therapy with amiloride.*

Interventions
Preparation and administration
- Administer with meals to prevent nausea. Warn patients to avoid excessive ingestion of potassium-rich foods or potassium-containing salt substitutes. (See *Taking amiloride at home.*)

Monitoring and supportive care
- Amiloride may cause severe hyperkalemia in diabetic patients following I.V. glucose tolerance testing; the drug is discontinued at least 3 days before testing.
- Keep in mind that renal and hepatic function test results may be transiently abnormal in nondiabetic patients.

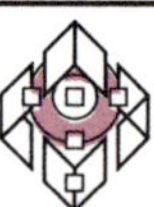

MedTest

1. In a patient receiving amiloride, monitor:
   a. heart rate and rhythm.
   b. blood pressure.
   c. serum creatinine level.
   d. serum potassium level.

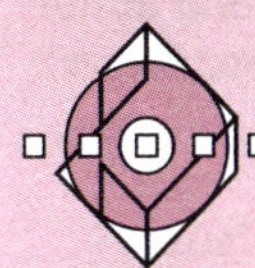

Patient-teaching checklist

Taking amiloride at home

In addition to explaining the drug's action and dosage, teach the patient who will continue amiloride therapy after discharge to follow these important guidelines.

Take your medication correctly
☐ Take amiloride with meals to prevent nausea.
☐ Take the drug early in the day to prevent interruption of sleep caused by frequent urination at night.

Know when to call your doctor
☐ Amiloride can cause dehydration, so monitor your fluid volume by weighing yourself daily.
☐ A 2-lb (1-kg) weight increase or increasing difficulty breathing is most likely caused by fluid accumulation. Report these symptoms to your doctor immediately.
☐ Avoid potassium-rich foods such as bananas, potassium-containing salt substitutes, and potassium supplements, unless otherwise instructed by your doctor.
☐ Report weakness, cramps, numbness, tingling or prickling sensations, diarrhea, or an irregular heartbeat to your doctor immediately. These may be symptoms of an abnormally high potassium level caused by amiloride.

Minimize adverse reactions
☐ Remember to change positions slowly (especially from lying flat to sitting upright) and dangle your legs over the bedside for a few minutes before standing to minimize the dizziness that may be caused by amiloride. Lie down immediately if dizziness or faintness occurs.
☐ Protect your skin from sunlight as much as possible because amiloride may cause photosensitivity. Severe sunburn may result from even brief exposure to sunlight. Wear protective clothing such as a hat. Use a sunblock with a skin protection factor (SPF) of at least 15 to protect your skin and lips.

---

2. Amiloride exerts its diuretic effects by acting on the:
   a. distal renal tubule to inhibit sodium reabsorption.
   b. proximal part of the ascending loop of Henle to inhibit sodium reabsorption.
   c. distal renal tubule to inhibit aldosterone.
   d. cortical diluting segment of the nephron.

3. Dietary guidelines for the patient taking amiloride include:
   a. reduction of fat intake to 30% of diet.
   b. moderation in the use of potassium-rich foods.

c. restriction of fluid intake to 1 liter/day.

d. ingestion of oranges, bananas, tomatoes, and dates.

Amiodarone hydrochloride

Also known by the brand name Cordarone, amiodarone is a benzofuran derivative that's classified therapeutically as a ventricular and supraventricular antiarrhythmic. It's available in 100- and 200-mg tablets. Amiodarone's use is somewhat limited by its severe adverse effects.

Pharmacokinetics

• *Absorption:* Slow and variable. Bioavailability ranges from 22% to 86%. Peak plasma levels occur 3 to 7 hours after oral administration; however, onset of action may be delayed from 2 to 3 days to 2 to 3 months — even with loading doses.

• *Distribution:* Widespread, because the drug accumulates in adipose tissue and in organs with marked perfusion, such as the lungs, liver, and spleen. It's also highly protein-bound (96%). The therapeutic serum level probably ranges from 1 to 2.5 mcg/ml.

• *Metabolism:* Extensively in the liver to a pharmacologically active metabolite, desethyl amiodarone.

• *Excretion:* Primarily hepatic. Patients with impaired renal function don't require dosage reduction because no renal excretion occurs. The drug's elimination half-life ranges from 40 to 50 days.

Indications, dosage, and action

Ventricular and supraventricular arrhythmias, including recurrent supraventricular tachycardia, atrial fibrillation and flutter

• *Adult dosage:* Loading dose of 800 to 1,600 mg P.O. daily for 1 to 3 weeks until initial therapeutic response occurs. Maintenance dosage is 200 to 600 mg P.O. daily.

• *Pediatric dosage:* 10 mg/kg P.O. per day or 800 mg/1.73 m^2 of body surface area (BSA) P.O. per day for 10 days or until response is seen; then 5 mg/kg or 400 mg/1.73 m^2 of BSA. Usual maintenance dosage is 2.5 mg/kg or 200 mg/1.73 m^2 of BSA per day.

• *Antiarrhythmic action:* Although amiodarone has mixed class Ic and class III antiarrhythmic effects, the drug generally is considered a class III agent that widens the action potential duration (repolarization inhibition). Amiodarone increases the effective refractory period in the atria, ventricles, AV node, His-Purkinje system, and bypass tracts and slows conduction in the atria, AV node, His-Purkinje system, and ventricles; sinus node automaticity decreases. Amiodarone also noncompetitively blocks alpha- and beta-adrenergic receptors. Clinically, it has little, if any, negative inotropic effect. Coronary and peripheral vasodilation may occur with long-term therapy.

Contraindications and cautions

• Avoid using amiodarone in patients with preexisting sinus node dysfunction and bradycardia causing syncope or second- or third-degree AV block (unless the patient has an artificial pacemaker) because of its po-

tent effects on the AV conduction system.
• Use with caution in patients with CHF because of possible adverse hemodynamic effects.
• Also use cautiously in patients with liver disease because hepatic metabolism may be reduced.
• Administer cautiously to patients with hypokalemia because the drug may be ineffective.
• Amiodarone should be discontinued if signs of pulmonary toxicity or epididymitis occur.
• Use with caution in elderly patients because they may experience ataxia.
• Amiodarone is excreted in breast milk and shouldn't be used in breast-feeding women.
• Pregnancy risk category C

Life-threatening adverse reactions

• Arrhythmias or exacerbated arrhythmias, CHF
• Severe pulmonary toxicity (10% incidence of fatality) with high doses
• Overt liver disease

Common adverse reactions

• Pulmonary toxicity (10% to 17% incidence in patients with ventricular arrhythmias given doses of about 400 mg/day), pulmonary inflammation or fibrosis
• Malaise, peripheral neuropathy, extrapyramidal symptoms, fatigue, ataxia, dizziness, paresthesia (20% to 40% incidence — may respond to dose reduction)
• Nausea, vomiting, anorexia, constipation (25% incidence, usually dur-

ing high-dose administration); altered liver enzyme levels, hepatic dysfunction
• Corneal microdeposits (in nearly all patients receiving drug for more than 6 months), visual disturbances
• Hyperthyroidism (usually dose related)
• Dermatologic reactions (15% incidence), with photosensitivity as most common reaction (10% incidence)

Infrequent adverse reactions

• Exacerbated arrhythmias (2% to 5%), bradycardia, hypotension, edema, CHF, cardiac conduction abnormalities
• Headache, insomnia, sleep disturbances
• Abdominal pain; abnormal taste, smell, and salivation
• Hypothyroidism, hyperthyroidism, gynecomastia
• Blue-gray skin pigmentation, flushing
• Decreased lipid levels

Interactions

• *Antiarrhythmics, phenothiazine, tricyclic antidepressants:* May cause additive effects that lead to a prolonged QT interval, possibly resulting in torsades de pointes.
• *Digoxin, phenytoin, procainamide, quinidine:* Concomitant use may lead to increased serum levels of these drugs, with enhanced effects.
• *Warfarin:* Concomitant use prolongs PT as a result of enhanced drug displacement from protein-binding sites.

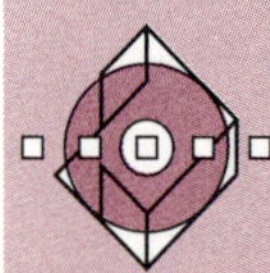

Taking antiarrhythmics at home

In addition to explaining the drug's action and dosage, teach the patient who will continue antiarrhythmic therapy after discharge to follow these important guidelines.

Take your medication correctly
☐ Take the drug as prescribed even when you're feeling better.

Know when to call your doctor
☐ Notify your doctor immediately if you experience chest pain, difficulty breathing, coughing, or any other abnormal respiratory symptoms while taking this drug.

Minimize adverse reactions
☐ Schedule frequent rest periods throughout the day if you experience fatigue or dizziness as a result of antiarrhythmic therapy.
☐ Avoid driving or other potentially hazardous activities until the adverse CNS effects of the drug are known.

Other instructions
☐ Don't take any other medication before checking with your doctor or pharmacist.
☐ See your doctor regularly as scheduled because antiarrhythmic therapy requires close follow-up and regular diagnostic studies (such as ECGs and serum electrolyte tests) to monitor its therapeutic effects.

Interventions

Preparation and administration
• The loading dose is divided into three equal doses and given with meals to minimize GI intolerance.
• The maintenance dose may be given once daily, but it may be divided into two doses taken with meals if GI intolerance occurs. (See *Taking antiarrhythmics at home.*)

Monitoring and supportive care
• Monitor blood pressure and heart rate and rhythm frequently for significant changes.
• Perform continuous ECG monitoring at the beginning of drug therapy and whenever dosage is changed. Notify the doctor of any significant changes.
• Periodically monitor liver and thyroid function test results.
• Monitor serum electrolytes, particularly potassium and magnesium levels.
• Monitor for signs and symptoms of pneumonitis, such as exertional dyspnea, nonproductive cough, and pleuritic chest pain. Also monitor results of pulmonary function tests and chest X-rays.
• Reassure the patient that adverse reactions are more prevalent with high doses but usually resolve within about 4 months after drug therapy stops.

Safety tip. Pulmonary toxicity is more common when daily dosages exceed 400 mg. Amiodarone should be discontinued if pulmonary complications occur. You may then be asked to treat the patient with corticosteroids.
• Digoxin, quinidine, phenytoin, procainamide, and warfarin dosages

may be reduced during amiodarone therapy to avoid toxicity.

• Remind the patient to avoid sunlight and to wear protective clothing and sunblock while outdoors. Amiodarone causes photosensitivity, which may persist for several months after therapy is stopped.

• Also warn the patient that the drug may cause a blue-gray skin discoloration, especially in areas exposed to the sun.

• Although corneal microdeposits typically appear 1 to 4 months after therapy begins, only 2% to 3% of patients have visual disturbances. Periodic ophthalmologic evaluations should be performed to assess the patient for corneal microdeposits.

• Know that children receiving amiodarone concomitantly with digoxin may experience more acute interactions.

• Children may also experience faster onset of action and shorter duration of effect than adults.

• Be aware that amiodarone alters thyroid function test results, causing increased serum thyroxine and decreased triiodothyronine levels. However, most patients maintain normal thyroid function during therapy.

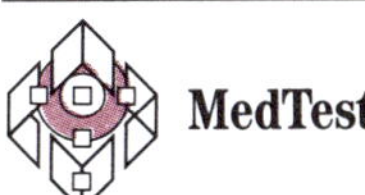 **MedTest**

1. Amiodarone is excreted mainly through the:
    a. respiratory tract.
    b. skin.
    c. biliary tree.
    d. kidneys.

2. To assess for visual disturbances:
    a. recommend weekly, then monthly, eye examinations.
    b. check the patient's vision monthly using a Snellen chart.
    c. inspect the patient's eyes weekly with an ophthalmoscope.
    d. use fluorescein dye to look for corneal lesions.

3. To assess for the most significant adverse reaction to amiodarone, monitor your patient for:
    a. exertional dyspnea, nonproductive cough, and pleuritic pain.
    b. any changes in blood pressure and heart rate and rhythm.
    c. nausea and vomiting.
    d. sunburn with blistering and tingling.

Amlodipine besylate

Known by the brand name Norvasc, amlodipine is a calcium channel blocker that's available in 2.5-, 5-, and 10-mg tablets.

Pharmacokinetics

• *Absorption:* Peak plasma concentrations are seen in 6 to 12 hours.

• *Distribution:* Absolute bioavailability has been estimated to be between 64% and 90%, with approximately 93% of the circulating drug bound to plasma proteins. Steady-state plasma levels are reached after 7 to 8 days of consecutive therapy.

• *Metabolism:* By the liver to inactive metabolites.

• *Excretion:* By the kidneys, with 10% of the parent compound and 60% of the metabolites excreted in urine.

Indications, dosage, and action
Hypertension
• *Adult dosage:* Initially, 5 mg P.O. daily; maximum dosage is 10 mg once daily. Titrate over 7 to 14 days.

Small, fragile, or elderly patients or those with hepatic insufficiency, 2.5 mg daily.
• *Action:* A calcium ion antagonist, amlodipine inhibits the influx of calcium into vascular smooth muscle, causing vasodilation, a reduction in peripheral vascular resistance, and decreased blood pressure. Amlodipine doesn't affect cardiac muscle.

Chronic stable angina or vasospastic angina (Prinzmetal's or variant angina)
• *Adult dosage:* 5 to 10 mg daily; usual dosage is 10 mg daily.

Small, fragile, or elderly patients or those with hepatic insufficiency, 5 mg daily.
• *Action:* Dilates coronary arteries and arterioles, increasing coronary blood flow. Also reduces total peripheral resistance (afterload), thus reducing myocardial oxygen demand.

Contraindications and cautions
• Use cautiously in patients receiving other vasodilators, especially those with severe aortic stenosis.
• Use cautiously in patients with CHF.
• Because this drug is metabolized by the liver, also use with caution in patients with hepatic disease.
• Pregnancy risk category C

Life-threatening adverse reactions
None reported

Common adverse reactions
• Edema (with 10-mg dose only)
• Headache

Infrequent adverse reactions
• Edema (with 2.5- and 5-mg doses only), dizziness, flushing, palpitations, angina, MI, CHF
• Somnolence, fatigue
• Nausea, abdominal pain

Interactions
None noted

Interventions
Preparation and administration
• Give amlodipine without regard to meals. (See *Taking calcium channel blockers at home.*)

Monitoring and supportive care
• Obtain a baseline blood pressure measurement; then monitor blood pressure frequently during initiation of therapy. Because drug-induced vasodilation has a gradual onset, acute hypotension is rare.
• Some patients, especially those with severe obstructive CAD, have developed increased frequency, duration, or severity of angina or even acute MI after initiation of calcium channel blocker therapy or when dosage is increased. Monitor the patient carefully.
• Notify the doctor of signs of CHF, such as increased shortness of breath, cough, weight gain, or ankle or hand swelling.

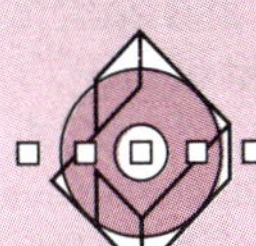

Patient-teaching checklist

Taking calcium channel blockers at home

In addition to explaining the drug's action and dosage, teach the patient who will continue calcium channel blocker therapy after discharge to follow these important guidelines.

General guidelines
☐ Take the drug as prescribed even when you're feeling better.
☐ Check your blood pressure frequently. Notify your doctor if any changes occur.
☐ If you're taking the drug for angina, you may continue to take your prescribed nitrate medication for acute angina episodes.

Know when to call your doctor
☐ Notify your doctor immediately if you experience chest pain, shortness of breath, or palpitations. If you have angina, report increased frequency, duration, or severity of angina.
☐ Alert your doctor if you notice fluid retention, as exhibited by a weight gain of 2 lb (1 kg) or more, swelling of your hands or ankles, or shortness of breath.

Minimize adverse reactions
☐ Lie down immediately if dizziness occurs.
☐ Check with your doctor or pharmacist before taking any OTC medications.
☐ Schedule frequent rest periods throughout the day if you're becoming easily fatigued.
☐ Avoid driving, operating machinery, or other hazardous activities requiring skill and coordination if you're experiencing dizziness.
☐ Follow dietary restrictions to minimize fluid retention.

• Sublingual nitroglycerin may be taken as needed for anginal symptoms without fear of interactions. If the patient continues nitrate therapy during titration of amlodipine dosage, urge continued compliance.

• Be aware that dosage adjustments are necessary in patients with hepatic, but not renal, failure because the drug is metabolized primarily by the liver.

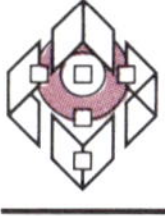

MedTest

1. Amlodipine is classified pharmacologically as:
    a. an ACE inhibitor.
    b. a beta-adrenergic blocker.
    c. a calcium channel blocker.
    d. a sympathomimetic agent.

2. Dosage reductions of amlodipine may be required for patients with:
   a. renal failure.
   b. diabetes mellitus.
   c. CHF.
   d. hepatic failure.

3. Administer amlodipine:
   a. with meals to reduce GI symptoms.
   b. early in the day to prevent insomnia.
   c. at bedtime to encourage rest.
   d. once daily, without regard to meals.

Amrinone lactate

Also known by the brand names Inocor and Inocor Lactate Injection, amrinone is a bipyridine derivative that's therapeutically classified as an inotropic vasodilator. It's available in 5-mg/ml ampules for injection.

Pharmacokinetics

• *Absorption:* Onset of action occurs in 2 to 5 minutes with I.V. administration, with peak effects in about 10 minutes. Cardiovascular effects may persist for 1 to 2 hours.
• *Distribution:* Protein binding ranges from 10% to 49%. Therapeutic steady-state serum levels range from 0.5 to 7 mcg/ml (ideal concentration is 3 mcg/ml).
• *Metabolism:* In the liver.
• *Excretion:* In the urine. Elimination half-life is about 4 hours but may be prolonged in patients with CHF.

Indications, dosage, and action
Short-term management of CHF
• *Adult dosage:* Initially, 0.75 mg/kg by I.V. bolus over 2 to 3 minutes; then begin maintenance infusion of 5 to 10 mcg/kg/minute. Additional bolus of 0.75 mg/kg may be given 30 minutes after therapy starts. Maximum daily dosage is 10 mg/kg.
• *Action:* Produces inotropic action by increasing cellular levels of cyclic adenosine monophosphate. Produces vasodilation through a direct relaxant effect on vascular smooth muscle, decreasing preload and afterload.

Contraindications and cautions
• Don't give amrinone to patients with known hypersensitivity to amrinone or sulfites (sodium metabisulfite is used as a preservative).
• Amrinone should not be used in place of surgery in patients with severe aortic or pulmonic valve disease.
• Use amrinone with caution in patients with hypertrophic cardiomyopathy because it may exacerbate outflow tract obstruction.
• Also use cautiously in patients recovering from acute MI because drug may be arrhythmogenic.
• Use with caution in patients with hepatic disease because drug may be hepatotoxic.
• Use cautiously in patients with renal impairment because amrinone may accumulate.
• Be aware that amrinone may be excreted in breast milk and is not recommended for breast-feeding women.
• Pregnancy risk category C

Life-threatening adverse reactions
- Arrhythmias
- Thrombocytopenia
- Anaphylaxis

Common adverse reactions
None noted

Infrequent adverse reactions
- Arrhythmias, hypotension
- Nausea, vomiting, cramps, anorexia, dyspepsia, diarrhea, hepatotoxicity
- Reversible thrombocytopenia
- Burning at injection site
- Fever, chest pain, hypersensitivity reactions (pericarditis, ascites, myositis, vasculitis, pleuritis)

Interactions
- *Disopyramide:* May cause severe hypotension.

Interventions
Preparation and administration
- Administer the drug as supplied or dilute it in 0.45% or 0.9% NaCl solution to a concentration of 1 to 3 mg/ml. (See *Amrinone combinations to avoid.*)

Monitoring and supportive care
- Monitor the patient's blood pressure and heart rate throughout infusion. If his blood pressure decreases but he's asymptomatic, slow the infusion and monitor him closely. However, if his blood pressure drops and he becomes symptomatic, if he develops new arrhythmias, or if existing arrhythmias worsen, the infusion should be stopped. The dosage may need to be reduced.

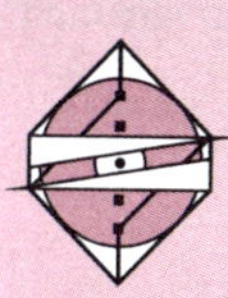

Incompatibility warning
Amrinone combinations to avoid

You should never dilute amrinone with solutions containing dextrose because the drug will slowly lose potency over 24 hours, with no visible change in color or texture. Amrinone may, however, be administered (diluted or undiluted) into running dextrose infusions through a Y-connector or directly into the tubing.

Also remember that furosemide cannot be administered through I.V. lines containing amrinone because a precipitate will form immediately, compromising amrinone's effectiveness.

- Monitor the patient's platelet count. A count below 150,000/mm^3 usually necessitates dosage reduction.
- Monitor hepatic enzyme and electrolyte levels (especially potassium). Amrinone may increase serum hepatic enzyme levels and decrease serum potassium levels.
- Also monitor liver function test results to detect hepatic damage (rare).
- Amrinone overdose may lead to severe hypotension. Treatment may include administration of a vasopressor and cautious fluid volume replacement.
- Know that amrinone is prescribed primarily for patients who haven't responded to therapy with digitalis

glycosides, diuretics, inotropics, and vasodilators.

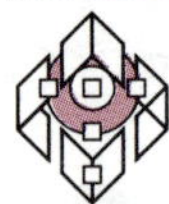 **MedTest**

1. Amrinone produces its vasodilating effect by:
   a. beta blockade.
   b. alpha-adrenergic activity.
   c. direct effect on vascular smooth muscle.
   d. calcium channel blockade.

2. Amrinone's main use is for short-term management of:
   a. angina.
   b. CHF.
   c. ventricular irritability.
   d. peripheral vascular occlusions.

3. While monitoring your patient's blood pressure during amrinone infusion, you note a gradual, asymptomatic decrease. You then:
   a. slow the administration rate and continue careful monitoring.
   b. stop the drug immediately.
   c. prepare to administer norepinephrine.
   d. notify the cardiologist and await further instructions.

Atenolol

Also known by the brand name Tenormin, atenolol is a cardioselective beta$_1$-adrenergic blocker. It's therapeutically classified as an antihypertensive and antianginal agent. The drug is available in 25-, 50- and 100-mg tablets and in vials for injection containing 5 mg/10 ml.

Pharmacokinetics
• *Absorption:* 50% to 60% is absorbed. Onset occurs within 60 minutes, with peak effect at 2 to 4 hours. Antihypertensive effect lasts about 24 hours.
• *Distribution:* Distributed into most tissues and fluids except the brain and CSF. The drug is 5% to 15% protein-bound.
• *Metabolism:* Minimal.
• *Excretion:* Approximately 50% is excreted unchanged in urine; remainder is excreted as unchanged drug and metabolites in feces. In patients with normal renal function, elimination half-life is 6 to 7 hours.

Indications, dosage, and action
Hypertension
• *Regular adult dosage:* Initially, 25 to 50 mg P.O. as a single daily dose. Dosage may be increased to 100 mg/day after 7 to 14 days. Dosages higher than 100 mg/day are unlikely to produce further benefit.
• *Dosage in renal failure:* In patients with creatinine clearance of 15 to 35 ml/minute, 50 mg per day; in patients with creatinine clearance below 15 ml/minute, 50 mg on alternate days; in patients undergoing hemodialysis, 50 mg after each treatment.
• *Action:* Blocks beta$_1$-adrenergic receptors, thus decreasing cardiac output, sympathetic outflow from the CNS, and renin release.

Angina pectoris
• *Adult dosage:* 50 mg P.O. once daily; may be increased to 100 mg/day after 7 days for optimal effect. Maximum daily dosage is 200 mg.
• *Action:* Decreases myocardial contractility and heart rate, thus reducing myocardial oxygen consumption.

Reduction of mortality in acute MI
• *Adult dosage:* 5 mg I.V. over 5 minutes, followed by another 5 mg I.V. 10 minutes later. In patients who tolerate the full I.V. dose, 50 mg P.O. 10 minutes after final I.V. dose, then an additional 50 mg P.O. 12 hours later. Thereafter, 100 mg P.O. daily as a single dose or 50 mg b.i.d. for at least 7 days.
• *Action:* How atenolol improves survival in patients with MI is unknown.

Contraindications and cautions
• Avoid use in patients with overt cardiac failure or second- or third-degree AV block unless a pacemaker is in place. Don't use in cardiogenic shock because the drug may worsen this condition.
• Use cautiously in elderly patients and patients with impaired renal function because drug elimination may be impaired.
• Also use cautiously in patients with reduced myocardial contractility because beta-adrenergic blockade may precipitate or worsen CHF.
• Use cautiously in patients with diabetes mellitus or hyperthyroidism because atenolol may mask tachycardia (but not dizziness or sweating) caused by hypoglycemia or hyperthyroidism.

• Use with caution in patients with bronchospastic diseases, such as asthma or emphysema, because dosages exceeding 100 mg/day may inhibit the bronchodilating effects of endogenous catecholamines.
• Be aware that safety during breast-feeding hasn't been established.
• Pregnancy risk category C

Life-threatening adverse reactions
• VT, cardiac arrest, CHF
• Bronchospasm

Common adverse reactions
• Bradycardia (18% in patients with MI), hypotension (25% in MI), ECG changes, VT (16% in MI), supraventricular tachycardia, cold extremities
• Dyspnea
• Dizziness, tiredness (26%), depression (12%)

Infrequent adverse reactions
• Heart block, atrial fibrillation, atrial flutter
• Wheezing, bronchospasm
• Lethargy, vertigo, light-headedness, drowsiness, fatigue
• Diarrhea, nausea
• Impotence

Interactions
• *Alpha-adrenergic agents, indomethacin, NSAIDs:* Decreased antihypertensive effect. Monitor blood pressure and adjust dosage.
• *Antihypertensives:* Enhanced antihypertensive effect. Use together cautiously.
• *Calcium channel blockers:* Additive effect. Use together cautiously.

• *Digitalis glycosides:* Excessive bradycardia. Use together cautiously.
• *Insulin, oral antidiabetic drugs:* Can alter dosage requirements in previously stabilized diabetics. Observe patient carefully.

Interventions
Preparation and administration
• Give a single oral dose at the same time each day. Atenolol may be taken without regard to meals. (See *Taking beta-adrenergic blockers at home,* page 63.)

Safety tip. Always check the patient's apical pulse before giving this drug; if his pulse rate is less than 60 beats/minute, withhold the dose and call the doctor immediately.
• You can mix I.V. doses with D_5W or 0.9% NaCl solution. The solution is stable for 48 hours after mixing.

Monitoring and supportive care
• Monitor for clinical signs of overdose, including hypotension, bradycardia, and heart failure, and report such signs immediately.

Safety tip. Although atenolol masks tachycardia associated with hypoglycemia and hyperthyroidism, it doesn't mask CNS symptoms such as dizziness, headache, restlessness, or mental status changes, so monitor for these symptoms.
• Abrupt withdrawal may precipitate thyroid storm in hyperthyroid patients and may exacerbate angina in patients with MI or angina. The drug should be withdrawn gradually over a 2-week period.

• Know that atenolol also may cause changes in exercise tolerance.
• Be aware that atenolol has reportedly elevated platelet count as well as serum levels of potassium, uric acid, transaminase, ALP, LD, creatinine, and BUN.

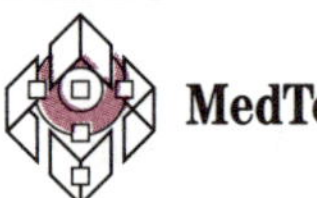 **MedTest**

1. Before giving each dose of atenolol you should:
   a. check the patient's blood pressure.
   b. check his blood glucose level.
   c. check his potassium level.
   d. check the patient's apical pulse.

2. Atenolol's negative inotropic and chronotropic action, which decreases myocardial contractility and heart rate to reduce myocardial oxygen consumption, make it useful in treating:
   a. hypertension.
   b. chronic stable angina.
   c. CHF
   d. acute MI.

3. Which of the following adverse reactions is most common in patients taking atenolol?
   a. Impotence
   b. Dizziness
   c. Bronchospasm
   d. Nausea

Atropine sulfate

A belladonna alkaloid, atropine is therapeutically classified as an antiarrhythmic and a vagolytic. It's available for injection in vials containing 0.05, 0.1, 0.3, 0.4, 0.5, 0.8, 1, and 1.2 mg/ml. An anticholinergic (parasympatholytic) agent with many uses, atropine is the mainstay of drug treatment for bradyarrhythmias.

Pharmacokinetics

- *Absorption:* Effects on heart rate peak within 4 minutes after I.V. administration. With endotracheal administration, atropine is well absorbed from the bronchial tree.
- *Distribution:* Only 18% of the drug binds with plasma protein; it enters the CNS.
- *Metabolism:* Metabolized in the liver to several metabolites.
- *Excretion:* 30% to 50% of a dose is excreted unchanged by the kidneys. Small amounts may be excreted in the feces. Elimination is biphasic, with a terminal half-life of about 12½ hours.

Indications, dosage, and action
Symptomatic bradycardia, bradyarrhythmias (junctional or escape rhythm)
- *Adult dosage:* Usually 0.5 to 1 mg by I.V. push; repeat q 5 minutes to a maximum of 2 mg. May be given by endotracheal tube at doses 2 to 2½ times the I.V. dose.
- *Pediatric dosage:* 0.01 mg/kg up to maximum 0.4 mg I.V.; or 0.3 mg/m^2; may repeat q 4 to 6 hours.

- *Action:* Blocks acetylcholine's vagal effects on the SA and AV nodes, thereby increasing SA and AV node conduction velocity and heart rate. Also increases the sinus node discharge rate and decreases the AV node's effective refractory period.

Contraindications and cautions
- Use cautiously in patients with acute MI because the drug increases heart rate and myocardial oxygen consumption. It may promote arrhythmias, including ventricular fibrillation, VT, and atrial fibrillation.
- Also use cautiously in patients with acute angle-closure glaucoma, obstructive uropathy, GI obstruction, myasthenia gravis, paralytic ileus, intestinal atony, unstable CV status from acute hemorrhage, or toxic megacolon because the drug may worsen these disorders.
- Give cautiously to patients with Down's syndrome because they are more sensitive to the drug.
- Administer carefully to men with benign prostatic hyperplasia; urine retention may occur.
- Pregnancy risk category C

Life-threatening adverse reactions
- Extreme tachycardia, angina (with doses greater than 2 mg)

Common adverse reactions
- Tachycardia (possibly extreme), palpitations, angina
- Headache, insomnia, dizziness, restlessness
- Dry mouth, constipation
- Blurred vision, mydriasis (with 2-mg dose)

Infrequent adverse reactions
• Ataxia, disorientation, hallucinations, delirium, coma, excitement, agitation, confusion (especially in elderly patients)
• Thirst, nausea, vomiting
• Urine retention
• Photophobia (with 1-mg dose)
• Leukocytosis
• Hot, flushed skin
• Fever

Interactions
• *Amantadine, antiarrhythmics, antiparkinsonian agents, glutethimide, meperidine, phenothiazines, tricyclic antidepressants:* Increased anticholinergic effects. Use together cautiously.
• *Antacids:* Decreased absorption of anticholinergics. Separate administration times by at least 1 hour.
• *Digoxin:* Increased digoxin levels if slow-dissolving digoxin tablets are used.
• *Ketoconazole, levodopa:* Decreased absorption. Avoid concomitant use.
• *Methotrimeprazine:* May produce extrapyramidal symptoms. Monitor patient carefully.
• *Potassium chloride wax-matrix tablets:* Increased risk of mucosal lesions. Use cautiously.

Interventions
Preparation and administration
• Inject directly into a large vein or I.V. tubing over 1 to 2 minutes.
• Be aware that the drug may cause paradoxical initial bradycardia with I.V. administration (especially with doses less than 0.5 mg), which usually disappears within 2 minutes.

Monitoring and supportive care
• Observe for tachycardia, which may precipitate ventricular fibrillation in a patient with a cardiac disorder.
• Clinical signs of overdose, such as extreme tachycardia and delirium, reflect excessive anticholinergic activity. Report these signs immediately and prepare to treat with physostigmine salicylate and general supportive measures.
• Keep in mind that high doses may cause fever, urine retention, and CNS effects, including hallucinations and confusion (anticholinergic delirium).
• Closely monitor the patient's intake and output; atropine may cause urine retention and hesitancy. If possible, have the patient void before taking the drug.

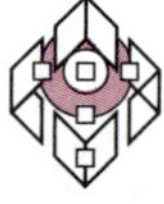 **MedTest**

1. For symptomatic bradycardia, give I.V. doses of atropine:
   a. by rapid injection into a vein.
   b. by diluting the drug in 50 ml of D_5W and infusing it over 15 to 20 minutes.
   c. into a large vein or I.V. tubing over 1 to 2 minutes.
   d. q 5 to 10 minutes to a total of 6 mg.

2. The antidote for atropine overdose is:
   a. protamine sulfate.
   b. physostigmine salicylate.
   c. phenylephrine hydrochloride.
   d. paramethasone acetate.

3. If an I.V. line isn't in place and atropine is required for immediate treatment of symptomatic bradycardia, the next best route for rapid absorption is:

   a. S.C. injection.
   b. I.M. injection.
   c. direct intracardiac injection.
   d. endotracheal insufflation.

Benazepril hydrochloride

Also known by its brand name Lotensin, benazepril is an ACE inhibitor that's classified therapeutically as an antihypertensive. It's available in 5-, 10-, 20- and 40-mg tablets.

Pharmacokinetics
- *Absorption:* After oral administration, at least 37% of benazepril is absorbed from the GI tract. Peak plasma concentrations occur in 2 to 4 hours.
- *Distribution:* Highly (97%) bound to plasma proteins.
- *Metabolism:* By the liver to its active metabolite, benazeprilat.
- *Excretion:* Mostly excreted in urine, with biliary elimination accounting for only 12% of excretion. Its elimination half-life is 10 to 11 hours.

Indications, dosage, and action
Hypertension
- *Adult dosage:* Initially, 10 mg daily. Usual dosage is 20 to 40 mg once daily or b.i.d.; doses above 80 mg/day have not been evaluated.

- *Dosage in hypovolemia, renal failure, or in patients receiving diuretics:* Initial dose is 5 mg.
- *Action:* Inhibits ACE activity, resulting in a decreased rate of conversion of angiotensin I to angiotensin II, a potent vasoconstrictor. Reduced formation of angiotensin II decreases peripheral vascular resistance (afterload) and aldosterone secretion. This results in reduced sodium and water retention and decreased blood pressure.

Vasodilation and CHF
- *Adult dosage:* Initially, 5 mg P.O. daily; maintenance dosage is 5 to 10 mg daily in a single dose.
- *Action:* Reduces afterload, resulting in increased cardiac output; PAWP and pulmonary vascular resistance also decrease, resulting in improved cardiac output.

Contraindications and cautions
- Don't give benazepril to patients with a history of angioedema.
- Use cautiously in patients with impaired renal or hepatic function and in diabetic patients.
- Avoid use during pregnancy because ACE inhibitors can cause fetal or neonatal injury or death. When pregnancy is detected, ACE inhibitors should be discontinued as soon as possible.
- Advise lactating women to avoid breast-feeding. Minimal amounts of unchanged benazepril and benazeprilat are excreted in breast milk.
- Pregnancy risk category C (first trimester); D (second and third trimesters)

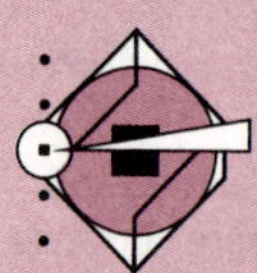

Life-threatening hazards of multidrug therapy with benazepril

Interacting drug	Effects
Potassium-sparing diuretics (such as spironolactone)	Increase risk of hyperkalemia
Potassium supplements (such as potassium chloride)	Increase risk of hyperkalemia
Salt substitutes containing potassium	Increase risk of hyperkalemia

Life-threatening adverse reactions
- MI
- Hypersensitivity reactions

Common adverse reactions
- Headache

Infrequent adverse reactions
- Symptomatic hypotension, orthostatic hypotension, syncope, angina, arrhythmias, chest pain, palpitations, edema
- Dry, persistent, tickling, nonproductive cough; dyspnea
- Dizziness, postural dizziness, fatigue, somnolence, light-headedness, anxiety, amnesia, depression, insomnia, malaise, nervousness, neuralgia, neuropathy, paresthesia, tremor, vertigo
- Nausea, vomiting, abdominal pain, anorexia, constipation, diarrhea, dry mouth, dyspepsia, dysphagia, gastroenteritis, increased salivation, taste disturbance
- Impotence
- Epistaxis
- Rash, dermatitis, pruritus, photosensitivity, purpura
- Angioedema, arthralgia, arthritis, increased sweating, myalgia, weight gain, asthenia

Interactions
- *Diuretics, other antihypertensives:* Risk of excessive hypotension; diuretic may be discontinued or benazepril dose may be reduced.
- *Lithium:* Possible increased serum lithium levels and lithium toxicity; monitor carefully.

For dangerous interactions, see *Life-threatening hazards of multidrug therapy with benazepril.*

Interventions
Preparation and administration
- Administer the drug without regard to meals. (See *Taking ACE inhibitors at home.*)

Monitoring and supportive care
- Take blood pressure at peak drug levels (2 to 6 hours after a dose) and at trough levels (just before a dose)

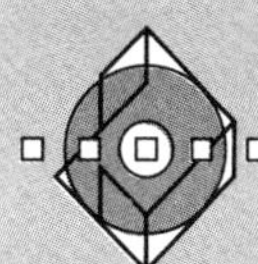

Patient-teaching checklist

Taking ACE inhibitors at home

In addition to explaining the drug's action and dosage, teach the patient who will continue ACE inhibitor therapy after discharge to follow these important guidelines.

Take your medication correctly
☐ Take this drug exactly as prescribed even when you're feeling better.
☐ Check your blood pressure frequently. Notify your doctor about any significant change.

Know when to call your doctor
☐ Notify your doctor immediately or go to the nearest hospital for emergency treatment if you develop swelling of your face, eyes, lips, or tongue or experience difficulty in breathing.
☐ Report any signs or symptoms of infection (sore throat or fever), easy bruising, or bleeding to your doctor because ACE inhibitors can impair your body's ability to prevent infection or bleeding.

Minimize adverse reactions
☐ Rise slowly (especially from lying flat to sitting upright) and dangle your legs over the bedside for a few minutes before standing to minimize possible light-headedness caused by this drug. Lie down immediately if faintness or dizziness occurs.
☐ Drink plenty of fluids. Remember that inadequate fluid intake, vomiting, diarrhea, and excessive perspi-

ration can lead to light-headedness and fainting. Use caution in hot weather, while exercising, and if your stomach is upset. If you aren't able to maintain an adequate fluid intake, notify your doctor.
☐ ACE inhibitors may cause a dry, persistent, tickling, nonproductive cough, which doesn't indicate a serious condition and is reversible when therapy is discontinued. If it becomes troublesome, notify your doctor.
☐ Don't use salt substitutes as part of your diet plan for blood pressure control unless otherwise instructed. Salt substitutes contain potassium which, when used with ACE inhibitors, may cause potentially fatal hyperkalemia (elevated potassium levels).

Other instructions
☐ Follow dietary restrictions to minimize fluid retention.
☐ Check with your doctor or pharmacist before taking any OTC medications.
☐ If you're pregnant or plan to become pregnant, notify your doctor immediately. ACE inhibitors can cause fetal harm if taken during pregnancy.

to verify adequate blood pressure control.

• Severe hypotension can occur when benazepril is given with diuretics. If possible, diuretic therapy should be discontinued 2 to 3 days before starting benazepril. If benazepril doesn't adequately control blood pressure, the diuretic may be reinstituted with care.

• Assess renal and hepatic function before and periodically throughout therapy. Also monitor CBC and serum potassium levels.

Safety tip. Be aware that light-headedness can occur, especially during the first few days of therapy. Inadequate fluid intake, vomiting, diarrhea, and excessive perspiration can lead to light-headedness and syncope. Carefully monitor intake and output, assess for dizziness, and institute safety measures such as raising siderails on the bed.

• Other ACE inhibitors have been associated with agranulocytosis and neutropenia. Tell the patient to immediately report any signs of infection (sore throat or fever), easy bruising, or bleeding.

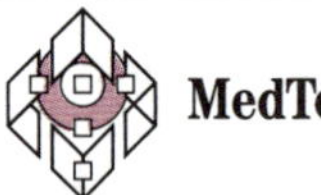 **MedTest**

1. Benazepril is effective in treating CHF because it:
    a. increases aldosterone secretion.
    b. decreases prostaglandin synthesis.
    c. reduces afterload and pulmonary vascular resistance.
    d. decreases plasma renin activity.

2. To verify adequate blood pressure control in the patient receiving benazepril, check the patient's blood pressure:
    a. when giving each dose.
    b. daily when the patient rises.
    c. when the patient is supine, sitting, and standing.
    d. at peak and trough drug level times.

3. A clinically insignificant adverse effect that benazepril, like other ACE inhibitors, causes is:
    a. seizures.
    b. a dry, persistent, tickling, nonproductive cough.
    c. symptomatic hypotension.
    d. nausea, vomiting, and diarrhea.

Bepridil hydrochloride

Also known by its brand name, Vascor, bepridil is a calcium channel blocker that's classified therapeutically as an antianginal. It's available in 200-, 300-, and 400-mg tablets.

Pharmacokinetics

• *Absorption:* Peak concentrations occur in 2 to 3 hours.
• *Distribution:* Over 99% of this drug is plasma protein–bound.
• *Metabolism:* In the liver.
• *Excretion:* 70% is excreted in urine, and 22% is excreted in feces as metabolites. Elimination half-life averages 42 hours (range is 26 to 64 hours).

Indications, dosage, and action
Chronic stable angina in patients unresponsive to other antianginals
• *Adult dosage:* Initially, 200 mg P.O. daily; adjust dosage according to patient tolerance and response. Maximum daily dosage is 400 mg. Most patients receive 300 mg daily.
• *Action:* Blocks calcium ion influx into cardiac and vascular smooth muscle cells. Decreases heart rate and peripheral resistance (afterload), reducing myocardial oxygen consumption.

Contraindications and cautions
• Be aware that bepridil is contraindicated in patients with a history of serious ventricular arrhythmias, SSS, second- or third-degree AV block (except those with a functioning ventricular pacemaker), hypotension (below 90 mm Hg systolic), uncompensated cardiac insufficiency, or drug-induced or congenital QT-interval prolongation.
• Use with caution in patients with left bundle-branch heart block or sinus bradycardia.
• Use cautiously in elderly patients and in patients with renal or hepatic disorders.
• Use cautiously in breast-feeding women. Bepridil is excreted in breast milk.
• Pregnancy risk category C

Life-threatening adverse reactions
• Ventricular arrhythmias
• Agranulocytosis

Common adverse reactions
• Prolonged QT interval, palpitations (with 300-mg dose)
• Dyspnea (with 300-mg dose)
• Headache, nervousness, tremor (with 200-mg dose), dizziness (15% incidence with 300-mg dose to 27% with 400-mg dose), drowsiness (with 300- or 400-mg dose)
• GI distress (with 200-mg dose), nausea (26% with 300-mg dose; 18% with 400-mg dose), diarrhea (with 300- and 400-mg doses), anorexia (with 400-mg dose)
• Tinnitus (with 300-mg dose)
• Asthenia

Infrequent adverse reactions
• Edema, CHF, vasodilation, sinus tachycardia, sinus bradycardia, hypertension
• Rhinitis, cough, pharyngitis
• Paresthesia, insomnia, syncope, depression, vertigo, akathisia
• Dry mouth, anorexia, abdominal pain, constipation, taste change, flatulence, gastritis, increased appetite, elevated hepatic enzyme levels
• Impotence, decreased libido
• Blurred vision
• Rash, sweating, skin irritation
• Flulike syndrome, superinfection, fever, pain, myalgic asthenia

Interactions
See *Hazards of multidrug therapy with bepridil*, page 90.

Interventions
Preparation and administration
• Know that the patient may take bepridil without regard to meals.
• Remind him to notify the doctor immediately if he experiences persist-

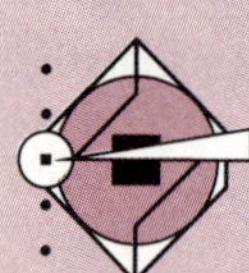

Interactions alert

Hazards of multidrug therapy with bepridil

Interacting drug	Effects
Antiarrhythmics (such as quinidine and procainamide)	Prolong the QT interval
Digitalis glycosides	Increase digoxin levels and may increase AV nodal depression
Potassium-wasting diuretics (such as furosemide)	Cause hypokalemia and may lead to ventricular arrhythmias
Tricyclic antidepressants (such as amoxapine and desipramine)	Prolong the QT interval

ent infections, unusual bleeding, or other serious adverse reactions. (See *Taking calcium channel blockers at home,* page 77.)

Monitoring and supportive care
• Monitor serum potassium levels and correct hypokalemia before initiating therapy.
• Monitor the QT and QT_c intervals before and during therapy. Reduced dosage is required if QT or QT_c prolongation occurs. If prolongation persists, withhold the dose and notify the doctor.
• Assess the patient for any unusual bruising or bleeding or any signs of infection (for example, sore throat or fever). If infection is suspected, obtain a WBC count.
• Know that increased ALT levels and abnormal liver function test results may also occur with this drug.

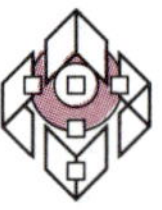

MedTest

1. Bepridil is pharmacologically classified as:
   a. an adrenergic agent.
   b. a beta blocker.
   c. a calcium channel blocker.
   d. a local anesthetic.

2. Bepridil's main use is in the treatment of:
   a. hypertension.
   b. hypotension.
   c. arrhythmias.
   d. angina.

3. When initiating bepridil therapy, closely monitor the patient's:
   a. WBC count.
   b. serum creatinine levels.
   c. liver function studies.
   d. QT and QT_c intervals.

Betaxolol hydrochloride

Known by the brand name Kerlone, betaxolol is a beta-adrenergic blocker classified therapeutically as an antihypertensive agent. It's available in 10- and 20-mg tablets.

Pharmacokinetics

- *Absorption:* A small first-pass effect reduces bioavailability by about 10%. Absorption is not affected by food.
- *Distribution:* Peak plasma concentrations occur in about 3 hours. The drug is 50% bound to plasma proteins.
- *Metabolism:* Hepatic; about 85% of the drug is recovered in the urine as metabolites.
- *Excretion:* Primarily renal (about 80%). Elimination half-life is 14 to 22 hours. Elimination half-life is prolonged in patients with hepatic disease, but clearance is not affected and, therefore, dosage adjustment is unnecessary.

Indications, dosage, and action
Hypertension
- *Adult dosage:* Initially, 10 mg P.O. once daily. Full antihypertensive effect should be seen in 7 to 14 days. If necessary, double dosage to 20 mg P.O. once daily.
- *Action:* The cardioselective beta$_1$-adrenergic blocking effects of betaxolol slow the heart rate, decrease the force of myocardial contractility, and decrease cardiac output to lower blood pressure.

Contraindications and cautions

- Be aware that betaxolol is contraindicated in patients with bronchial asthma, severe COPD, sinus bradycardia, second- or third-degree AV block, CHF, cardiac failure, cardiogenic shock, or restricted pulmonary function because betaxolol may worsen these symptoms or conditions.
- Use betaxolol with extreme caution in patients with diabetes mellitus because the drug may mask some signs of hypoglycemia, such as tachycardia.
- Know that beta blockers may also mask tachycardia associated with hyperthyroidism. In patients suspected of having thyrotoxicosis, betaxolol should be withdrawn gradually to avoid thyroid storm.
- Use cautiously in patients with angle-closure glaucoma (give with a miotic).
- Use with caution in patients with myasthenia-like symptoms such as muscle weakness.
- Use cautiously in patients with CHF controlled by digitalis glycosides and diuretics or those with a history of CHF. Such patients may have no overt symptoms but may exhibit signs of cardiac decompensation with oral beta-blocker therapy.
- Use with caution in patients with bronchospastic disease. High doses of betaxolol can cause bronchospasm.
- Know that rapid withdrawal of the drug can precipitate angina pectoris in patients with unrecognized CAD.
- Use with caution in elderly patients with cardiac or pulmonary disease.

• Use with caution in breast-feeding women. Betaxolol is excreted in breast milk.
• Pregnancy risk category C

Life-threatening adverse reactions
• CHF
• Bronchospasm

Common adverse reactions
• Bradycardia (increased incidence in patients age 65 and over), chest pain (when receiving 20- to 40-mg doses)
• Headache, insomnia (when receiving 20- to 40-mg doses), dizziness (when receiving 20- to 40-mg doses), fatigue (when receiving 20- to 40-mg doses)
• Nausea (when receiving 20- to 40-mg doses)
• Arthralgia and myalgia (when receiving 20- to 40-mg doses)

Infrequent adverse reactions
• Symptomatic bradycardia, palpitations, edema, peripheral vascular insufficiency, hypotension, worsening of angina, CHF, syncope, orthostatic hypotension, conduction disturbances
• Dyspnea, wheezing, pharyngitis, rhinitis, upper respiratory infection
• Depression, nervousness, anxiety, insomnia, paresthesia, lethargy
• Dyspepsia, diarrhea, dry mouth, anorexia, constipation
• Impotence
• Rash, fever

Interactions
• *Catecholamine-depleting drugs, reserpine:* May have an additive effect when administered with a beta blocker.
• *Lidocaine:* Beta blockers may enhance lidocaine's effects. Use cautiously.

For dangerous interactions, see *Life-threatening hazards of multidrug therapy with betaxolol.*

Interventions
Preparation and administration
• Obtain a baseline assessment of the patient's blood pressure and apical pulse before beginning therapy.
• Betaxolol may be taken without regard to meals. (See *Taking beta-adrenergic blockers at home,* page 63.)

Monitoring and supportive care
• Monitor blood glucose levels closely; beta blockade may inhibit glycogenolysis and some signs and symptoms of hypoglycemia.

Safety tip. CNS symptoms of hypoglycemia are not masked by betaxolol, so assess the patient for dizziness, headache, restlessness, or mental status changes.
• Before surgery, advise the anesthesiologist that the patient is receiving a beta blocker.
• Know that withdrawal of beta blockers before surgery is controversial.
• Be aware that dosage adjustments in patients with renal failure are usually not necessary, but therapy should begin with 5 mg daily. Dosage may be increased at 2-week intervals in increments of 5 mg/day to a total of 20 mg/day.

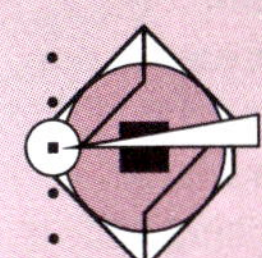

Life-threatening hazards of multidrug therapy with betaxolol

Interacting drug	Effects
Calcium channel blockers (such as verapamil)	Increase risk of profound hypotension, left ventricular failure, and AV conduction disturbances, especially if given I.V.
General anesthetics (such as halothane)	May increase antihypertensive effects

• To withdraw the drug, dosage should be reduced gradually over at least 2 weeks.

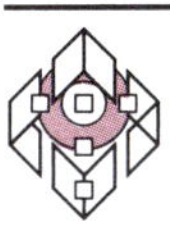

MedTest

1. The cardioselective beta$_1$-adrenergic blocking action of betaxolol is helpful in managing hypertension because it:
   a. decreases peripheral arterial resistance.
   b. slows heart rate and decreases cardiac output.
   c. directly dilates cardiac and peripheral arterioles.
   d. decreases aldosterone secretion, reducing sodium and water retention.

2. A life-threatening adverse reaction to betaxolol is:
   a. bronchospasm.
   b. cardiac arrest.
   c. seizures.
   d. CVA.

3. When discontinuing betaxolol, the patient should be told to:
   a. stop taking the drug.
   b. go to half doses for 1 week, and then stop the drug.
   c. go to half doses for 3 days, then quarter doses for 3 days, and then stop the drug.
   d. reduce dosage gradually, over at least 2 weeks.

Bretylium tosylate

Also known by the brand names Bretylate and Bretylol, bretylium tosylate is an adrenergic blocker that's classified therapeutically as a ventricular antiarrhythmic agent. It's available in vials containing 50 mg/ml and in premixed bags of D$_5$W containing 2 or 4 mg/ml. It can be administered by I.M. or I.V. injection.

Pharmacokinetics
• *Absorption:* After I.M. or I.V. administration, onset begins within 20 to

60 minutes, with peak effects in 6 to 9 hours.
- *Distribution:* Only about 1% to 10% is plasma protein–bound.
- *Metabolism:* No metabolites have been identified.
- *Excretion:* Excreted in the urine mostly as unchanged drug; elimination half-life ranges from 5 to 10 hours (longer in patients with renal impairment). Duration of effect ranges from 6 to 24 hours.

Indications, dosage, and action
Ventricular fibrillation
- *Adult dosage:* 5 mg/kg undiluted by rapid I.V. injection. If necessary, increase dose to 10 mg/kg undiluted and repeat q 15 to 30 minutes until 30 mg/kg have been given.

Unstable VT and other ventricular arrhythmias
- *Adult dosage:* Initially, 500 mg diluted in 50 ml of D₅W or 0.9% NaCl solution, infused I.V. over more than 8 minutes at 5 to 10 mg/kg. Dose may be repeated in 1 to 2 hours. Thereafter, infused q 6 to 8 hours diluted in 500 ml of D₅W or 0.9% NaCl solution at 1 to 2 mg/minute.

I.M. injection — 5 to 10 mg/kg undiluted. Repeat in 1 to 2 hours if needed. Thereafter, repeat q 6 to 8 hours.
- *Pediatric dosage:* 2 to 5 mg/kg I.M. as a single dose. Alternatively, give 5 mg/kg I.V. Follow with 10 mg/kg I.V. if fibrillation persists.
- *Action:* Bretylium prolongs the action potential duration and effective refractory period. It normalizes conduction between ischemic and non-

ischemic myocardium. Initially, bretylium causes an increase in norepinephrine release; subsequent depletion of norepinephrine stores causes a persistent adrenergic blockade, with decreased blood pressure and heart rate.

Contraindications and cautions
- Be aware that bretylium is contraindicated in patients with arrhythmias induced by digitalis glycosides because it may worsen these arrhythmias.
- Use with extreme caution in patients with fixed cardiac output and pulmonary hypertension because of the risk of severe and sudden drop in blood pressure.
- Don't give I.M. to treat life-threatening ventricular fibrillation because bretylium may not reach therapeutic levels for 6 to 9 hours.
- Pregnancy risk category C

Life-threatening adverse reactions
None noted

Common adverse reactions
- Severe orthostatic hypotension (50%)

Infrequent adverse reactions
- Bradycardia, anginal pain, transient arrhythmias, transient hypertension, mild orthostatic hypotension
- Vertigo, dizziness, light-headedness, syncope (usually secondary to hypotension)
- Severe nausea, vomiting

Interactions
• *All antihypertensives:* May potentiate hypotension. Monitor blood pressure.
• *Digitalis glycosides:* Bretylium may exacerbate VT associated with digitalis toxicity.
• *Other antiarrhythmics:* Additive or antagonistic antiarrhythmic effects. Monitor for additive toxicity.
• *Sympathomimetics:* Bretylium may potentiate the action of pressor amines (sympathomimetics) when used together during early catecholamine release.

Interventions
Preparation and administration
• When administering by direct I.V. injection, use a 20G to 22G needle and inject over about 1 minute into the vein or an I.V. line containing a free-flowing, compatible solution.
• When administering by continuous infusion, use diluted solution of 500 ml of D_5W or 0.9% NaCl solution and administer at a rate of 1 to 2 mg/minute.
• When infusing drug intermittently, infuse ordered dose over 10 to 30 minutes.
• For I.M. injection, don't exceed a 3-ml volume in any one site, and rotate sites to prevent tissue damage.

Monitoring and supportive care
• Monitor for hypotension. If supine systolic pressure falls to less than 75 mm Hg, report it to the doctor and be prepared to treat with vasopressors (such as dopamine or norepinephrine). Volume expanders and position changes also may be effective.

◈ **Safety tip.** Monitor heart rate and rhythm and blood pressure continuously throughout therapy for any significant changes.
• The initial release of norepinephrine caused by bretylium may induce transient hypertension and arrhythmias. Monitor the patient closely.
• Tell the patient to remain supine and to avoid sudden postural changes until tolerance to hypotension develops.
• Avoid initiating bretylium therapy concomitantly with digitalis glycoside therapy, if possible. Don't use in digitalized patients unless the arrhythmia is life-threatening, not caused by digitalis, and unresponsive to other drugs.
• Observe for increased anginal pain in susceptible patients.
• Because bretylium is excreted by the kidneys, patients with renal impairment require dosage modification.
• Be aware that this drug isn't a first-line agent in treating cardiac arrest, according to the American Heart Association's ACLS guidelines. With ventricular fibrillation, the drug should follow lidocaine; with VT, it should follow lidocaine or procainamide. Use with other CPR measures, such as countershock, epinephrine, and sodium bicarbonate. VT and other ventricular arrhythmias respond to the drug less rapidly than ventricular fibrillation does, requiring 20 minutes to 2 hours.
• Be aware that the drug is ineffective against atrial arrhythmias.

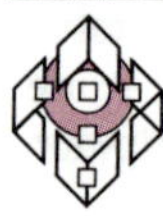

MedTest

1. Following I.V. administration of bretylium, suppression of VT and other ventricular arrhythmias usually occurs within:
  a. 2 to 5 minutes.
  b. 20 minutes to 2 hours.
  c. 3 to 5 hours.
  d. 6 to 9 hours.

2. When administering bretylium, monitor the patient's heart rate and rhythm and blood pressure:
  a. before giving the drug.
  b. q 2 to 5 minutes during administration.
  c. continuously throughout therapy.
  d. immediately following administration of the drug.

3. Bretylium should be avoided if the patient is already receiving:
  a. a digitalis glycoside.
  b. a beta blocker.
  c. a calcium channel blocker.
  d. other antiarrhythmic drugs.

Bumetanide

Also known by the brand name Bumex, bumetanide is a loop diuretic that's available in 0.5-, 1-, and 2-mg tablets, and in vials of 0.25 mg/ml for injection.

Pharmacokinetics

• *Absorption:* 85% to 95% of an oral dose is absorbed; food delays absorption. I.M. dose is completely absorbed. Diuresis usually begins 30 to 60 minutes after oral administration and 40 minutes after I.M. administration; peak diuresis occurs 1 to 2 hours after either. Diuresis begins a few minutes after I.V. administration and peaks in 15 to 30 minutes.
• *Distribution:* 92% to 96% protein-bound.
• *Metabolism:* By the liver to at least five inactive metabolites.
• *Excretion:* About 80% of bumetanide is excreted in urine; 10% to 20%, in feces. Elimination half-life ranges from 3.1 to 3.4 hours; duration of effect is 2 to 4 hours.

Indications, dosage, and action
Edema in CHF and in hepatic and renal disease
• *Adult dosage:* 0.5 to 2 mg P.O. once daily. If diuresis is inadequate, give a second or third dose at 4- to 5-hour intervals. For parenteral use, the initial dose is 0.5 to 1 mg I.V. or I.M. If response is still inadequate, give a second or third dose at 2- to 3-hour intervals. Maximum dosage is 10 mg/day.
• *Pediatric dosage:* 0.015 to 0.1 mg/kg I.M. or I.V., given daily. If given every other day, double the daily dosage. Use with extreme caution in neonates because drug contains 1% benzyl alcohol as a preservative.
• *Action:* Inhibits sodium and chloride reabsorption in the proximal part of the ascending loop of Henle, promoting the excretion of sodium, water, chloride, and potassium; produces renal and peripheral vasodilation and may temporarily increase the glomerular filtration rate and decrease peripheral vascular resistance.

Contraindications and cautions

• Avoid use in patients with anuria or electrolyte depletion and in hepatic coma; the drug may aggravate these underlying conditions.
• Don't give to patients with increasing BUN or creatinine levels or oliguria, despite its use as a diuretic in patients with renal impairment.
• Use with caution in patients with hepatic cirrhosis and ascites because electrolyte alterations may precipitate hepatic encephalopathy.
• Use cautiously in patients receiving digitalis glycosides because bumetanide-induced hypokalemia may predispose them to digitalis toxicity.
• Use with caution in patients allergic to sulfonamides.

Safety tip. Administer I.V. bumetanide slowly to decrease the risk of ototoxicity.
• Monitor elderly and debilitated patients closely; reduced dosages may be indicated.
• Don't give bumetanide to breast-feeding women.
• Pregnancy risk category C

Life-threatening adverse reactions

• Profound electrolyte and volume depletion, dehydration

Common adverse reactions

• Asymptomatic hyperuricemia (18.4%); hypochloremic alkalosis (14.9%); fluid and electrolyte imbalances, including hyponatremia and hypokalemia (14.7%); azotemia and increased serum creatinine levels; hyperglycemia and impaired glucose tolerance

Infrequent adverse reactions

• Volume depletion and dehydration, orthostatic hypotension, ECG changes
• Dizziness, headache, weakness
• Nausea, abdominal pain
• Transient deafness
• Transient thrombocytopenia and leukopenia
• Hypocalcemia and hypomagnesemia, changes in LD levels
• Urticaria, rash, pruritus
• Muscle pain (cramping) and tenderness

Interactions

• *Aminoglycoside antibiotics:* Potentiated ototoxicity. Use together cautiously.
• *Antihypertensive agents:* Increased risk of hypotension. Use with caution.
• *Indomethacin and other NSAIDs, probenecid:* Inhibited diuretic response. Use cautiously.
• *Lithium:* Bumetanide may reduce renal clearance of lithium and increase lithium levels; lithium dosage may require adjustment.
• *Ototoxic or nephrotoxic drugs:* Concomitant administration may result in enhanced toxicity.
• *Potassium-depleting drugs, such as amphotericin B and corticosteroids:* May cause severe potassium loss. Monitor patient's potassium levels.

Interventions
Preparation and administration
• Give I.V. bumetanide slowly, over 1 or 2 minutes. For intermittent infusion, give diluted drug through an intermittent infusion device or piggy-

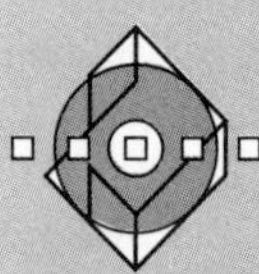

Patient-teaching checklist

Taking loop diuretics at home

In addition to explaining the drug's action and dosage, teach the patient who will continue diuretic therapy after discharge to follow these important guidelines.

General guidelines
☐ Take the diuretic as prescribed even when you're feeling better.
☐ Weigh yourself daily to monitor fluid volume. Also inspect your hands and ankles for swelling (evidence of fluid retention).

Know when to call your doctor
☐ Report any weight gain of 2 lb (1 kg) or more per day and ankle or hand swelling.
☐ Be aware of and report any indications of low potassium levels, such as fatigue, anorexia, and muscle weakness and cramping.
☐ Notify your doctor if you experience severe or continuing nausea, vomiting, or diarrhea to prevent the loss of too much water and potassium.

Watch your diet
☐ Eat foods high in potassium, if ordered, because loop diuretics cause potassium to be lost in the urine.

Also follow a low-sodium diet to minimize fluid retention.

Minimize adverse reactions
☐ Remember to change positions slowly (especially from lying down to sitting upright) and dangle your legs over the bedside for a few minutes before standing. These actions will minimize the dizziness caused by the drug. If dizziness or faintness occurs, lie down immediately.
☐ Avoid driving or operating machinery if you experience dizziness. Also limit alcohol intake and strenuous exercise in warm weather because you are more likely to feel dizzy.
☐ Monitor your blood glucose levels closely if you are a diabetic because this drug can increase your blood glucose level.
☐ Be alert for signs and symptoms of digoxin toxicity if you're taking this drug with digoxin. Store these drugs separately to avoid the risk of dosage error.

---

back it into an I.V. line containing a free-flowing compatible solution (such as D_5W, 0.9% NaCl solution, or lactated Ringer's solution). Infuse at the prescribed rate within 24 hours. Continuous infusion isn't needed.

• Give in the morning to prevent nocturia. If a second dose is necessary, give it in the early afternoon. Tell the patient to take the drug with food or milk if he experiences nausea. (See *Taking loop diuretics at home.*)

Monitoring and supportive care
• Monitor serum electrolyte, BUN, CO_2, and serum creatinine levels frequently. Also watch for signs of dehydration or hypotension. The drug should be discontinued if dehydration or hypotension occurs, or if BUN and serum creatinine levels rise.
• Monitor for clinical manifestations of overdose, including ototoxicity or profound electrolyte and volume depletion, which may cause circulatory collapse.
• Monitor serum potassium levels and watch for signs of hypokalemia (for example, muscle weakness and cramps). Supplemental potassium or potassium-sparing diuretics may be used to prevent hypokalemia and metabolic alkalosis in these patients.
• Consult with the doctor and the dietitian to provide a high-potassium diet, if indicated. Foods rich in potassium include citrus fruits, tomatoes, bananas, dates, and apricots.
• Monitor blood glucose levels in patients with diabetes. Severe hyperglycemia may be treated with oral antidiabetic agents.
• Monitor blood uric acid levels, especially in patients with a history of gout.
• Know that bumetanide therapy alters electrolyte balance and liver and renal function tests.

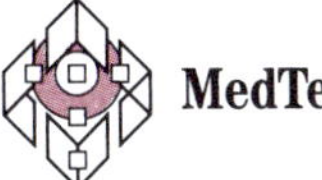 **MedTest**

1. Bumetanide should be used with caution in patients allergic to:
   a. penicillins.
   b. aminoglycosides.
   c. cephalosporins.
   d. sulfonamides.

2. The doctor has indicated a change in dosage from once a day to b.i.d. The patient's second dose should be given:
   a. in the early afternoon.
   b. with his evening meal.
   c. h.s.
   d. at midnight.

3. Assess (and include in your patient teaching) symptoms of hypokalemia, such as:
   a. muscle weakness and cramps.
   b. transient deafness.
   c. dry mucous membranes.
   d. nausea and diarrhea.

Captopril

Also known by the brand name Captoten, captopril is an ACE inhibitor that's classified therapeutically as an antihypertensive and used in the adjunctive treatment of CHF. It's available in 12.5-, 25- (37.5-mg in Canada), 50-, and 100-mg tablets.

Pharmacokinetics
• *Absorption:* Food may reduce absorption by up to 40%. Antihypertensive effect begins in 15 minutes; peak blood levels occur in 1 hour. Maximum therapeutic effect may require several weeks.
• *Distribution:* 25% to 30% protein-bound.
• *Metabolism:* 50% is metabolized in the liver.

• *Excretion:* Captopril and its metabolites are excreted primarily in urine. Duration of effect is usually 2 to 6 hours, increasing with higher doses. Elimination half-life is less than 3 hours.

Indications, dosage, and action
Mild to severe hypertension
• *Adult dosage:* Initially, 25 mg P.O. b.i.d. or t.i.d.; dosage may be increased to 50 mg t.i.d. after 1 to 2 weeks if blood pressure isn't satisfactorily controlled. Maximum dosage is 150 mg t.i.d. (450 mg/day).
• *Antihypertensive action:* Captopril competitively inhibits ACE activity, resulting in a decreased rate of conversion of angiotensin I to angiotensin II, which is a potent vasoconstrictor. Reduced formation of angiotensin II decreases afterload and aldosterone secretion. This, in turn, reduces sodium and water retention and lowers blood pressure.

CHF
• *Adult dosage:* Initially, 25 mg P.O. t.i.d.; may be increased to 50 mg t.i.d. to a maximum of 450 mg/day. In patients taking diuretics, initial dosage is 6.25 to 12.5 mg t.i.d.
• *Cardiac load reduction:* Captopril decreases afterload, resulting in increased cardiac output; PAWP and pulmonary vascular resistance also decrease, resulting in improved cardiac output and exercise tolerance in patients with CHF.

Contraindications and cautions
• Use cautiously in elderly patients or patients with impaired renal function.
• Use cautiously in patients with autoimmune diseases and in patients taking drugs that suppress immune function. Such patients are at increased risk for developing neutropenia, especially if they have impaired renal function.
• Know that elderly patients may need lower doses because of impaired drug clearance. They also may be more sensitive to captopril's antihypertensive effects.
• Use this drug with caution in breast-feeding women. Captopril is distributed into breast milk.
• Be aware that captopril is contraindicated during pregnancy because ACE inhibitors can cause fetal and neonatal injury or death. These problems haven't been detected when fetal exposure has been limited to the first trimester. When pregnancy is detected, ACE inhibitors should be discontinued as soon as possible.
• Pregnancy risk category C (in first trimester), D (in second and third trimesters)

Life-threatening adverse reactions
• Neutropenia, agranulocytosis
• Angioedema of tongue, glottis, or larynx, resulting in airway obstruction

Common adverse reactions
None noted

Infrequent adverse reactions
• Tachycardia, hypotension, angina pectoris, CHF, pericarditis, MI, Raynaud's phenomenon
• Persistent cough
• Dizziness, fainting

• Anorexia, transient elevation of liver enzyme levels
• Proteinuria, nephrotic syndrome, membranous glomerulopathy, renal failure (in patients with preexisting renal disease or those receiving high doses), urinary frequency, impotence
• Loss of taste
• Leukopenia, neutropenia, agranulocytosis, pancytopenia, positive antinuclear antibody titers, eosinophilia
• Hyperkalemia
• Rash, pruritus, flushing or pallor, photosensitivity
• Fever, angioedema of the face and extremities

Interactions

• *Antacids:* Decreased absorption. Separate administration times.
• *Antihypertensive agents, diuretics:* Risk of hypotension. Monitor blood pressure closely.
• *Digitalis glycosides:* May increase serum digoxin concentration by 15% to 30%.
• *Insulin, oral antidiabetic agents:* Risk of hypoglycemia when therapy is initiated. Monitor blood glucose levels closely.
• *NSAIDs:* May reduce antihypertensive effect. Monitor blood pressure closely.
• *Potassium-sparing diuretics, potassium supplements:* Increased risk of hyperkalemia. Monitor serum potassium levels closely.

Interventions
Preparation and administration
• Give captopril 1 hour before meals; food reduces absorption. (See *Taking ACE inhibitors at home,* page 87.)

Monitoring and supportive care
• Monitor the patient's blood pressure and pulse rate frequently.
• Usually, diuretic therapy is discontinued 2 to 3 days before beginning ACE inhibitor therapy to reduce the risk of hypotension; if the drug doesn't adequately control blood pressure, diuretics may be reinstated. Thiazide diuretics, in particular, may enhance captopril's effects.
• Monitor serum potassium levels because of the potential for potassium retention, particularly with concurrent use of potassium-sparing diuretics.
• Assess for and tell the patient to report feelings of light-headedness, dizziness, or faintness, especially in the first few days, so that the dosage can be adjusted.

Safety tip. If the patient experiences dizziness, institute appropriate safety measures, such as installing side rails on the bed and restricting the patient's activity.
• Be aware that captopril may cause false-positive results for urinary acetone; it also may cause hyperkalemia and transiently elevated liver enzyme levels.

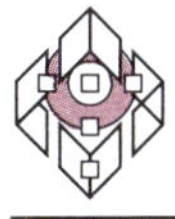 **MedTest**

1. Patients taking captopril should have which serum electrolyte monitored, and why?
   a. Potassium, because captopril can cause hyperkalemia
   b. Sodium, because the drug can cause hyponatremia

c. Chlorides, because this drug can cause hyperchloremia
d. Potassium, because captopril can cause hypokalemia

2. Captopril's antihypertensive action occurs in part because the drug:
   a. inhibits antidiuretic hormone production.
   b. increases aldosterone secretion.
   c. decreases plasma renin activity.
   d. reduces sodium and water retention.

3. A possible life-threatening adverse effect of captopril is:
   a. agranulocytosis.
   b. hepatic toxicity.
   c. renal toxicity.
   d. neurologic hyperactivity.

Cholestyramine

Also known by the brand names Cholybar, Questran, and Questran-Light, cholestyramine is an anion exchange resin that's classified therapeutically as an antilipemic and bile acid sequestrant agent. It's available in a 4-g bar, a 378-g can of powder, 9-g single-dose packets (Questran), and 5-g single-dose packets (Questran-Light). Each scoop of powder or single-dose packet contains 4 g of cholestyramine resin.

Pharmacokinetics
• *Absorption:* Cholestyramine isn't absorbed. Cholesterol levels may begin to decrease 24 to 48 hours after the start of therapy and continue to drop for up to 12 months.
• *Distribution:* None.

• *Metabolism:* None.
• *Excretion:* Insoluble cholestyramine with bile acid complex is entirely excreted in feces.

Indications, dosage, and action
Primary hyperlipidemia and hypercholesterolemia and elevated serum cholesterol levels
• *Adult dosage:* 4 g before meals and h.s., not to exceed 32 g daily. Can be given in two divided doses.
• *Pediatric dosage:* Ages 6 to 12, 80 mg/kg or 2.35 g/m^2 t.i.d. Safe dosage hasn't been established for children under age 6.
• *Action:* Bile is normally excreted into the intestine to facilitate absorption of fat and other lipid materials. Cholestyramine binds with bile acid, forming an insoluble compound. With less bile available in the digestive system, more cholesterol is used by the liver to replace its supply of bile acids, and serum cholesterol levels decrease.

Contraindications and cautions
• Avoid use in patients with complete biliary obstruction and in patients hypersensitive to any of the drug's components.
• Don't give cholestyramine powder to patients with tartrazine allergies; the powder form contains tartrazine (FD&C Yellow No. 5).
• Because Questran-Light contains aspartame, avoid use in patients with phenylketonuria or hypersensitivity to aspartame.
• Use cautiously in patients with malabsorption syndrome, whose condition may deteriorate from further de-

creased absorption of fats, folic acid, and vitamins A, D, E, K.
• Use cautiously in patients predisposed to constipation and conditions aggravated by constipation, such as severe, symptomatic CAD. The resin increases the risk of fecal impaction.
• Be aware that patients over age 60 are more likely to experience adverse GI and nutritional reactions.
• Use with caution in pregnant women because impaired maternal absorption of vitamins and other nutrients is a potential threat to the fetus.
• Use with caution in breast-feeding women.
• Know that children may be at greater risk of hyperchloremic acidosis during cholestyramine therapy.
• Pregnancy risk category C

Life-threatening adverse reactions
None noted

Common adverse reactions
• Constipation (related to dose and age; more common in patients over age 60)

Infrequent adverse reactions
• Fecal impaction, aggravation of hemorrhoids, abdominal discomfort, flatulence, nausea, vomiting, steatorrhea
• Deficiencies of vitamins A, D, E, and K from decreased absorption; hyperchloremic acidosis with long-term use or very high doses
• Rash; irritation of skin, tongue, and perianal area

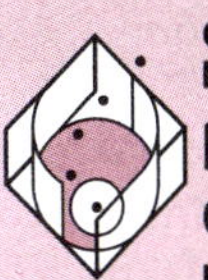

Making cholestyramine more palatable

To increase compliance in the patient who is having difficulty taking cholestyramine because of its consistency or taste, tell him to mix the entire next-day's dose in 90 to 180 ml (3 to 6 oz) of milk, fruit juice, or another beverage and then refrigerate it until needed. As an alternative, suggest to the patient that he try administering the drug in a beverage that masks its taste, such as coffee or tea.

Interactions
• *Acetaminophen, beta-adrenergic blockers, corticosteroids, coumarin anticoagulants, digitalis glycosides, fat-soluble vitamins (A, D, E, and K), iron preparations, thiazide diuretics, thyroid hormone:* Cholestyramine may substantially decrease absorption. Separate administration times by at least 2 hours.
• *Warfarin:* The binding potential of cholestyramine may decrease the anticoagulant effects of warfarin; however, concurrent depletion of vitamin K may either negate this effect or increase anticoagulant activity. Carefully monitor PT.

Interventions
Preparation and administration
• To mix, sprinkle powder in a beverage or on a wet food, let it stand a few minutes, and then stir it to obtain a uniform suspension. (See *Making cholestyramine more palatable,*

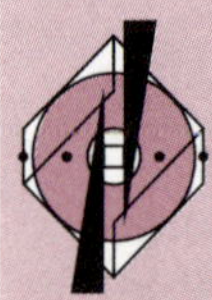

Administration guidelines
Giving cholestyramine in powder form

Several forms of cholestyramine may be administered as a powder. Ask the patient which beverage or wet food he'd prefer, and then mix the powder by following these steps.

- Sprinkle the powder on the surface of the preferred beverage (90 to 180 ml) or wet food, such as applesauce or crushed pineapples.
- Let the powder stand a few minutes, and then stir it to obtain a uniform suspension.
- Be cautious in mixing the powder with carbonated beverages; this may result in excessive foaming. To minimize this foaming, use a large glass and mix slowly. Advise the patient not to drink the dose too quickly to avoid swallowing air.

and *Giving cholestyramine in powder form.*)

Safety tip. Give other drugs at least 1 hour before or at least 4 hours after cholestyramine because cholestyramine blocks their absorption.

Monitoring and supportive care
- Monitor serum cholesterol and triglyceride levels frequently during the first few months of therapy and periodically thereafter. In some patients, the initial decrease is followed by a return to baseline cholesterol levels or elevated levels.
- Monitor bowel function. Treat constipation promptly by encouraging a diet high in fiber and fluids or by adding a stool softener.
- Cholestyramine should be discontinued if constipation continues even after a reduction in dosage, if a paradoxical increase in serum cholesterol level occurs, or if clinical response is inadequate after 3 months of therapy.
- Encourage the patient to adopt a healthier lifestyle that includes exercise and dietary modifications. (See *Taking cholestyramine at home.*)
- Be aware that cholestyramine therapy alters serum concentrations of ALP, AST, chloride, phosphorus, potassium, calcium, and sodium. Impaired calcium absorption may lead to osteoporosis.

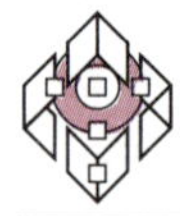

MedTest

1. Administer cholestyramine powder in a fluid volume of at least:
    a. 30 ml.
    b. 90 ml.
    c. 120 ml.
    d. 240 ml.

2. The adverse reaction that the patient is most likely to experience and that would require assessment and intervention is:
    a. diarrhea.

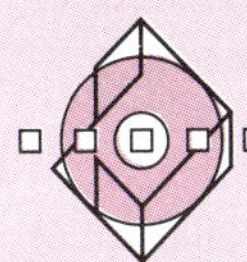

Patient-teaching checklist

Taking cholestyramine at home

In addition to explaining the drug's action and dosage, teach the patient who will continue cholestyramine therapy after discharge to follow these important guidelines.

Take your medication correctly
☐ Take this drug before meals and at bedtime.
☐ Never take the powder form dry because it may cause you to choke. Instead, mix it in a beverage or wet food.
☐ Chew each bite of the chewable bar form well before swallowing.
☐ Take cholestyramine as prescribed even when you're feeling better.
☐ Continue taking the drug even if unpleasant adverse reactions occur; when you stop taking it, your serum cholesterol level may increase again.

Know when to call your doctor
☐ Make sure you discuss any adverse effects with your doctor.
☐ Notify your doctor if severe constipation occurs.

Other instructions
☐ Adopt a healthier lifestyle to correct any cardiac risk factors, such as obesity (lose weight), a diet high in saturated fats and cholesterol (reduce or eliminate these foods), smoking (engage in a stop-smoking program), and a sedentary lifestyle (exercise regularly). These risk factors not only predispose you to cardiac disorders but may also reduce the drug's effectiveness.
☐ Take preventive measures to minimize constipation, such as drinking plenty of fluids, increasing the amount of fiber in your diet, and exercising.
☐ Take other medications in your prescribed regimen at least 1 hour before or 4 to 6 hours after cholestyramine (longer if possible).
☐ Comply with scheduled tests to measure serum cholesterol and triglyceride levels.

b. vomiting.
c. steatorrhea.
d. constipation.

3. Cholestyramine therapy puts the patient at risk for deficiencies of vitamins:
  a. A, D, E, and K.
  b. B_1, B_2, B_6, and B_{12}.
  c. B complex and C.
  d. A, C, and K.

Clofibrate

Also known by the brand name Atromid-S, clofibrate is a fibric acid derivative that's classified therapeutically as an antilipemic agent. It's available in 500-mg capsules.

Pharmacokinetics
• *Absorption:* Slow; peak plasma concentration occurs 2 to 6 hours after a single dose.
• *Distribution:* The active metabolite, clofibric acid, is highly protein-bound.
• *Metabolism:* Clofibrate is hydrolyzed by serum enzymes to clofibric acid, which is metabolized by the liver into active metabolites.
• *Excretion:* About 20% of clofibric acid is excreted unchanged in urine; 70% is eliminated in urine as conjugated metabolites. Elimination half-life ranges from 6 to 25 hours and is prolonged in patients with renal impairment or cirrhosis. Serum triglyceride levels decrease in 2 to 5 days, with peak clinical effect in 21 days.

Indications, dosage, and action
Hyperlipoproteinemia
• *Adult dosage:* 2 g P.O. daily in two to four divided doses. Some patients may respond to lower doses as assessed by serum lipid monitoring.
• *Action:* May lower serum triglyceride levels by accelerating the catabolism of VLDLs; lowers serum cholesterol levels by inhibiting cholesterol biosynthesis.

Contraindications and cautions
• Be aware that clofibrate is contraindicated in patients with renal or hepatic dysfunction because it increases the incidence of adverse reactions.
• Know that this drug is also contraindicated in patients with primary biliary cirrhosis because it may paradoxically raise their cholesterol levels.
• Use cautiously in patients with a history of peptic ulcer disease.
• Know that clofibrate shouldn't be used in pregnant or lactating patients because fetal and infant drug concentrations may exceed maternal ones. Recommend an alternative feeding method during therapy.
• Pregnancy risk category C

Life-threatening adverse reactions
• Cardiac arrhythmias
• Thrombotic-embolic phenomena
• Hepatic cancer
• Rhabdomyolysis (with preexisting renal insufficiency)
• Toxic epidermal necrolysis

Common adverse reactions
• Nausea

Infrequent adverse reactions
• Increased risk of angina, arrhythmias, intermittent claudication
• Drowsiness, headache, fatigue, weakness
• Transient and reversible elevations of liver function test results, diarrhea, vomiting, dyspepsia, stomatitis, flatulence, gastritis, hepatomegaly, twofold increase in risk of gallstones during long-term therapy
• Decreased libido, sexual dysfunction, renal dysfunction (hematuria, proteinuria, dysuria, and anuria)
• Leukopenia, agranulocytosis, eosinophilia
• Rash, urticaria, pruritus, dry skin, alopecia, dry, brittle hair
• Flulike syndrome with weakness and muscle aches, weight gain, and polyphagia

Interactions

- *Cholestyramine:* Concomitant administration decreases clofibrate's absorption rate.
- *Furosemide, oral anticoagulants, sulfonylureas:* May increase the action of these drugs by displacing them from plasma protein–binding sites. Monitor for toxicity.
- *Lovastatin, pravastatin, simvastatin:* Risk of myositis, rhabdomyolysis, and renal failure. Avoid concomitant use.
- *Oral contraceptives, rifampin:* May antagonize clofibrate's lipid-lowering effect. Monitor serum lipids.
- *Probenecid:* Increased clofibrate effect. Monitor for toxicity.

Interventions

Preparation and administration

- Administer with food to minimize GI discomfort. (See *Taking clofibrate at home*, page 108.)

Monitoring and supportive care

- Monitor serum cholesterol and triglyceride levels regularly during therapy to gauge drug's therapeutic effectiveness.
- Also monitor serum levels of amylase, CK, ALT, and AST because clofibrate therapy may increase them. Drug may decrease plasma beta-lipoprotein and plasma fibrinogen concentrations.
- The drug should be discontinued if liver function tests show significant abnormalities, if serum amylase level increases, if a paradoxical increase in cholesterol or LDL levels occurs, or if no therapeutic response occurs after 3 months of therapy.

- Monitor renal function, blood counts, and serum electrolyte and blood glucose levels.
- Observe the patient for serious adverse reactions, such as thrombophlebitis, pulmonary embolism, angina, and arrhythmias, and notify the doctor immediately if you detect any.
- Know that clofibrate shouldn't be used indiscriminately. Studies suggest that clofibrate may increase the risk of gallstones, cancer, postcholecystectomy complications, and pancreatitis.
- Know that this drug may also be used to treat patients with type IV or V hyperlipidemia. Such patients typically have serum triglyceride levels over 2,000 mg/dl.

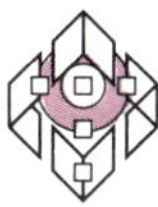 **MedTest**

1. Clofibrate is contraindicated in patients with hepatic or renal dysfunction because of potential:
   a. drug accumulation, increasing the incidence of adverse reactions.
   b. accelerated metabolism or excretion, interfering with the drug's action.
   c. drug accumulation, increasing the desired action and requiring a lower dose.
   d. delayed metabolism or excretion, increasing drug interactions.

2. Administer clofibrate:
   a. without regard to meals.
   b. 30 minutes to 1 hour before meals to enhance absorption.

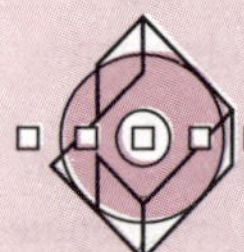

Patient-teaching checklist

Taking clofibrate at home

In addition to explaining the drug's action and dosage, teach the patient who will continue clofibrate therapy after discharge to follow these important guidelines.

Take your medication correctly
☐ Take clofibrate with food or immediately after meals to reduce the risk of an upset stomach.
☐ Take clofibrate as prescribed, even when you're feeling better, but don't exceed the prescribed dosage.
☐ Continue taking the drug even if unpleasant adverse reactions occur; when you stop taking it, your blood lipid levels may increase again. But make sure you discuss any adverse reactions with your doctor.

Know when to call your doctor
☐ Remember to report the following symptoms to your doctor immedi-ately: flulike symptoms, chest pain, irregular heartbeat, shortness of breath, and severe stomach pain with nausea or vomiting.

Modify your lifestyle
☐ Take steps to correct any cardiac risk factors, such as obesity (lose weight and adhere to a low-fat, low-cholesterol diet), smoking (engage in a stop-smoking program), and a sedentary lifestyle (begin an exercise program). These factors may reduce the drug's effectiveness.

---

c. with meals to minimize GI discomfort.
d. 1 to 2 hours after meals to avoid interfering with nutrient absorption.

3. Which of the following should be monitored frequently during clofibrate therapy?
a. Serum CK and transaminase levels
b. Serum amylase, cholesterol, and triglyceride levels
c. Serum amylase and lipase levels
d. Plasma beta-lipoprotein and fibrinogen levels

Clonidine hydrochloride

Known by the brand names Catapres, Catapres-TTS, and Dixarit (in Canada), clonidine is a centrally acting antiadrenergic agent that's classified therapeutically as an antihypertensive agent. It's available in 0.1-, 0.2-, and 0.3-mg tablets. The Catapres-TTS patch is available in three forms: TTS-1, which releases 0.1 mg/24 hours; TTS-2, which releases 0.2 mg/24 hours; and TTS-3, which releases 0.3 mg/24 hours.

Pharmacokinetics
• *Absorption:* Well absorbed from the GI tract. Blood pressure begins to decline in 30 to 60 minutes, with peak effect occurring in 2 to 4 hours. Clonidine is also well absorbed after transdermal administration; therapeutic plasma levels are achieved 2 to 3 days after initial application. (See *Using a clonidine patch,* page 110.)
• *Distribution:* Widespread throughout the body.
• *Metabolism:* In the liver, where nearly 50% is transformed into inactive metabolites.
• *Excretion:* Approximately 65% is excreted in urine; 20% in feces. The elimination half-life ranges from 6 to 20 hours in patients with normal renal function. After oral administration, effects persist 8 hours; after transdermal use, effects last 7 days.

Indications, dosage, and action
Essential, renal, and malignant hypertension
• *Adult dosage:* Initially, 0.1 mg P.O. b.i.d.; then increase by 0.1 to 0.2 mg daily or every few days until desired response is achieved. Usual dosage range is 0.2 to 1.2 mg daily in divided doses. Maximum effective dosage is 2.4 mg/day. If transdermal patch is used, apply one patch to area of intact skin q 7 days, remembering to remove old patch.
• *Action:* Decreases sympathetic outflow from the CNS by an action on central alpha-adrenergic receptors. Initially, may stimulate peripheral alpha-adrenergic receptors, producing transient vasoconstriction.

Contraindications and cautions
• Be aware that the transdermal form of clonidine is contraindicated in patients with hypersensitivity to any component of the patch's adhesive layer.
• Know that clonidine is also contraindicated in breast-feeding women because it is excreted in breast milk.
• Use cautiously in elderly patients and in patients with severe coronary insufficiency, diabetes mellitus, MI, CV disease, chronic renal failure, a history of depression, or those taking other antihypertensives.
• Pregnancy risk category C

Life-threatening adverse reactions
• Severe rebound hypertension

Common adverse reactions
• Drowsiness (33%), dizziness (16%), sedation, weakness
• Constipation, nausea and vomiting, dry mouth (40%)
• Contact dermatitis from transdermal patch (25% to 50%)

Infrequent adverse reactions
• Orthostatic hypotension, palpitations and tachycardia, bradycardia
• Nervousness and agitation, headache, depression, insomnia, bizarre dreams, fatigue
• Anorexia and malaise; mild, transient abnormalities in liver function tests
• Decreased sexual activity, impotence, loss of libido, nocturia, difficulty urinating, urine retention, gynecomastia

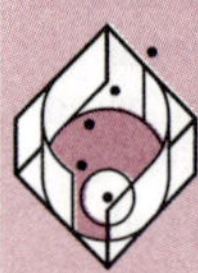

Compliance builder

Using a clonidine patch

To increase compliance in the patient who resists taking oral clonidine or has difficulty remembering to take it, ask the doctor about switching to the clonidine patch. This patch requires only a weekly application and usually adheres despite showering and other routine daily activities.

Tell the patient that an adhesive overlay is available to provide additional skin adherence, if necessary.

• Transient glucose intolerance (after large doses)
• Rash, pruritus, urticaria, angioedema, alopecia, myalgia, arthralgia

Interactions
• *Alcohol and other CNS depressants:* Enhanced CNS depression. Use together cautiously.
• *MAO inhibitors, tolazoline, and tricyclic antidepressants:* May decrease antihypertensive effect. Use together cautiously.
• *Propranolol and other beta blockers:* Paradoxical hypertensive response.

Interventions
Preparation and administration
• Always give the last dose h.s. to minimize the effects of orthostatic hypotension. (See *Taking clonidine at home.*)

Monitoring and supportive care
• Monitor pulse rate and blood pressure frequently.
• Monitor the patient's weight daily at the initiation of therapy to assess for fluid retention.
• Be aware that the transdermal patch provides antihypertensive activity for up to 7 days. Since therapeutic plasma levels are not achieved until 2 to 3 days after initial application, the patient may need oral antihypertensive therapy during this interim period.
• Give 4 to 6 hours before scheduled surgery. Discontinuing clonidine for surgery isn't recommended.
• Don't discontinue abruptly; this may cause severe rebound hypertension. Dosage should be reduced gradually over 2 to 4 days.
• In patients receiving both clonidine and a beta blocker, the beta blocker should be withdrawn gradually before the clonidine to minimize adverse reactions.
• Tirate dosages in patients with renal impairment. They may respond to smaller dosages of clonidine.
• Be aware that clonidine may be used to lower blood pressure quickly in some hypertensive emergencies.
• Know that clonidine has been used investigationally to prevent migraines, treat severe dysmenorrhea and menopausal flushing, and to rapidly detoxify patients who are withdrawing from opiates.
• Be aware that clonidine has also been used investigationally in smoking cessation therapy; it may suppress the craving for nicotine.
• Clonidine may decrease urinary excretion of vanillylmandelic acid and

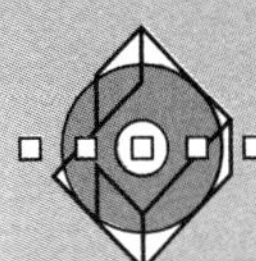

Patient-teaching checklist

Taking clonidine at home

In addition to explaining the drug's action and dosage, teach the patient who will continue clonidine therapy after discharge to follow these important guidelines.

Take your medication correctly

☐ Take your last oral dose immediately before bedtime.

☐ Apply the transdermal patch to a clean, dry, hairless area of intact skin on your upper arm or torso once every 7 days. The area should be free of scars or irritation.

☐ Remember to place the transdermal patch at a different site each week to avoid skin irritation and possible overdose. Also remember to remove the old patch before applying a new one.

☐ After removing a used patch, fold the patch in half with the sticky sides together. Make sure to dispose of it out of the reach of children.

☐ Take clonidine as prescribed even when you're feeling better. The transdermal patch may take 2 to 3 days to produce optimal effects, so you may need to take tablets as prescribed in the interim.

☐ Never trim or cut the transdermal patch to adjust the dosage. Check with your doctor if you think the medicine isn't working as it should.

☐ Continue taking the drug even if unpleasant adverse reactions occur, because abrupt discontinuation can cause severe hypertension. But make sure you discuss any adverse reactions with your doctor.

Minimize adverse reactions

☐ Be aware that this drug can cause drowsiness, but tolerance will develop. Avoid driving and other potentially hazardous activities while drowsiness persists.

☐ Dizziness or even fainting may occur if you drink alcohol, stand for long periods of time, exercise excessively, or are exposed to hot weather. Take precautions to avoid or limit these factors.

☐ Remember to change positions slowly (especially from lying flat to sitting upright) and to dangle your legs over the bedside for a few minutes before standing. These actions will minimize dizziness. Lie down immediately if dizziness or faintness occurs.

Other instructions

☐ Increase the fiber content of your diet, exercise regularly, and maintain adequate fluid intake to combat the constipating effects of this drug.

☐ Use sugarless gum or candy, take small sips of water, or suck on ice chips to relieve a dry mouth.

☐ Report any weight gain of more than 5 lb (2.3 kg) per week to your doctor.

catecholamines; it may slightly increase blood or serum glucose levels and may cause a weakly positive Coombs' test.

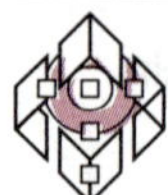 **MedTest**

1. When clonidine is prescribed in a transdermal patch, it should be applied:
   a. b.i.d.
   b. daily.
   c. weekly.
   d. monthly.

2. Patients taking clonidine should report any weight gain in excess of:
   a. 1 lb (0.5 kg) per week.
   b. 2 lb (1 kg) per week.
   c. 5 lb (2.3 kg) per week.
   d. 10 lb (5 kg) per week.

3. If your patient is taking oral clonidine b.i.d., the last dose should be taken:
   a. in the early afternoon.
   b. with his evening meal.
   c. 12 hours after the first dose.
   d. h.s.

Colestipol hydrochloride

Also known by the brand name Colestid, colestipol is an anion exchange resin that's classified therapeutically as an antilipemic agent. It's available as granules in 5-g packets and in 500-mg bottles.

Pharmacokinetics
- *Absorption:* Not absorbed. Cholesterol levels may decrease in 24 to 48 hours, with the peak effect occurring at 1 month.
- *Distribution:* None.
- *Metabolism:* None.
- *Excretion:* In feces.

Indications, dosage, and action
Primary hypercholesterolemia
- *Adult dosage:* 5 to 30 g P.O. daily in two to four divided doses.
- *Pediatric dosage:* 10 to 20 g or 500 mg/kg daily in two to four divided doses.
- *Action:* Bile acid is normally excreted into the intestine to facilitate the absorption of fats and other lipids. Colestipol binds with bile acid, forming an insoluble compound that is excreted in feces. The liver must then synthesize new bile acid from cholesterol, resulting in reduced LDL levels.

Contraindications and cautions
- Be aware that colestipol is contraindicated in patients with biliary obstruction or atresia because the drug is ineffective in these patients.
- Know that it is also contraindicated in patients with primary biliary cirrhosis because the cholesterol levels of these patients may be further increased.
- Use colestipol cautiously in patients with constipation because of the risk of fecal impaction.
- Use with caution in patients with malabsorption syndrome, whose condition may deteriorate from further decreased absorption of fats and fat-soluble vitamins A, D, E, and K.

• Use with caution in pregnant women because impaired maternal absorption of vitamins and other nutrients is a potential threat to the fetus.
• Use cautiously in elderly patients, who are more likely to experience adverse GI and nutritional reactions.
• Be aware that safety in children hasn't been established, but the drug has been used in a limited number of children with hypercholesterolemia.
• Be aware that safety in breast-feeding women hasn't been established. Another feeding method should be recommended during colestipol therapy.
• Pregnancy risk category C

Life-threatening adverse reactions
None noted

Common adverse reactions
• Constipation (may be dose related)

Infrequent adverse reactions
• Shortness of breath
• Headache, dizziness, fatigue, weakness
• Abdominal discomfort, flatulence, nausea, vomiting, diarrhea, steatorrhea, fecal impaction, aggravation of hemorrhoids, anorexia
• Deficiency of vitamin A, D, E, and K from decreased absorption; hyperchloremic acidosis with long-term use or very high doses
• Rashes; sore skin, tongue, and perianal skin

Interactions
• *Orally administered drugs, especially chenodiol, digitalis glycosides, penicillin G, tetracycline, and thiazide diuretics:* Colestipol impairs ab-

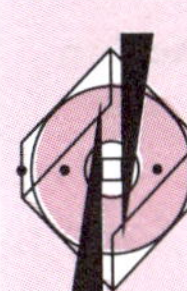

Administration guidelines
Giving colestipol in granule form

Follow these steps to administer colestipol granules:
• Sprinkle granules on the surface of the patient's preferred beverage (at least 90 ml) or wet food, such as applesauce, pulpy fruit, thin soup, or hot cereal.
• Let stand a few minutes; then stir it to obtain a uniform suspension.
• Mixing colestipol with carbonated beverages may result in excessive foaming. To minimize foaming, use a large glass and stir slowly.
• To make sure that the entire dose is ingested, rinse the container and have the patient drink this fluid.

sorption, thus decreasing their therapeutic effect. Give these drugs at least 1 hour before or 4 to 6 hours after colestipol; dosage adjustments of these drugs may be necessary when colestipol is withdrawn, to prevent high-dose toxicity.

Interventions
Preparation and administration
• To mix, sprinkle granules on the patient's preferred beverage or wet food, and let it stand for a few minutes. If a liquid is used, have the patient drink the dose; then add water to the container, swirl it, and have him drink that as well. This will ensure that he ingests the entire dose. (See *Giving colestipol in granule form,* above, and *Taking colestipol at home,* page 114.)

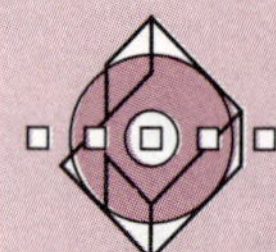

Taking colestipol at home

In addition to explaining the drug's action and dosage, teach the patient who will continue colestipol therapy after discharge to follow these important guidelines.

Take your medication correctly
☐ Never take granules dry because they may make you choke. Instead, mix them in the beverage or wet food of your choice.
☐ Add a small amount of liquid to the glass after ingesting the mixed amount, swirl it, and then drink this residue to ensure ingestion of the entire dose.
☐ Drink the dose slowly to prevent swallowing air.
☐ Take colestipol as prescribed even when you're feeling better.
☐ Take other drugs at least 1 hour before or 4 to 6 hours after taking colestipol to avoid blocking their absorption.

Know when to call your doctor
☐ Continue taking the drug even if unpleasant adverse reactions occur; if you stop taking it, your blood cholesterol level may increase again. Be sure to discuss any adverse reactions with your doctor.

Other instructions
☐ Correct cardiac risk factors, such as obesity, smoking, and a sedentary lifestyle, to enhance your quality of life and cardiac health.
☐ Adopt a low-fat, low-cholesterol diet because colestipol is more effective when used in conjunction with dietary restrictions. Also make sure your diet is high in fiber and vitamins A, D, E, and K.
☐ Take preventive measures to minimize constipation, such as drinking plenty of fluids (if not contraindicated), exercising, and increasing the amount of fiber in your diet. Notify your doctor if severe constipation occurs.
☐ Comply with scheduled tests that measure serum cholesterol and triglyceride levels to monitor the effectiveness of colestipol.

• Know that palatability may be enhanced if the next daily dose is mixed and refrigerated the previous evening. (See *Mixing colestipol with beverages.*)
• Administer all other medications at least 1 hour before or 4 to 6 hours after colestipol to avoid blocking their absorption.
• Be aware that the patient's total pharmaceutical regimen may need to be adjusted during the course of his coletipol therapy in order to ensure desired effects. His regimen may also

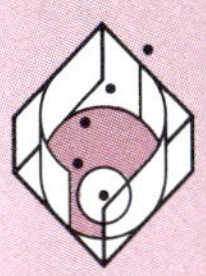

Mixing colestipol with beverages

To increase compliance in the patient who resists taking colestipol because of its consistency and taste, tell him to mix the entire next-day's dose in 90 to 180 ml of milk (3 to 6 oz), fruit juice, or some other noncarbonated beverage, and then to refrigerate it. This should make the drug more palatable the following morning.

need to be adjusted after therapy to prevent toxicities.

Monitoring and supportive care

• Monitor serum cholesterol and triglyceride levels frequently during the first few months of therapy and periodically thereafter.
• Be aware that in some patients receiving long-term colestipol therapy, the initial decrease in cholesterol levels may be followed by a return to baseline levels within 1 month after cessation of therapy.
• Monitor the patient's bowel elimination habits. Manage constipation by increasing fluid and dietary fiber intake or adding a stool softener.
• Monitor levels of digitalis glycosides and other drugs to ensure appropriate dosages during and after colestipol therapy.
• Monitor for signs of vitamin A, D, E, or K deficiency.

• The drug may be discontinued if constipation worsens after a dosage reduction, if a paradoxical increase in the serum cholesterol level occurs, or if the patient experiences an inadequate clinical response after 1 to 3 months of treatment.
• Know that colestipol alters serum levels of ALP, AST, chloride, phosphorus, potassium, and sodium.

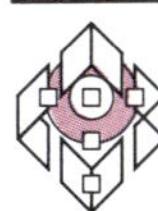

MedTest

1. In order to ensure that your patient receives his entire dose of colestipol:
    a. dilute the entire dose in at least 90 ml of fluid.
    b. dilute the entire dose in a full glass of water.
    c. mix the next daily dose the evening before and refrigerate it.
    d. follow the dose with additional liquid swirled in the same glass.

2. Peak decreases in cholesterol levels occur in:
    a. 24 to 48 hours.
    b. 1 week.
    d. 2 weeks.
    d. 1 month.

3. If constipation worsens after dosage reduction:
    a. increase intake of fluids.
    b. increase dietary fiber.
    c. stop the colestipol.
    d. add a stool softener to the patient's regimen.

Diazoxide

Also known by the brand name Hyperstat I.V., diazoxide is a thiazide-derivative vasodilator that's classified therapeutically as an antihypertensive agent. It's available for injection in vials containing 300 mg/20 ml.

Pharmacokinetics
- *Absorption:* Onset occurs within 5 minutes of I.V. administration.
- *Distribution:* Concentrates in the kidneys, liver, and adrenal glands. Crosses the placenta and blood-brain barrier. About 90% protein-bound.
- *Metabolism:* Metabolized partially in the liver to inactive metabolites.
- *Excretion:* Diazoxide and its metabolites are excreted slowly by the kidneys. The duration of the antihypertensive effect averages 3 to 12 hours.

Indications, dosage, and action
Hypertensive crisis
- *Adult and pediatric dosage:* 1 to 3 mg/kg I.V. (to a maximum of 150 mg) q 5 to 15 minutes until an adequate reduction in blood pressure is achieved. Repeat q 4 to 24 hours p.r.n. Drug also may be given by continuous I.V. infusion (7.5 to 30 mg/minute), but switch to oral antihypertensive as soon as possible.
- *Action:* Directly relaxes arteriolar smooth muscle, causing vasodilation and diminishing peripheral vascular resistance, thus reducing blood pressure.

Contraindications and cautions
- Don't use in patients with known hypersensitivity to other thiazide derivatives.
- Don't use in coarctation of the aorta or an AV shunt.
- Use cautiously in patients who may be harmed by sodium and water retention.
- Use cautiously in impaired cerebral, cardiac, or renal function because the drug may abruptly reduce blood pressure.
- Use cautiously in elderly patients; they may have a more pronounced hypotensive response.
- Use carefully in children.
- Because the drug appears in breast milk, avoid use in breast-feeding women.
- Pregnancy risk category C

Life-threatening adverse reactions
- Myocardial ischemia leading to serious arrhythmias or MI, severe hypotension

Common adverse reactions
- Orthostatic hypotension, sodium and water retention, sweating, flushing, warmth, angina, myocardial ischemia, MI, arrhythmias, ECG changes
- Headache, light-headedness, euphoria
- Abdominal discomfort
- Leukopenia
- Transient hyperglycemia, hyperuricemia
- Local inflammation and pain with extravasation, allergic reactions, such as rash and fever

Infrequent adverse reactions
- Dyspnea, coughing or choking sensation
- Cerebral infarction, cerebral ischemia, dizziness, lethargy, weakness

- Nausea and vomiting, acute pancreatitis

Interactions
- *Antidiabetic agents, insulin:* May alter insulin and oral antidiabetic requirements in previously stable diabetic patients.
- *Beta blockers, hydralazine and other antihypertensive agents, nitrates, thiazide diuretics:* May cause severe hypotension. Use together cautiously.
- *Other diuretics:* Concomitant use with diuretics may potentiate hyperglycemic, hyperuricemic, or antihypertensive effects of diazoxide.
- *Phenytoin:* Concomitant use may increase metabolism and decrease the plasma–protein binding of phenytoin.
- *Warfarin:* May displace warfarin or other highly protein-bound substances from binding sites.

Interventions
Preparation and administration
- Protect solutions from light, heat, or freezing; don't administer solutions that have darkened or that contain particulate matter.
- Give this drug by I.V. bolus or by infusion until blood pressure is reduced adequately.

Monitoring and supportive care
- After I.V. injection, monitor blood pressure and the ECG continuously. Keep the patient supine or in Trendelenburg's position during the infusion and for 1 hour after it. Notify the doctor immediately if severe hypotension develops.

⬥ **Safety tip.** Keep norepinephrine available for emergency treatment of severe hypotension.
- In patients with CAD, monitor for ischemic ECG changes and for arrhythmias.
- Monitor the patient's fluid intake and output carefully and weigh him daily, reporting increases of more than 3 lb (about 1.5 kg). If fluid or sodium retention develops, the doctor may order diuretics.
- Before discontinuing close monitoring for hypotension, check the patient's standing blood pressure.
- Monitor the I.V. site for infiltration or extravasation.
- Tell the patient to report any adverse reactions immediately.
- Monitor all patients' daily blood glucose and electrolyte levels, watching diabetic patients closely for severe hyperglycemia or HNKS. Also monitor daily urine glucose and ketone levels.
- Keep in mind that diazoxide inhibits glucose-stimulated insulin release and may cause false-negative insulin response to glucagon.
- Check serum uric acid levels frequently.
- Explain to the patient that orthostatic hypotension can be minimized by rising slowly and avoiding sudden position changes.
- Know that oral diazoxide is only used to treat hypoglycemia resulting from hyperinsulinism; it's not used to treat functional hypoglycemia. It may be used temporarily to control preoperative or postoperative hypoglycemia in patients with hyperinsulinism. Significant hypotension doesn't occur after oral administra-

tion in doses used to treat hypoglycemia.

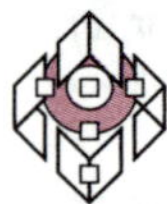 **MedTest**

1. Following administration of I.V.
diazoxide, the maximum hypotensive
effect should occur within:
   a. 60 seconds.
   b. 5 minutes.
   c. 30 minutes.
   d. 1 hour.

2. How long should you keep the patient in a supine position following
administration of diazoxide?
   a. 1 hour.
   b. 2 hours.
   c. 6 hours.
   d. 12 hours.

3. In addition to closely monitoring
your patient's blood pressure during
and following administration of
diazoxide, your follow-up care includes close monitoring of:
   a. hemoglobin and hematocrit levels.
   b. cardiac rate and rhythm.
   c. serum chloride levels.
   d. intake, output, and body
   weight.

Digoxin

Also known by the brand names
Lanoxicaps, Lanoxin, and Novo-
digoxin (in Canada), digoxin is a digitalis glycoside that's classified therapeutically as an antiarrhythmic and
inotropic agent. It's available in

0.125-, 0.25-, and 0.5-mg tablets; 0.05-,
0.1-, and 0.2-mg capsules; an elixir of
0.05 mg/ml; and unit-dose ampules
for injection containing 0.05 mg/ml
(in Canada), 0.1 mg/ml (pediatric),
and 0.25 mg/ml.

Pharmacokinetics

• *Absorption:* 60% to 85% with tablet
or elixir administration, 90% to 100%
with capsule administration, and
about 80% with I.M. administration.
   Onset with oral administration occurs in 30 minutes to 2 hours, with
peak effects in 6 to 8 hours. With I.M.
administration, onset occurs in 30
minutes with peak effects in 4 to 6
hours. With I.V. administration, onset
occurs in 5 to 30 minutes with peak
effects in 1 to 5 hours.
• *Distribution:* Crosses the blood-
brain barrier and placenta; 20% to
30% is bound to plasma proteins. The
usual therapeutic range for steady-
state serum levels is 0.5 to 2 ng/ml.
Toxic symptoms are more frequent
and serious with levels above
2.5 ng/ml.
• *Metabolism:* In most patients, a
small amount is metabolized in the
liver and intestine by bacteria. This
metabolism may be substantial in
some patients. The drug undergoes
variable enterohepatic recirculation.
Metabolites have minimal cardiac activity.
• *Excretion:* Mostly by kidneys as unchanged drug. Some patients excrete
a substantial amount of metabolized
or reduced dose. In patients with renal failure, most of dose is excreted
in bile. In healthy patients, elimination half-life is 30 to 40 hours. In pa-

tients lacking functioning kidneys, elimination half-life is at least 4 days.

Indications, dosage, and action
CHF, atrial fibrillation and flutter, PAT
Dosages differ depending on the drug's form.
Tablets and elixir
• *Adult dosage:* For rapid digitalization, 0.75 to 1.25 mg P.O. over 24 hours in two or more divided doses q 6 to 8 hours. For slow digitalization, 0.125 to 0.5 mg daily for 5 to 7 days. Maintenance dosage is 0.125 to 0.5 mg daily.
• *Pediatric dosage:* Administer loading dose according to age, as described below. For all ages, maintenance dose is 20% to 33% of total loading dose.

Ages 10 and older: For rapid digitalization, 0.75 to 1.25 mg P.O. over 24 hours in two or more divided doses q 6 to 8 hours. For slow digitalization, 0.125 to 0.5 mg daily for 5 to 7 days.

Ages 5 to 10: 20 to 35 mcg/kg P.O. over 24 hours in two or more divided doses q 6 to 8 hours.

Ages 2 to 5: 30 to 40 mcg/kg P.O. over 24 hours in two or more divided doses q 6 to 8 hours.

Ages 1 month to 2 years: 35 to 60 mcg/kg P.O. over 24 hours in two or more divided doses q 6 to 8 hours.

Premature infants and neonates: 20 to 35 mcg/kg P.O. over 24 hours in two or more divided doses q 6 to 8 hours.

Capsules and injection
• *Adult dosage:* For rapid digitalization, 0.4 to 0.6 mg P.O. or I.V. initially, followed by 100 to 300 mcg q 6 to 8 hours, as needed and tolerated, for 24 hours. For slow digitalization, 0.05 to 0.35 mg daily in one or two divided doses for 7 to 22 days as needed until therapeutic serum levels are reached. Maintenance dosage is 0.05 to 0.35 mg daily in one or two divided doses.
• *Pediatric dosage:* Loading dose is based on the child's age and is administered in three or more divided doses over the first 24 hours. Initial dose should be 50% of the total dosage; subsequent doses are given q 4 to 8 hours as needed and tolerated. Maintenance dosage is 25% to 35% of the total loading dose, given daily as a single dose to children ages 10 and older, or divided and given in two or three equal doses daily to children younger than age 10.

Ages 10 and over: For rapid digitalization, 8 to 12 mcg/kg P.O. or I.V. over 24 hours, divided as above.

Ages 5 to 10: For rapid digitalization, 15 to 30 mcg/kg P.O. over 24 hours, divided as above.

Ages 2 to 5: For rapid digitalization, 25 to 35 mcg/kg P.O. or I.V. over 24 hours, divided as above.

Ages 1 month to 2 years: For rapid digitalization, 30 to 50 mcg/kg I.V. over 24 hours, divided as above.

Neonates: For rapid digitalization, 20 to 30 mcg/kg I.V. over 24 hours, divided as above.

Premature infants: For rapid digitalization, 15 to 25 mcg/kg I.V. over 24 hours, divided as above. Maintenance dosage is 20% to 30% of the total digitalizing dose, divided and given in two or three equal doses daily. (Capsules are not used in children younger than age 2.)

• *Inotropic action:* Digoxin inhibits sodium-potassium movement by combining with adenosine triphosphatase, an enzyme involved in myocardial sodium balance. This action may indirectly alter calcium availability to muscle cells, which increases the force and velocity of myocardial contraction. In patients with CHF, the increased cardiac output reduces sympathetic tone and slows heart rate.

• *Antiarrhythmic action:* Digoxin has direct and indirect effects on the SA and AV nodes. It slows heart rate and conduction velocity through the AV node, and prolongs the effective refractory period of the AV node.

Contraindications and cautions

• Don't use in ventricular fibrillation.
• Use with extreme caution in patients with idiopathic hypertrophic cardiomyopathy because the drug may cause increased obstruction of left ventricular outflow.
• Use carefully in patients with incomplete AV block who don't have a pacemaker because the drug may induce advanced or complete AV block.
• Because the drug increases the risk of arrhythmias, use with care in patients with severe pulmonary disease, hypoxia, myxedema, WPW syndrome, acute MI, severe heart failure, frequent PVCs or VT, acute myocarditis, or an otherwise damaged myocardium.
• Use cautiously in patients with sinus node disease because the drug may worsen sinus bradycardia or SA block.
• Use cautiously in chronic constrictive pericarditis. Patients may respond unfavorably.
• Use cautiously in low cardiac output states caused by valvular stenosis, chronic pericarditis, or chronic cor pulmonale because the drug may decrease heart rate and cardiac output.
• Closely watch patients with conditions that increase cardiac sensitivity to digitalis glycosides, including hypokalemia, COPD, and acute hypoxemia.
• Use I.V. digoxin with care in patients with hypertension because I.V. administration may increase blood pressure.
• Know that hypothyroid patients are very sensitive to digitalis glycosides. Hyperthyroid patients, on the other hand, may need larger doses.
• Use cautiously in elderly patients because of reduced renal clearance; dosage may need to be adjusted to prevent accumulation.
• Because it's excreted in human milk, use with caution in breast-feeding women.
• Pregnancy risk category C

Life-threatening adverse reactions

• Increased severity of CHF and arrhythmias

Common adverse reactions

• Arrhythmias, hypotension, bradycardia
• Fatigue, generalized weakness, agitation
• Anorexia, nausea, vomiting

- Yellow-green halos around visual images, blurred vision, light flashes, photophobia, diplopia

Infrequent adverse reactions
- Hallucinations, headache, malaise, dizziness, vertigo, stupor, paresthesia
- Diarrhea
- Gynecomastia

Interactions
- *Aminosalicylic acid, antacids containing aluminum or magnesium, cholestyramine, colestipol, cytotoxic agents, dietary bran, kaolin-pectin, metoclopramide, radiation therapy*: May decrease absorption of oral digoxin. Monitor for decreased effect and low blood levels.
- *Anticholinergics:* May increase digoxin absorption of oral tablets. Monitor blood levels and observe for toxicity.
- *I.V. calcium, thiazides:* Hypercalcemia, hypokalemia, and hypomagnesemia, predisposing patient to digitalis toxicity. Monitor serum calcium, potassium, and magnesium levels.

For dangerous interactions, see *Hazards of multidrug therapy with digoxin,* page 122.

Interventions
Preparation and administration
- Obtain baseline heart rate and rhythm and blood pressure, and check serum electrolyte levels before giving initial dose.
- Question patient about use of digitalis glycosides within the previous 2 weeks before administering a loading dose. The loading dose is always divided over the first 24 hours unless the clinical situation indicates otherwise.
- Before giving each dose, check apical pulse rate and rhythm for a full minute. Record and report any significant changes to the doctor. Check blood pressure and obtain a 12-lead ECG reading.

Safety tip. Excessive slowing of the pulse rate (60 beats/ minute or less) may be a sign of digitalis toxicity. Withhold the drug dose and notify the doctor.
- Infuse I.V. drug doses slowly over at least 5 minutes.
- Digoxin solution is also available in soft capsules (Lanoxicaps). Because these capsules are better absorbed than tablets, dose is usually slightly smaller.

Safety tip. When changing from oral tablets or elixir to liquid-filled capsules or parenteral therapy, the dosage should be reduced by 20% to 25%. When changing from liquid-filled capsules to parenteral therapy, dosage is about equivalent.

Monitoring and supportive care
- Monitor ECG and serum levels of digoxin, calcium, potassium, and magnesium.
- Monitor for signs of toxicity. Ask the patient about changes in eating patterns, nausea, vomiting, anorexia, visual disturbances, and other evidence of toxicity. (See *Taking digoxin at home,* page 123.) The drug should be discontinued if signs of toxicity develop.
- Monitor serum drug levels. Therapeutic levels range from 0.5 to 2 ng/ml. Blood must be drawn at least 4 hours, and preferably 6 to 8

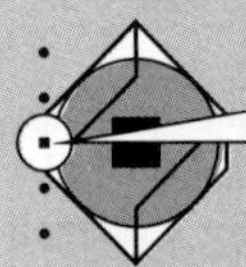

Interactions alert

Hazards of multidrug therapy with digoxin

Interacting drug	Effects
Amphotericin B (antifungal agent)	Depletes total body potassium levels, possibly leading to digoxin toxicity
Antiarrhythmics (such as amiodarone, procainamide, propafenone, quinidine, and verapamil)	May be synergistic, causing additive cardiac effects (50% to 100% increase in serum digoxin levels)
Calcium salts (such as calcium chloride, calcium gluceptate, and calcium gluconate) given I.V.	Are synergistic; potentially life-threatening arrhythmias may occur if used together
Corticosteroids (such as prednisone)	May deplete total body potassium levels, possibly leading to digoxin toxicity
Corticotropin	Depletes total body potassium levels, potentially causing digoxin toxicity
Diuretics (such as bumetanide, ethacrynic acid, furosemide, bumetanide, and thiazides such as chlorothiazide)	May cause electrolyte disturbances, causing fatal cardiac arrhythmias
Edetate disodium (heavy metal antagonist)	Depletes total body potassium levels, possibly leading to digoxin toxicity
Rauwolfia alkaloids (such as reserpine)	Increase risk of life-threatening arrhythmias
Sodium polystyrene sulfonate (potassium-removing resin)	Depletes total body potassium levels, possibly leading to digoxin toxicity
Succinylcholine (skeletal muscle relaxant)	Elevates serum potassium, which may result in GI and cardiac toxicity
Sympathomimetics (such as ephedrine, epinephrine, isoproterenol)	Increase risk of life-threatening arrhythmias

hours, after the last dose to allow levels to equilibrate. Cardiac signs of digoxin toxicity commonly precede other signs. Most common are ventricular arrhythmias or AV conduction disturbances. Digoxin-induced VT may lead to fatal ventricular fibrillation or asystole.

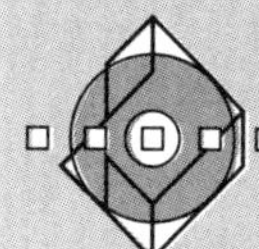

Patient-teaching checklist

Taking digoxin at home

In addition to explaining the drug's action and dosage, teach the patient who will continue digoxin therapy after discharge to follow these important guidelines.

Take your medication correctly

□ Take your pulse rate before each dose. If you detect any significant increase or decrease in rate (especially if your heart rate slows to less than 60 beats/minute) or if your pulse becomes increasingly irregular, notify your doctor before taking your next dose.

□ Don't take more digoxin than your doctor prescribed and don't miss any doses. However, if you do miss a dose and you remember it within 12 hours, take it as soon as you remember. Otherwise, wait until your next scheduled dose. Never double your dose to make up for a missed dose.

□ Measure the liquid form of digoxin only with the specially marked dropper included in the packet. Remember that the medicine is to be taken by mouth, even if it comes in a dropper bottle.

□ Take digoxin as prescribed even when you're feeling well.

Know when to call your doctor

□ Don't stop taking digoxin suddenly without consulting your doctor because a serious change in your heart function may occur. However, notify your doctor immediately if you experience GI upset (such as a change in appetite, nausea, vomiting, or diarrhea), visual disturbances (such as yellow-green halos, blurred vision, light flashes, light sensitivity, or double vision), changes in mental status (such as agitation, hallucinations, malaise, or dizziness), or an irregular pulse. These adverse reactions may indicate that you've developed a toxic reaction to digoxin.

Other instructions

□ Include potassium-rich foods, such as bananas or oranges, in your daily diet unless otherwise instructed.

□ Comply with scheduled follow-up doctor visits and periodic laboratory tests to evaluate the effectiveness of digoxin.

□ Check with the doctor or pharmacist before taking OTC medications. If you see more than one doctor, make sure all of them know you're taking digoxin because this drug interacts with many other drugs.

□ Store digoxin at room temperature and protect it from moisture, direct light, and heat.

• Treat life-threatening digoxin toxicity with digoxin-specific antibody fragments (digoxin immune FAB). Each 40 mg of digoxin immune FAB binds about 0.6 mg of digoxin in the bloodstream.

• Know that GI absorption may be reduced in patients with CHF.

• Generally, the digoxin dose should be reduced and the serum level monitored if the patient is receiving digoxin concomitantly with amiodarone, diltiazem, flecainide, nifedipine, verapamil, or quinidine. Also monitor the patient for signs of digoxin toxicity.

• Because digoxin may cause post-cardioversion asystole, it's usually withheld for 1 or 2 days before elective cardioversion in patients with atrial fibrillation.

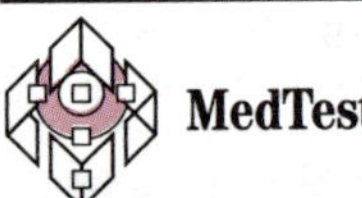 **MedTest**

1. Of the following oral and parenteral administration forms of digoxin, which is most completely absorbed?
- **a.** I.M. injection
- **b.** Tablet
- **c.** Elixir
- **d.** Capsule

2. How long does it customarily take to achieve steady-state levels of digoxin?
- **a.** 24 to 48 hours
- **b.** 3 to 5 days
- **c.** 7 days or more
- **d.** 2 to 3 weeks

3. When taking the patient's apical pulse for a full minute before administering the dose, monitor carefully for:
- **a.** a rate of 60 beats/minute or less.
- **b.** a previously noted pulse deficit.
- **c.** a rate of 100 beats/minute or more.
- **d.** significant changes.

Digoxin immune FAB

Also known by the brand name Digibind, digoxin immune FAB is an antibody fragment that's classified therapeutically as a digitalis glycoside antidote. It's available in a 40-mg vial for injection.

Pharmacokinetics
• *Absorption:* Peak serum concentrations occur at the completion of I.V. infusion.
• *Distribution:* After I.V. administration, the drug appears to distribute rapidly throughout extracellular space, into both plasma and interstitial fluid. It's not known if this drug crosses the placental barrier or is distributed into breast milk.
• *Metabolism:* Unknown.
• *Excretion:* In urine via glomerular filtration. Drug has a serum half-life of 15 to 20 hours.

Indications, dosage, and action
Potentially life-threatening digoxin or digitoxin intoxication
• *Adult and pediatric dosage:* Administer I.V. over 30 minutes or as a bolus if cardiac arrest is imminent. Dosage varies according to the amount of drug to be neutralized; 60 mg will bind 1 mg of digoxin or digitoxin. Average dose is 10 vials (400 mg). However, if neither a serum digoxin level nor an estimated ingestion amount is known, administer 20 vials (800 mg). See package insert for complete, specific instructions.

- *Action:* Specific antigen-binding fragments bind to molecules of free digoxin or digitoxin in extracellular fluid and intravascularly. This prevents and reverses the pharmacologic and toxic effects of the digitalis glycoside. Digitalis toxicity begins to subside within 30 minutes after completion of a 15- to 30-minute I.V. infusion of digoxin immune FAB. Reversal of toxicity is usually complete within 2 to 6 hours.

Contraindications and cautions

- Be aware that no contraindications or systemic allergic reactions have been reported; however, patients sensitive to ovine or sheep products may be intolerant of digoxin immune FAB. Skin testing is recommended in these high-risk patients.
- Use cautiously in patients with low cardiac output and CHF because the condition may worsen from the subsequent decrease in effective inotropic concentrations of digoxin.
- Know that VT may develop in patients with preexisting atrial fibrillation because of the reversal of the glycoside effects on the AV node.
- Be aware that renal impairment may delay elimination of FAB-digoxin complex for 1 week or longer.
- Use cautiously in breast-feeding women.
- Pregnancy risk category C

Life-threatening adverse reactions

- CHF, arrhythmias from hypokalemia or from arrhythmias otherwise suppressed by digoxin
- Hypersensitivity, anaphylactic reaction

Common adverse reactions

(Adverse reactions are related more to the withdrawal of the digitalis glycosides than to a direct effect of the antibody fragment.)
- Diminished cardiac output, increased ventricular rate in the presence of preexisting atrial fibrillation
- Hypokalemia

Interactions

- *Digitalis glycosides:* Drug causes binding of digitalis glycosides, reducing their effectiveness. Before redigitalization, elimination of digoxin immune FAB, which takes several days, should be complete.

Interventions
Preparation and administration
- Patients with sensitivity or allergy to sheep or ovine products should be pretreated with an antihistamine, such as diphenhydramine, and a corticosteroid. (See *Reconstituting and skin testing for digoxin immune FAB,* page 126.)

Safety tip. Small doses (2 mg or less) may require diluting the reconstituted solution with 36 ml of sterile 0.9% NaCl solution for injection to produce a 1-mg/ml solution.
- Use this antidote only for life-threatening overdose in patients in shock or cardiac arrest; with ventricular arrhythmias; with progressive bradycardia, such as severe sinus bradycardia; or with second- or third-degree AV block unresponsive to atropine.
- Check serum digoxin or digitoxin levels before giving the antidote because they may be difficult to interpret after therapy. Total serum levels

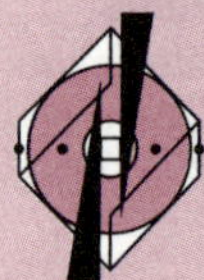

Reconstituting and skin testing for digoxin immune FAB

Follow the instructions below to reconstitute and administer digoxin immune FAB and to test the patient's skin for a possible allergic reaction.

Reconstitution
- Refrigerate the powder for reconstitution until ready for use.
- Reconstitute each 40-mg vial with 4 ml of sterile water for injection. (Be aware that the dose depends on the amount of digoxin to be neutralized. Each 40-mg vial binds approximately 0.6 mg of digoxin or digitoxin; the average dose is 10 vials, or 400 mg.) Mix gently.
- Use the reconstituted product immediately. However, it may be stored for up to 4 hours in the refrigerator if absolutely necessary.
- Infuse the drug I.V. through a 0.22-micron filter over 30 minutes or as a bolus injection when cardiac arrest is imminent.

Skin testing
Skin testing may be necessary for high-risk patients (such as those sensitive to sheep or ovine products). Use one of these two methods:
- *Interdermal test.* Dilute 0.1 ml of reconstituted solution in 9.9 ml of sterile 0.9% NaCl solution; then withdraw and inject 0.1 ml of this solution intradermally. Inspect the site after 20 minutes for signs of erythema or urticaria.
- *Scratch test.* Dilute as for intradermal test. Place one drop of diluted solution on the skin and make a ¼" scratch through the drop with a sterile needle. Inspect the site after 20 minutes for signs of erythema or urticaria.

If results are positive with either test, avoid using digoxin immune FAB.

---

may rise after treatment, but this reflects FAB-bound (inactive) digoxin.
- Keep medications and equipment for CPR readily available during administration of digoxin immune FAB for patients who respond poorly to withdrawal from digoxin's inotropic effects. Dopamine, dobutamine, or vasodilators may be used.
- Infants may require smaller doses; the manufacturer recommends reconstituting as directed and administering with a tuberculin syringe.

Monitoring and supportive care
- Closely monitor temperature, blood pressure, ECG, and serum potassium levels before, during, and after administration. Check serum potassium levels repeatedly, because severe digitalis intoxication can cause life-threatening hyperkalemia and

reversal by digoxin immune FAB may lead to rapid hypokalemia.

• Monitor the patient's clinical status. Improvement in cardiac arrhythmias, neurologic and GI symptoms, and visual disturbances indicate effective treatment.

• In patients with CAD, assess for increasing angina.

• Know that suicidal ingestion often involves more than one medication. Be alert for signs of other drug toxicities.

• Use in infants and small children hasn't produced adverse effects. However, monitor for volume overload in small children.

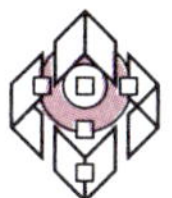 **MedTest**

1. While the dosage of digoxin immune FAB varies according to the amount of drug to be neutralized, the average dose is about 400 mg or 10 vials. This will bind approximately:
    a. 1 mg of digoxin or digitoxin.
    b. 3 mg of digoxin or digitoxin.
    c. 6 mg of digoxin or digitoxin.
    d. 10 mg of digoxin or digitoxin.

2. How long after the 15- to 30-minute infusion of digoxin immune FAB will toxicity begin to subside?
    a. within 30 minutes.
    b. within 1 hour.
    c. within 2 hours.
    d. within 6 hours.

3. Use digoxin immune FAB:
    a. whenever the patient shows any signs or symptoms of digitalis toxicity.

b. when the serum digoxin level exceeds 4 ng/ml.
c. for any patient who may have overdosed on digoxin.
d. for life-threatening overdoses only.

Diltiazem hydrochloride

Also known by the brand names Cardizem, Cardizem CD, Cardizem SR, and Dilacor XR, diltiazem is a calcium channel blocker that's classfied therapeutically as an antianginal agent. It's available in 30-, 60-, 90-, and 120-mg tablets; in sustained-release (12-hour) capsules (Cardizem SR) of 60, 90, and 120 mg; in dual-release (24-hour) capsules (Cardizem CD) of 120, 180, 240, and 300 mg; in extended-release (24-hour) capsules (Dilacor XR) of 180 and 240 mg; and in vials for injection containing 5 mg/ml.

Pharmacokinetics

• *Absorption:* About 80% absorbed rapidly from the GI tract, but only about 40% enters the systemic circulation because of significant first-pass effect in the liver. After tablet ingestion, peak serum levels occur in about 2 to 3 hours.
• *Distribution:* 70% to 85% of circulating diltiazem is bound to plasma proteins.
• *Metabolism:* Metabolized by the liver to active and inactive metabolites.
• *Excretion:* About 35% in urine and about 65% in bile as unchanged drug and inactive and active metabolites.

Elimination half-life is 3 to 9 hours. Half-life may increase in elderly patients; however, renal dysfunction doesn't appear to affect half-life.

Indications, dosage, and action
Prinzmetal's or variant angina, or chronic stable angina
• *Adult dosage:* 30 mg P.O. q.i.d. a.c. and h.s. Dosage may be increased gradually to 360 mg/day, in divided doses three to four times a day. Alternatively, use dual-release capsules (Cardizem CD). The usual initial dosage is 120 or 130 mg once daily. Increase dosage gradually once q 1 to 2 weeks to a maximum of 480 mg daily.
• *Action:* Decreases myocardial oxygen demand and cardiac workload by reducing heart rate, relieving coronary artery spasm (through coronary artery vasodilation), increasing coronary artery blood flow, and dilating peripheral vessels. These effects relieve ischemia and pain.

Hypertension
• *Adult dosage:* 60 to 120 mg P.O. b.i.d. (Cardizem SR); or 180 to 480 mg (Cardizem CD or Dilacor XR) once a day. Adjust dosage according to patient response. Maximum antihypertensive effect is usually evident after 14 days. Usual dosage range is 240 to 360 mg daily for Cardizem CD and 180 to 480 mg daily for Dilacor XR.
• *Action:* By dilating systemic arteries and arterioles, diltiazem decreases total peripheral resistance and afterload, reducing blood pressure.

Atrial fibrillation and flutter, PSVT
• *Adult dosage:* 0.25 mg/kg I.V. as a bolus injection over 2 minutes. Repeat after 15 minutes if response is not adequate. May be followed by continuous infusion of 5 to 15 mg/hour.
• *Action:* Diltiazem prolongs AV conduction time and AV node refractoriness, thereby slowing ventricular response.

Contraindications and cautions
• Because of the drug's antihypertensive effect, don't use diltiazem in severe hypotension (systolic blood pressure below 90 mm Hg) or cardiogenic shock.
• Don't use in second- or third-degree AV block or SSS (unless a pacemaker is in place) because of the drug's effect on the cardiac conduction system.
• Use cautiously in CHF, impaired ventricular function, or conduction abnormalities because the drug may worsen these conditions.
• Use cautiously in elderly patients and in patients with impaired liver function because elimination half-life may be prolonged.
• Because it's excreted in breast milk, avoid use in breast-feeding women.
• Pregnancy risk category C

Life-threatening adverse reactions
• Arrhythmias, CHF

Common adverse reactions
• Arrhythmias, flushing, hypotension

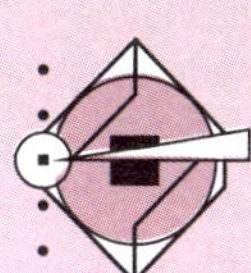

Life-threatening hazards of multidrug therapy with diltiazem

Drug interaction	Effects
Beta blockers (such as propranolol)	May cause combined effects that result in CHF, conduction disturbances, arrhythmias, and hypotension
Cyclosporine (immunosuppressant)	May cause increased serum cyclosporine levels and subsequent cyclosporine-induced nephrotoxicity
Digoxin	May result in excessive bradycardia or conduction abnormalities because diltiazem increases serum digoxin levels by 20% to 40%

• Fatigue, drowsiness, nervousness, depression, insomnia, confusion, akathisia, headache
• Nausea, vomiting, constipation, transient elevation of liver enzymes
• Nocturia, polyuria
• Photosensitivity

Infrequent adverse reactions
• Edema, bradycardia, conduction abnormalities (first-degree AV block), sweating
• Dyspnea
• Headache, dizziness, asthenia
• Rash, pruritus

Interactions
• *Cimetidine:* May inhibit diltiazem metabolism. Monitor for toxicity.
• *Furosemide:* Forms a precipitate when mixed with diltiazem injection. Administer through separate I.V. lines.

For dangerous interactions, see *Life-threatening hazards of multidrug therapy with diltiazem.*

Interventions
Preparation and administration
• Obtain a baseline assessment of the patient's blood pressure and apical pulse rate. Also obtain baseline information regarding frequency of angina before initiating therapy and monitor it during dosage adjustments.

Safety tip. If systolic blood pressure is less than 90 mm Hg, or heart rate is less than 50 beats/minute, withhold the dose and notify the doctor.

Monitoring and supportive care
• Assist patients with ambulation during initiation of diltiazem therapy because dizziness may occur.

• If nitrate therapy is prescribed during diltiazem therapy, urge the patient to continue compliance. If he experiences increased fatigue, tell him to space administration of the two drug doses.
• Headache is a common adverse effect with once-a-day dosing. Administer with aspirin (if not contraindicated) or acetaminophen at the beginning of therapy.
• If diltiazem is added to the therapy of patients receiving digoxin, monitor serum digoxin levels. Observe patients closely for signs of toxicity, especially elderly patients, those with unstable renal function, and those with serum digoxin levels in the upper therapeutic range. Tell patient taking the tablet form of diltiazem to take the drug before meals and at bedtime. If he's taking the capsule (extended-release) form, remind him to swallow the drug whole without crushing or chewing it. (See *Taking calcium channel blockers at home,* page 77.)
• Know that the extended-release formulations Dilacor XR and Cardizem SR are not interchangeable with each other or with the dual-release formulation Cardizem CD.

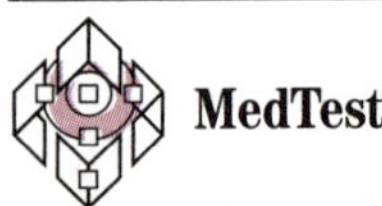 **MedTest**

---

1. Instruct patients to take sustained- and extended-release forms of diltiazem:
   a. q 6 or 12 hours.
   b. q 12 hours or daily.
   c. daily or every other day.
   d. every other day or weekly.

2. If a patient develops headaches during initial use of extended-release diltiazem, he should:
   a. notify his doctor immediately.
   b. stop taking diltiazem.
   c. take the drug with aspirin or acetaminophen, if not contraindicated.
   d. return to q.i.d. dosing.

3. If a patient experiences increased fatigue when taking diltiazem with nitrates, he should:
   a. space administration of the two drug doses.
   b. stop taking diltiazem.
   c. stop taking the nitrate.
   d. notify his doctor that his condition is worsening rather than improving.

Dipyridamole

Also known by the brand names Persantine, Pyridamole, Apo-Dipyridamole (in Canada), and Persantin 100 (in Australia), dipyridamole is a pyrimidine analogue that's classified therapeutically as a platelet-aggregation inhibitor. It's available in 25-, 50-, and 75-mg tablets, and in a 10-mg ampule for injection.

Pharmacokinetics
• *Absorption:* Variable and slow. Bioavailability ranges from 27% to 59%. Serum concentrations peak 2 to $2\frac{1}{2}$ hours after oral administration.
• *Distribution:* Small amounts cross the placenta. Protein binding is 91% to 97%.
• *Metabolism:* By the liver. It isn't known if metabolites are active.

• *Excretion:* Occurs via biliary excretion of glucuronide conjugates. Some dipyridamole and conjugates may undergo enterohepatic circulation and fecal excretion; a small amount is excreted in urine. Elimination half-life varies from 1 to 12 hours.

Indications, dosage, and action

Inhibition of platelet adhesion to prosthetic heart valves

• *Adult dosage:* 75 to 100 mg P.O. daily (combined with warfarin or aspirin).
• *Action:* Dipyridamole inhibits platelet adhesion by increasing effects of prostacyclin or by inhibiting phosphodiesterase.

Alternative to exercise in thallium imaging

• *Adult dosage:* 0.57 mg/kg infused I.V. at a constant rate. Mix to a total of 40 ml and give over 4 minutes at a rate of 10 ml/min. Don't give more than 60 mg.
• *Action:* Inhibits adenosine uptake leading to coronary vasodilation, primarily in normal arteries. If an artery is narrowed, a smaller increase in flow occurs. When thallium is administered, it goes preferentially to the normal arteries, resulting in an abnormal thallium distribution that demonstrates perfusion defects.

Contraindications and cautions

• Know that this drug is ineffective in acute angina and shouldn't be used as a substitute for appropriate treatment, such as nitroglycerin.
• Use cautiously in hypotension and in patients taking anticoagulants.
• Use I.V. dipyridamole cautiously in patients with a history of pulmonary disease (bronchospastic disease, asthma, or COPD).
• Pregnancy risk category C

Life-threatening adverse reactions

• ECG abnormalities, hypotension

Common adverse reactions

• Hypotension, blood pressure lability, hypertension with I.V. infusion, flushing, diaphoresis
• Dizziness, weakness, syncope
• Nausea, vomiting, diarrhea, constipation
• Local irritation with undiluted injection

Infrequent adverse reactions

• Angina
• Headache
• Liver dysfunction

Interactions

• *Theophylline:* Blocks the action of dipyridamole.

Interventions

Preparation and administration

• Give this drug at least 1 hour a.c. However, it may be administered with meals if the patient develops GI distress. (See *Taking dipyridamole at home,* page 132.)
• Dilute the I.V. form to at least a 1:2 ratio with 0.45% or 0.9% NaCl solution or D_5W to a total volume of 40 ml. Inject thallium within 5 minutes of dipyridamole.
• Be aware that patients receiving I.V. dipyridamole should avoid all xanthine-containing drugs for at least 36

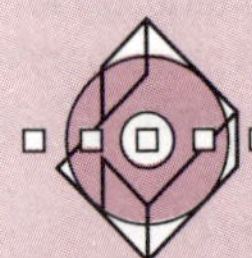

Patient-teaching checklist

Taking dipyridamole at home

In addition to explaining the drug's action and dosage, teach the patient who will continue dipyridamole therapy after discharge to follow these important guidelines.

Take your medication correctly
☐ Take dipyridamole 1 hour before meals with a full 8-oz glass of water or with meals or milk if GI upset occurs.
☐ Space doses evenly throughout the day.
☐ Take dipyridamole as prescribed even when you're feeling well.
☐ Continue taking the drug even if unpleasant adverse reactions occur. But make sure you discuss any adverse reactions, especially chest pain, with your doctor.

Minimize adverse reactions
☐ Remember to change positions slowly (especially from lying flat to sitting upright) and dangle your legs over the bedside for a few minutes before standing. This will help to minimize any drug-related dizziness, light-headedness, or fainting.
☐ Lie down immediately if dizziness or faintness occurs.
☐ Avoid driving or operating machinery until you've adjusted to the drug's effects.

Other instructions
☐ Check with your doctor or pharmacist before taking any OTC medications, especially aspirin or any combination containing aspirin.
☐ Store dipyridamole at room temperature and protect it from heat, direct light, and moisture.

hours prior to testing and should not drink coffee, tea, or other caffeine-containing soft drinks for 4 to 6 hours. Ensure that the patient takes nothing orally for 4 hours prior to the test.

Safety tip. Monitor blood pressure and ECG during and following administration of I.V. dipyridamole.

Monitoring and supportive care
• Monitor blood pressure. The drug should be discontinued if excessive hypotension occurs.

• Be alert for signs of bleeding and prolonged bleeding time, especially at high doses and during long-term therapy.
• When used as a stress test, total doses shouldn't exceed 60 mg.
• Dipyridamole shouldn't be used alone for the prophylaxis of thromboembolism in postoperative prosthetic valve patients; it may not be significantly better than aspirin alone.
• Be aware that dipyridamole's physiologic effects on platelet aggregation will cause an increase in bleeding time.

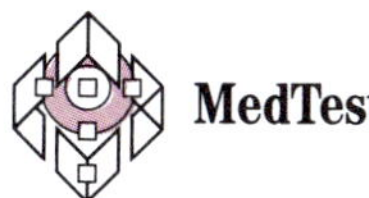

MedTest

1. The only FDA-approved use for oral dipyridamole is as:
  a. an antianginal agent.
  b. an antihypertensive agent.
  c. a vasodilator.
  d. a platelet adhesion inhibitor.

2. Given I.V. as part of a thallium scan in place of exercise, dipyridamole should be diluted to:
  a. 10 ml and administered over 2 minutes.
  b. 40 ml and administered over 10 minutes.
  c. 50 ml and administered over 30 minutes.
  d. 100 ml and administered over 60 minutes.

3. When administering I.V. dipyridamole, monitor the patient closely for:
  a. local irritation at the administration site.
  b. ectopic ventricular activity
  c. hypotension.
  d. rapid heart rate.

Disopyramide phosphate

Also known by the brand names Norpace, Norpace CR, Napamide, and Rythmodan-LA (in Canada), disopyramide phosphate is a pyridine derivative that's classified therapeutically as an antiarrhythmic agent. It's available in 100- and 150-mg capsules, 100- and 150-mg extended-release capsules, and (in Canada) 250-mg sustained-release tablets .

Pharmacokinetics
• *Absorption:* Rapid from the GI tract; 60% to 80% reaches systemic circulation. Onset usually occurs in 30 minutes; peak blood levels about 2 hours after administration of conventional capsules and 5 hours after administration of extended-release capsules.
• *Distribution:* 50% to 65% plasma protein–bound. Usual therapeutic serum level ranges from 2 to 4 mcg/ml, although some patients may require up to 7 mcg/ml. Levels above 9 mcg/ml are considered toxic.
• *Metabolism:* Metabolized in the liver to one major metabolite with little antiarrhythmic activity but more anticholinergic activity than the parent compound.
• *Excretion:* About 90% of an oral dose excreted in the urine as unchanged drug and metabolites. The usual elimination half-life is about 7 hours but lengthens in patients with renal or hepatic insufficiency. Duration of effect is usually 6 to 7 hours.

Indications, dosage, and action
PVCs, VT not needing cardioversion; converting atrial fibrillation and flutter to normal rhythm
• *Regular adult dosage:* Usual maintenance dosage is 150 to 200 mg P.O. q 6 hours; for patients who weigh less than 50 kg, dosage is 100 mg P.O. q 6 hours. You may also give sustained-release capsules q 12 hours.

• *Dosage in renal or hepatic impairment:* Patients with hepatic insufficiency or moderately impaired renal function should receive 100 mg P.O. q 6 hours or 200 mg (extended-release) q 12 hours. Patients with severely impaired renal function should receive only 100 mg (regular-release) at the following intervals: for patients with a creatinine clearance of 30 to 40 ml/minute, q 8 hours; for patients with a clearance of 15 to 30 ml/minute, q 12 hours; for those with a clearance of less than 15 ml/minute, q 24 hours.

• *Pediatric dosage:* For ages 12 to 18, 6 to 15 mg/kg/day. For ages 4 to 12, 10 to 15 mg/kg/day. For ages 1 to 4, 10 to 20 mg/kg/day. From birth to age 1, 10 to 30 mg/kg/day.

All children's dosages should be divided into equal amounts and given every 6 hours.

Extended-release capsules aren't recommended for use in children.

• *Action:* A class Ia antiarrhythmic agent, disopyramide depresses phase 0 of the action potential. It decreases myocardial excitability, conduction velocity, and contractility. Its anticholinergic activity may modify the drug's direct myocardial effects. In therapeutic doses, disopyramide reduces conduction velocity and suppresses ectopic pacemakers in the atria, ventricles, and His-Purkinje system.

Contraindications and cautions

• Don't use in second- or third-degree AV block (unless a pacemaker is in place) because of the risk of worsening AV block.

• Don't use in myasthenia gravis because the drug's anticholinergic effect may provoke a myasthenic crisis.

• Don't use in patients with untreated glaucoma or urine retention because of the drug's anticholinergic effect.

• Avoid use in uncompensated CHF and cardiogenic shock because of the drug's negative inotropic effect.

• Use cautiously in patients with SSS, WPW syndrome, or bundle-branch heart block because of the drug's unpredictable effects on AV conduction.

• Use with care in patients with cardiomyopathy because they may develop significant hypotension.

• Use with caution in elderly patients and patients with renal or hepatic insufficiency because decreased drug elimination may cause toxicity. Dosage adjustment may be necessary.

• The drug should be discontinued if hypotension, progressive heart failure, or AV block occurs; if the QRS complex widens by more than 25% over baseline; or if the QT interval lengthens more than 25% over baseline. If first-degree AV block develops, the dose should be decreased.

• Avoid use in breast-feeding women because drug is distributed in breast milk.

• Pregnancy risk category C

Life-threatening adverse reactions

• Arrhythmias, AV block, CHF, ventricular fibrillation, severe hypotension

• Myasthenic crisis in patients with myasthenia gravis

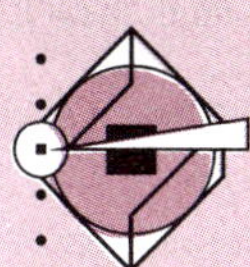

Interactions alert

Hazards of multidrug therapy with disopyramide

Interacting drug	Effects
Antiarrhythmics (such as bretylium)	May cause additive or antagonistic cardiac effects and additive toxicity
Warfarin (anticoagulant)	May cause anticoagulant effects, increasing risk of serious bleeding

Common adverse reactions
- Dizziness, agitation, fatigue, muscle weakness, headache
- Nausea, bloating and gas, abdominal pain, constipation, dry mouth (32%)
- Blurred vision; dry eyes, nose, and throat; change in intraocular pressure
- Urine retention and urinary frequency, urgency, and hesitancy

Infrequent adverse reactions
- Hypotension, edema, weight gain, chest pain, syncope
- Respiratory difficulty
- Depression, insomnia
- Anorexia, nausea, diarrhea, elevated liver enzymes, cholestatic jaundice
- Impotence
- Hypokalemia, increased cholesterol and triglyceride levels, hypoglycemia, elevated BUN and serum creatinine levels
- Rash
- Fever

Interactions
- *Anticholinergics:* Concomitant use may cause additive anticholinergic effects.
- *Hepatic enzyme inducers, phenytoin, rifampin:* Concomitant use may increase disopyramide metabolism.

For dangerous interactions, see *Hazards of multidrug therapy with disopyramide.*

Interventions
Preparation and administration
- Correct any underlying electrolyte abnormalities, especially hypokalemia, before administering this drug because disopyramide may be ineffective in such patients.
- Check the apical pulse before administering the drug. Notify the doctor if the pulse rate is slower than 60 beats/minute or faster than 120 beats/minute.
- When changing from immediate-release to sustained-release capsules, advise the patient to take a sustained-release capsule 6 hours after

taking the last immediate-release capsule.

• If the patient is taking the extended-release form of disopyramide, remind him to swallow the drug whole without crushing or chewing it. (See *Taking antiarrhythmics at home,* page 74.)

Monitoring and supportive care

Safety tip. Monitor blood pressure and cardiac rate and rhythm. You may need to reduce the dosage or discontinue therapy in hypotension, varying degrees of AV block, and QRS-complex and QT-interval changes.

• If the drug causes constipation, administer bulk laxatives and provide a diet high in fiber and fluids.

• Disopyramide may be prescribed for patients with heart failure who cannot tolerate quinidine or procainamide.

• Disopyramide is removed by hemodialysis. Dosage adjustments may be necessary in patients undergoing dialysis.

• Monitor pediatric and elderly patients closely for signs of toxicity; also monitor serum electrolyte and drug levels because a dosage reduction may be needed.

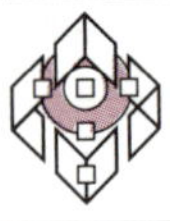 **MedTest**

1. Disopyramide is used to treat PVCs because it:
    a. increases AV conduction.
    b. reduces conduction velocity in the atria and ventricles.
    c. depresses myocardial contractility.
    d. suppresses automaticity.

2. Because of its anticholinergic effect, disopyramide must be used with caution or not at all in patients with:
    a. CHF.
    b. SSS or WPW syndrome.
    c. urine retention related to benign prostatic hyperplasia.
    d. renal or hepatic insufficiency.

3. The most common adverse reaction to disopyramide is:
    a. blurred vision.
    b. dry mouth.
    c. urinary hesitancy.
    d. dizziness.

Dobutamine hydrochloride

Also known by its brand name Dobutrex, dobutamine is a beta$_1$-adrenergic agonist that's classified therapeutically as an inotropic agent. It's available for injection and comes in 20-ml vials containing 12.5 mg/ml and in premixed containers of 500 mg in 250 ml of D$_5$W.

Pharmacokinetics

• *Absorption:* Onset occurs within 2 minutes, and peak concentrations within 10 minutes, of I.V. administration. Effects persist for a few minutes after administration is discontinued.

• *Distribution:* Widely distributed throughout the body.

• *Metabolism:* By the liver to inactive metabolites.
• *Excretion:* Mainly in urine as its metabolites.

Indications, dosage, and action
Short-term treatment of cardiac decompensation caused by depressed contractility
• *Adult dosage:* 2.5 to 10 mcg/kg/minute given I.V.; infusion rates up to 40 mcg/kg/minute may be needed, but this is rare. Titrate dosage carefully to the patient's response.
• *Action:* Selectively stimulates beta$_1$-adrenergic receptors to increase myocardial contractility and stroke volume, resulting in increased cardiac output. At therapeutic doses, dobutamine decreases afterload, reduces preload, and may facilitate AV node conduction.

Contraindications and cautions
• Don't use in patients with idiopathic hypertrophic cardiomyopathy or those who have a known hypersensitivity to the drug or any of its ingredients. This drug contains sodium bisulfate, which may trigger allergic reactions in patients with sulfite sensitivity.
• Use with extreme caution after MI because it may intensify or extend myocardial ischemia.
• Be aware that dobutamine increases AV conduction. When giving dobutamine to patients with atrial fibrillation, administer drugs that slow AV conduction, such as digitalis glycosides or diltiazem, before giving dobutamine.
• Know that lower doses are indicated for elderly patients, who may be more sensitive to the drug's effects.
• Avoid use in children.

• Because it's not known if dobutamine is excreted in breast milk, administer cautiously to breast-feeding women.
• Pregnancy risk category C

Life-threatening adverse reactions
• PVCs, other arrhythmias
• Anaphylactic reactions

Common adverse reactions
• Increased heart rate, hypertension, PVCs
• Tingling sensation, paresthesia, mild leg cramps
• Vomiting

Infrequent adverse reactions
• Angina, nonspecific chest pain, palpitations, precipitous hypotension
• Dyspnea
• Headache
• Nausea
• Decrease in serum potassium level
• Hypersensitivity reactions (skin, rash, fever, eosinophilia, bronchospasm)

Interactions
• *Nitroprusside:* Concomitant use may cause higher cardiac output and lower PAWP and is often used for these purposes.

For dangerous interactions, see *Life-threatening hazards of multidrug therapy with dobutamine,* page 138.

Interventions
Preparation and administration
• Hypovolemia should be corrected with appropriate plasma volume ex-

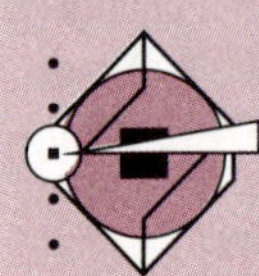

Interactions alert

Life-threatening hazards of multidrug therapy with dobutamine

Interacting drug	Effects
Beta blockers (such as propranolol)	Antagonize dobutamine's effect.
Guanadrel and guanethidine (antihypertensives)	May potentiate the pressor effects of dobutamine, possibly resulting in hypertension and cardiac arrhythmias
Inhalation hydrocarbon anesthetics (such as halothane and cyclopropane)	May trigger ventricular arrhythmias

panders before administration of dobutamine.
• Infuse the drug using a central venous catheter or into a large peripheral vein. Titrate the infusion to the patient's clinical status, as prescribed.

Safety tip. Use an infusion pump or other device to control the flow rate.
• Dilute concentrate for injection before administration. Compatible solutions include D_5W, 0.45% and 0.9% NaCl solution, and lactated Ringer's solution. The contents of one vial (250 mg) diluted with 1,000 ml of solution yields a concentration of 250 mcg/ml; diluted with 500 ml, a concentration of 500 mcg/ml; diluted with 250 ml, a concentration of 1,000 mcg/ml. The premixed solution contains 500 mg in 250 ml of D_5W, providing 2,000 mcg/ml (2 mg/ml).

• Concentration of infusion solution shouldn't exceed 5,000 mcg/ml (5 mg/ml).

Safety tip. Unless you're using a premixed solution, be sure to infuse a newly mixed solution within 24 hours.
• Be aware that pink discoloration of solution indicates slight oxidation but no significant loss of potency.
• Know that dobutamine is incompatible with sodium bicarbonate and certain other drugs. (See *Dobutamine combinations to avoid.*)

Monitoring and supportive care
• Monitor the ECG, blood pressure, cardiac output, and PAWP. Also monitor urine output.
• In patients with CAD, monitor for signs and symptoms of ischemia.
• Most patients experience an increase of 10 to 20 mm Hg in systolic blood pressure; some show an increase of 50 mm Hg or more. Most

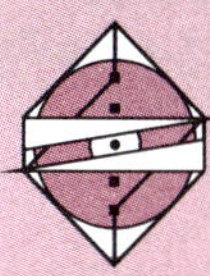

Incompatibility warning
Dobutamine combinations to avoid

Dobutamine is incompatible with sodium bicarbonate. When the two are mixed and left in contact longer than 3 to 4 hours, a precipitate forms, possibly blocking the flow of fluid. Dobutamine is also incompatible with heparin; again, precipitation occurs.

In addition, dobutamine is incompatible with hydrocortisone sodium, succinate, cefazolin, cefamandole, neutral cephalothin, penicillin, and ethacrynate sodium. With these drugs, however, no visible change occurs when mixed with dobutamine.

also experience an increase in heart rate of 5 to 15 beats/minute; some show increases of 30 or more beats/minute. PVCs may also occur in about 5% of patients. Dosage reduction may be necessary when these occur.

• Monitor serum electrolytes. The drug may lower serum potassium levels.

• Avoid extravasation, which may cause an inflammatory response.

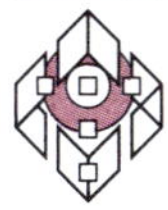

MedTest

1. Peak concentrations of I.V. dobutamine occur within:
  a. 2 minutes.
  b. 10 minutes.
  c. 30 minutes.
  d. 60 minutes.

2. Dobutamine increases myocardial contractility and stroke volume by stimulating:
  a. alpha-adrenergic receptors.
  b. $beta_1$-adrenergic receptors.
  c. $beta_2$-adrenergic receptors.
  d. dopaminergic receptors.

3. Most patients respond to dobutamine with an increase in:
  a. systolic blood pressure of 10 to 20 mm Hg.
  b. systolic blood pressure of 50 mm Hg or more.
  c. heart rate of 15 to 25 beats per minute.
  d. heart rate of 30 or more beats per minute.

Dopamine hydrochloride

Also known by the brand names Intropin, Dopastat, and (in Canada) Revimine, dopamine is an adrenergic agent that's classified therapeutically as an inotropic and a vasopressor. It's available in parenteral concentrates of 40, 80, and 160 mg/ml for injection; and in 0.8 mg/ml (200 or 400 mg), 1.6 mg/ml (400 or 800 mg) and 3.2 mg/ml (800 mg) in D_5W for parenteral infusion.

Pharmacokinetics
• *Absorption:* Onset after I.V. administration occurs within 5 minutes and lasts less than 10 minutes.

• *Distribution:* Doesn't cross the blood-brain barrier.
• *Metabolism:* Metabolized to inactive compounds in the liver, kidneys, and plasma by MAO and catechol-O-methyltransferase. About 25% is metabolized to norepinephrine within adrenergic nerve terminals.
• *Excretion:* In urine, mainly as its metabolites.

Indications, dosage, and action
Adjunctive treatment of shock
• *Adult dosage:* Initially 1 to 20 mcg/kg/minute I.V. Infusion rate may be increased by 1 to 4 mcg/kg/minute at 10- to 30-minute intervals until optimum response is achieved. In severely ill patients, infusion may begin at 5 mcg/kg/minute and gradually increase by increments of 5 to 10 mcg/kg/minute until the optimum response is achieved.

Short-term treatment of chronic CHF and reduced renal perfusion
• *Adult dosage:* Initially, 0.5 to 2 mcg/kg/minute I.V. Dosage may be increased until the desired renal response occurs. Average dosage is 1 to 3 mcg/kg/minute. Dosage over 5 mcg/kg/minute exceeds renal dosage and renal perfusion is no longer enhanced.
• *Action:* An immediate precursor of norepinephrine, dopamine stimulates dopaminergic, beta-adrenergic, and alpha-adrenergic receptors of the sympathetic nervous system. The main effects are dose dependent. It has a direct stimulating effect on $beta_1$-receptors (in I.V. dosages of 2 to 10 mcg/kg/minute), but little or no effect on $beta_2$-receptors. In I.V. dosages of 0.5 to 5 mcg/kg/minute, it acts on dopaminergic receptors, causing vasodilation in the renal, mesenteric, coronary, and intracerebral vascular beds (perhaps lowering blood pressure); in I.V. dosages above 10 mcg/kg/minute, it stimulates alpha-receptors resulting in increased peripheral resistance and renal vasoconstriction.

Contraindications and cautions
• Don't administer to patients with uncorrected tachyarrhythmias or ventricular fibrillation because of the drug's potential for severe cardiovascular effects.
• Administer commercially available dopamine solutions containing sulfites with extreme care to patients with known hypersensitivity to sulfites and to patients with asthma.
• Administer cautiously to patients with ischemic heart disease.
• Know that lower doses are indicated for the elderly, who may be more sensitive to the drug's effects.
• Pregnancy risk category C

Life-threatening adverse reactions
• Ventricular arrhythmias
• Anaphylactic reaction

Common adverse reactions
• Hypotension, ectopic beats, tachycardia, angina, palpitations
• Dyspnea
• Headache, anxiety
• Nausea, vomiting
• Local necrosis and sloughing of tissue (may occur with extravasation)

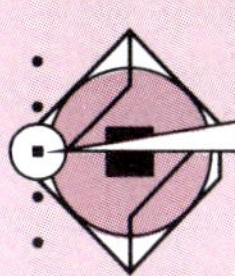

Interactions alert

Life-threatening hazards of multidrug therapy with dopamine

Interacting drug	Effects
Beta blockers (such as propranolol)	Antagonize the cardiac effects of dopamine
Digitalis glycosides (such as digitoxin and digoxin)	Increase risk of cardiac arrhythmias
General anesthetics (such as cyclopropane and halothane)	May cause ventricular arrhythmias and hypertension
I.V. phenytoin (anticonvulsant)	May cause hypotension and bradycardia
Levodopa (antiparkinsonian agent)	Increases risk of cardiac arrhythmias
MAO inhibitors (such as isocarboxazid)	May cause hypertensive crisis
Sympathomimetics (such as ephedrine, epinephrine, and isoproterenol)	Increase risk of cardiac arrhythmias

Infrequent adverse reactions

• Cardiac conduction abnormalities, widened QRS complex, bradycardia, hypertension, vasoconstriction
• Azotemia, hypokalemia
• Piloerection

Interactions

• *Alpha blockers:* May antagonize peripheral vasoconstriction caused by high doses of dopamine.
• *Ergot alkaloids, oxytoxics:* Extreme elevations in blood pressure. Avoid concurrent use.
• *Guanadrel, guanethidine, methyldopa, and trimethaphan:* Dopamine decreases antihypertensive effects of these agents.

For dangerous interactions, see *Life-threatening hazards of multidrug therapy with dopamine.*

Interventions
Preparation and administration
• Hypovolemia should be corrected with appropriate plasma volume expanders before administering dopamine.
• Administer by I.V. infusion using an infusion device to control flow rate.
• Administer dopamine into a large vein. Monitor continuously for free flow. Central venous access is recommended.

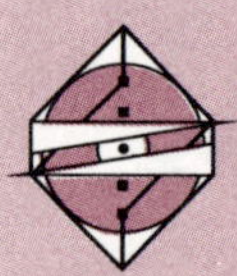

Incompatibility warning

Dopamine combinations to avoid

Dopamine is incompatible with iron salts and oxidizing agents. It's also incompatible with sodium bicarbonate and other alkaline solutions. When combined with sodium bicarbonate, dopamine slowly deteriorates without precipitation but with possible color changes. When dopamine is mixed with iron salts and oxidizing agents, no visible changes may occur.

Safety tip. Assess parenteral infusion sites carefully and frequently for signs of extravasation. If extravasation occurs, stop the infusion, call the doctor, and prepare to infiltrate the site promptly with 5 to 10 mg of phentolamine in 10 to 15 ml of sterile 0.9% NaCl solution for injection. Use a syringe with a fine needle, and infiltrate the area liberally.

• Mix with D₅W, 0.9% NaCl solution, or a combination of both. Unless using a premixed solution, mix the solution just before use. Don't mix with alkaline solutions. (See *Dopamine combinations to avoid.*)

• Don't mix other drugs in dopamine solutions.

Safety tip. Unless you're using a premixed solution, discard the solution after 24 hours, or earlier if it has discolored.

Monitoring and supportive care

• Most patients are satisfactorily maintained on less than 20 mcg/kg/minute.

Safety tip. Some patients may require dosages exceeding 20 mcg/kg/minute to obtain desired systolic pressure. The higher dosages, however, may affect their renal function. Make sure you check their urine output often to assess renal function. Know that higher dosages should be reduced once a patient's hemodynamic condition stabilizes.

• Monitor blood pressure, color and temperature of extremities during infusion and, if possible, cardiac output, cardiac rate and rhythm, CVP, and PAWP.

• If a disproportionate rise in the diastolic pressure (a marked decrease in pulse pressure) is observed in patients receiving dopamine, decrease the infusion rate and observe carefully for further evidence of predominant vasoconstrictor activity.

• Monitor patients with a history of occlusive vascular disease for decreased circulation to extremities.

• In patients with CAD, monitor for signs and symptoms of myocardial ischemia.

• Severe hypotension may result from abrupt withdrawal of the drug. Reduce the dosage gradually, while monitoring blood pressure closely.

• Know that dopamine may cause elevated urine catecholamine levels. It may also cause increased serum glucose levels, although the level usually doesn't rise above normal limits.

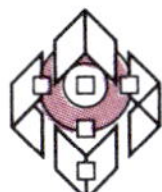 **MedTest**

1. Administer dopamine through a large vein to prevent extravasation and:
   a. local inflammation.
   b. local necrosis and tissue sloughing.
   c. petechiae from capillary injury.
   d. infiltration with local discomfort.

2. If extravasation does occur, you should:
   a. apply ice.
   b. apply heat.
   c. infiltrate the site with a phentolamine solution.
   d. administer a phentolamine solution through the I.V. tubing port.

3. Unless alpha-receptor stimulation and vasoconstriction is the desired response, decrease the infusion rate if the patient demonstrates:
   a. cool, pale extremities.
   b. a marked decrease in pulse pressure.
   c. a falling diastolic pressure.
   d. urine output of 30 ml/hour or more.

Enalaprilat and enalapril maleate

Also known by the brand names Vasotec, and (in Australia) Amprace and Renitec, enalapril is an ACE inhibitor that's classified therapeutically as an antihypertensive. It's avail-

able in 2.5-, 5-, 10-, and 20-mg tablets. The injectable form, enalaprilat, is available in 2-ml vials containing 1.25 mg/ml.

Pharmacokinetics
• *Absorption:* About 60% absorbed from the GI tract; blood pressure decreases within 1 hour, with peak antihypertensive effects in 4 to 6 hours.
• *Distribution:* Doesn't appear to cross the blood-brain barrier, but it does cross the placenta. Drug is 50% to 60% plasma-bound.
• *Metabolism:* Metabolized into the active metabolite enalaprilat.
• *Excretion:* About 94% in urine and feces as enalaprilat and enalapril. The total elimination half-life of enalaprilat is about 11 hours.

Indications, dosage, and action
Mild to severe hypertension
• *Regular adult dosage:* Initially, 5 mg P.O. once daily, then adjusted according to patient's response. Usual dosage range is 10 to 40 mg P.O. daily as a single dose or as two divided doses. Alternatively, patients temporarily unable to take P.O. medications may receive enalaprilat 0.625 to 1.25 mg I.V. q 6 hours, administered over a 5-minute period.
• *Dosage when converting from I.V. therapy to oral therapy:* Initially, 5 mg P.O. once a day. Dosage is adjusted according to response.
• *Dosage when converting from oral therapy to I.V. therapy:* 0.625 to 1.25 mg I.V. over 5 minutes q 6 hours. Higher dosages have not demonstrated greater efficacy.
• *Dosage in renal failure:* In patients with a creatinine clearance below

30 ml/minute, therapy should begin at 2.5 mg/day. Dosage is gradually titrated according to response. Patients undergoing hemodialysis should receive a supplemental dose of 2.5 mg on dialysis days.

• *Action:* Inhibits ACEs, preventing conversion of angiotensin I to angiotensin II, a potent vasoconstrictor. Reduced angiotensin II levels decrease peripheral arterial resistance (lowering blood pressure) and decrease aldosterone secretion (reducing sodium and water retention).

Adjunctive treatment of heart failure (with diuretics and digitalis glycosides)

• *Adult dosage:* Initially, 2.5 mg P.O. b.i.d. Dosage is adjusted based on clinical or hemodynamic response. Usual range is 5 to 20 mg daily in two divided doses; maximum dosage is 40 mg/day.

• *Action:* Enalapril reduces peripheral resistance and decreases afterload, which increases cardiac output.

Contraindications and cautions

• Use enalapril cautiously in collagen vascular disease or autoimmune diseases, and in patients taking drugs that may depress immune function or cause a decreased WBC count. Such patients are at increased risk for developing enalapril-induced neutropenia, especially if they also have renal impairment.

• Use cautiously in renal dysfunction because the drug may worsen this condition.

• Be aware that elderly patients may need lower doses because of impaired drug clearance.

• Because it's distributed into breast milk in trace amounts, avoid use in breast-feeding women.

• Enalapril is contraindicated during pregnancy because ACE inhibitors can cause fetal and neonatal injury or death. The drug should be discontinued as soon as possible. These problems haven't been detected when fetal exposure has been limited to the first trimester.

• Pregnancy risk category C (D in second and third trimesters)

Life-threatening adverse reactions

• MI
• Neutropenia, agranulocytosis
• Angioedema of tongue, glottis, and larynx; fetal and neonatal morbidity; anaphylactic reaction with hemodialysis patients

Common adverse reactions

• Hypotension
• Headache, insomnia, dizziness in patients with heart failure
• Decreased renal function (patients with bilateral renal stenosis or CHF)

Infrequent adverse reactions

• Orthostatic hypotension, hypotension
• Persistent cough, bronchitis, dyspnea, pneumonia
• Fatigue, asthenia, dizziness, vertigo
• Diarrhea, nausea, vomiting
• Urinary tract infection
• Thrombocytopenia, bone marrow depression
• Hyperkalemia
• Rash

Interactions
• *Aspirin, NSAIDs:* May reduce antihypertensive effect. Monitor patient's blood pressure.
• *Diuretics or other antihypertensive drugs:* Enalapril may increase antihypertensive effects of these agents.
• *Insulin, oral antidiabetic agents:* Risk of hypoglycemia, especially at initiation of enalapril therapy. Monitor blood glucose levels closely.
• *Lithium:* Lithium toxicity can result from decreased renal clearance. Monitor lithium levels.
• *Potassium supplements, potassium-sparing diuretics, salt substitutes:* Increased risk of hyperkalemia. Avoid these agents.

Interventions
Preparation and administration
• You may give enalapril before, during, or after meals. Food doesn't appear to affect its absorption. (See *Taking ACE inhibitors at home,* page 87.)
• Once-daily dosing is effective for most patients. You may give the drug in the morning or evening, at the patient's discretion.

Monitoring and supportive care
• Diuretic therapy should be discontinued 2 to 3 days before beginning enalapril therapy to reduce the risk of hypotension. If enalapril doesn't adequately control blood pressure, diuretics may be reinstated.
• Closely monitor patients treated for heart failure because hypotension may occur, especially after the initial dose. Observe the patient for at least 2 hours and then for at least 1 hour after his blood pressure has stabilized.
• You'll usually notice a response to I.V. enalaprilat in 15 minutes, but peak effects may not be seen for up to 4 hours.
• Monitor for signs and symptoms of neutropenia (sore throat and fever), and monitor WBC and differential counts before treatment and periodically thereafter as indicated. The drug should be discontinued if neutropenia occurs.
• Monitor intake and output and daily weight. Because proteinuria and nephrotic syndrome may occur in patients who are on enalapril therapy, monitor urine protein and specific gravity. The drug should be discontinued if renal failure occurs.
• Angioedema (including laryngeal edema) may occur, especially after the first enalapril dose. Assess for and advise the patient to report any signs or symptoms, such as swelling of his face, eyes, lips, or tongue or breathing difficulty.
• Assess for and advise the patient to report light-headedness, which is likely to occur during the first few days of therapy. The dosage may need to be adjusted.
• Assess for loss of taste, which may necessitate discontinuing the drug.
• Know that enalapril may elevate BUN and serum creatinine levels and, less commonly, liver enzyme and bilirubin levels; it may slightly decrease hemoglobin and hematocrit levels. Rare cases of thrombocytopenia and bone marrow depression also have been reported.

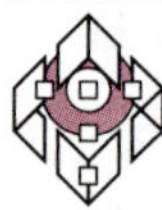

MedTest

1. The peak antihypertensive effect
of enalapril given P.O. occurs within:
    a. 1 hour.
    b. 4 to 6 hours.
    c. 12 to 24 hours.
    d. 2 to 3 days.

2. Enalapril should be administered:
    a. a.c.
    b. with meals.
    c. p.c.
    d. without regard to meals.

3. Enalapril may have to be discontinued if the patient experiences:
    a. light-headedness or dizziness.
    b. a sore throat or fever.
    c. loss of taste.
    d. a weight gain of more than 5 lb
    (2.3 kg) per week.

Epinephrine hydrochloride

Also known by the brand name Ad-
renalin Chloride, epinephrine is an
adrenergic that's classified therapeutically as a bronchodilator, vasopressor, and cardiac stimulant. It's available for parenteral injection and
comes in vials and ampules of
0.01 mg/ml (1:100,000), 0.1 mg/ml
(1:10,000), 0.5 mg/ml (1:2,000),
1 mg/ml (1:1,000); and in a 5-mg/ml
(1:200) parenteral suspension.

Pharmacokinetics
• *Absorption:* Rapid onset of action
after I.V. administration; 3- to 5-min-
ute onset after endotracheal administration. Drug peaks within 20 minutes. Duration is 20 to 30 minutes after I.V. dose; 1 to 3 hours after endotracheal dose.
• *Distribution:* Widely in the body.
• *Metabolism:* By MAO in sympathetic nerve endings, the liver, and other
tissues to inactive metabolites.
• *Excretion:* In urine, mainly as its
metabolites and conjugates.

Indications, dosage, and action
**Restoration of cardiac rhythm in
cardiac arrest and during CPR**
• *Adult dosage:* Initially, 0.5 to 1 mg
I.V. Range is 0.1 to 1 mg (1 to 10 ml
of a 1:10,000 solution). May be given
intracardiac if no I.V. route is available. Alternatively, may be given by
injection into the endotracheal tube;
however, dosage is 2 to 2½ times the
I.V. dose. May be repeated q 5 minutes if needed. Some clinicians advo-
cate higher dose (up to 0.1 mg/kg).
Initial dose may be followed by 1- to
4-mcg/minute I.V. infusion.
• *Pediatric dosage:* Initially, 0.01 mg/
kg (0.1 ml/kg of a 1:10,000 solution)
by I.V. bolus; may be repeated q 5 minutes if needed. Alternatively, 0.1 mcg/
kg/minute initially; may increase in
increments of 0.1 mcg/kg/minute to a
maximum of 1 mcg/kg/minute.

For neonates, give 0.01 to
0.03 mg/kg (0.1 to 0.3 ml/kg of a
1:10,000 solution) by I.V. bolus or
intratracheal injection. May be repeated q 5 minutes if needed.
• *Action:* Epinephrine stimulates al-
pha-, beta$_1$- and beta$_2$-adrenergic re-

ceptors. Alpha-adrenergic stimulation causes peripheral vasconstriction. $Beta_1$-adrenergic stimulation causes increased cardiac output and heart rate. $Beta_2$-receptor stimulation causes dilation of large blood vessels in skeletal muscle and bronchodilation.

Epinephrine increases cardiac output, but decreases cardiac efficiency. Myocardial oxygen consumption is also increased. Systolic blood pressure increases, but diastolic pressure may decrease because of the drug's effect on larger blood vessels.

Contraindications and cautions
• Avoid use in patients with organic heart disease, cardiac dilation, and arrhythmias (except during cardiac arrest) because it increases myocardial oxygen demand.
• Don't use in patients with organic brain damage or cerebral arteriosclerosis because of potential adverse CNS effects.
• Avoid use in patients with acute angle-closure glaucoma because the drug may worsen the condition.
• Use cautiously in elderly patients, diabetic patients, and those with CV diseases or hypertension, histories of sensitivity to sympathomimetics, Parkinson's disease (temporary increase in tremor or rigidity), psychoneurotic disorders, or hyperthyroidism.
• Use cautiously in patients with sulfite hypersensitivity; some epinephrine preparations contain sulfites.
• Be aware that epinephrine may delay the second stage of labor in pregnant women and may also cause anoxia in the fetus. However, epineph-

rine added to epidural anesthestics is safe.
• Because it's excreted in breast milk, avoid use in breast-feeding women.
• Pregnancy risk category C

Life-threatening adverse reactions
• MI, ventricular fibrillation
• Apnea
• CVA

Common adverse reactions
• Palpitations, tachycardia
• Headache, tremor, dizziness, lightheadedness, nervousness

Infrequent adverse reactions
• ECG changes, (decreased T-wave amplitude), angina, arrhythmias, syncope, hypertension
• Pulmonary edema, dyspnea
• Fear, anxiety, restlessness, sleeplessness, excitability, weakness, disorientation, impaired memory, hallucinations, suicidal tendencies
• Nausea, vomiting
• Sweating, pallor, contact dermatitis, extravasation injury (local necrosis at injection site)

Interactions
• *Antidiabetic agents:* Epinephrine raises blood glucose levels; dosage adjustments may be necessary.
• *Anticholinergics, antihistamines, thyroid hormones, tricyclic antidepressants:* May cause severe adverse cardiac effects when given with sympathomimetics. Avoid giving together.

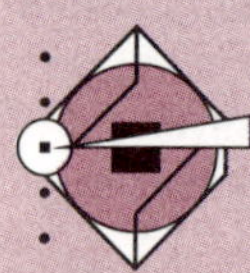

Interactions alert

Life-threatening hazards of multidrug therapy with epinephrine

Interacting drug	Effects
Alpha-adrenergic blocking agents (such as doxazosin)	May cause profound hypotension and tachycardia
Beta-adrenergic blocking agents (such as propranolol)	May cause severe vasoconstriction and reflex bradycardia
Cyclopropane or halogenated hydrocarbon general anesthetics (such as halothane)	Increase risk of life-threatening ventricular arrhythmias
Digitalis glycosides (such as digoxin)	Increase risk of life-threatening ventricular arrhythmias
Levodopa (antiparksonian agent)	Increases risk of life-threatening cardiac arrhythmias
MAO inhibitors (such as isocarboxazid)	Increase risk of hypertensive crisis

• *Doxapram, mazindol, methylphenidate:* Enhanced CNS stimulation or pressor effects.

• *Ergot alkaloids:* Enhanced vasoconstrictor activity and severe hypertension.

• *Phenothiazines:* Because phenothiazines block alpha-adrenergic receptors, don't use epinephrine to treat hypotension caused by phenothiazines because it may worsen hypotension.

• *Sympathomimetics:* Concomitant use with epinephrine may produce additive effects and toxicity.

For dangerous interactions, see *Life-threatening hazards of multidrug therapy with epinephrine.*

Interventions
Preparation and administration

Safety tip. To avoid hazardous medication errors, carefully check the type of solution prescribed and its concentration, dosage, and route before administration.

• Don't use a preparation that's discolored or contains a precipitate. Discard solutions after 24 hours or if they're discolored.

• Before withdrawing epinephrine suspension into a syringe, shake the vial or ampule thoroughly to disperse particles; then inject it promptly.

Safety tip. A tuberculin syringe may assure greater accuracy in measurement of parenteral doses.

• Don't mix with an alkaline solution such as sodium bicarbonate, or oxidiz-

ing agents such as nitrates, or nitrites. Use D₅W, 0.9% NaCl solution, or a combination of both. Mix just before use. Check with a pharmacist for specific compatability information before using with any drug or solution.
• Keep the solution in a light-resistant container.

Monitoring and supportive care
• Monitor vital signs and urine output. Epinephrine may widen pulse pressure.
• Place patients receiving I.V. epinephrine on a cardiac monitor. Keep resuscitation equipment available.
• When this drug is administered I.V., check the patient's blood pressure repeatedly during the first 5 minutes and then q 3 to 5 minutes until he's stable.
• Know that intracardiac administration requires external cardiac massage to move the drug into coronary circulation.
• In the event of a sharp blood pressure rise, rapid-acting vasodilators, such as nitrites or alpha-adrenergic blocking agents, should be given to counteract the marked pressor effect of large doses of epinephrine.
• Observe the patient closely for adverse reactions. If adverse reactions develop, the dosage may need to be adjusted or the drug discontinued.
• The drug's drying effect on bronchial secretions may make mucus plugs more difficult to dislodge. Institute a bronchial hygiene program, including postural drainage, breathing exercises, and adequate hydration. Monitor the amount, consistency, and color of sputum.

• Epinephrine may increase blood glucose levels. Closely observe patients with diabetes for hyperglycemia.
• Be aware that epinephrine raises serum lactic acid and BUN levels and interferes with tests for urinary catecholamines.

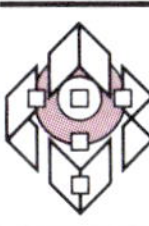 **MedTest**

1. In cardiac arrest, if an I.V. site is not available, the next best administration route for epinephrine is:
   a. intracardiac.
   b. subcutaneous.
   c. intramuscular.
   d. intratracheal.

2. While administering epinephrine I.V., you should monitor cardiac status continually and the patient's blood pressure:
   a. repeatedly during the first 5 minutes and then q 3 to 5 minutes until stable.
   b. q 2 minutes for 30 minutes, then q 5 minutes for 30 minutes, and then hourly.
   c. q 5 minutes for 1 hour, then q 15 minutes × 4, then q 30 minutes × 4, then hourly × 4, and then p.r.n.
   d. q 5 minutes × 4, then q 10 minutes × 4, then q 15 minutes × 4, then q 30 minutes × 4, then q 1 hour × 4, and then q 4 hours.

3. If epinephrine is administered by intracardiac injection, it will require:
   a. follow-up I.V. dosing as soon as a route is available.

b. external cardiac massage to move the drug into coronary circulation.

c. a 15-second break in CPR to allow the drug to reach coronary circulation.

d. follow-up S.C. doses (massaged well) q 5 minutes.

Esmolol

Also known by the brand name Brevibloc, esmolol is a $beta_1$-adrenergic blocker that's classified therapeutically as a class II antiarrhythmic agent. It's available for injection and comes in 10-ml ampules containing 250 mg/ml and in 10-ml vials containing 10 mg/ml.

Pharmacokinetics
- *Absorption:* Given by I.V. infusion.
- *Distribution:* Rapidly throughout the plasma. Drug is 55% protein-bound.
- *Metabolism:* Hydrolyzed rapidly by plasma esterases.
- *Excretion:* By kidneys as metabolites. Elimination half-life is about 9 minutes.

Indications, dosage, and action
Supraventricular tachycardia
- *Adult dosage:* The dosage range is 50 to 200 mcg/kg/minute; the average dose is 100 mcg/kg/minute. Individual dosage adjustment requires stepped titration, in which each step consists of a loading dose followed by a maintenance dose.

To begin treatment, administer a loading infusion of 500 mcg/kg/minute (0.5 mg/kg/minute) for 1 minute followed by a 4-minute maintenance infusion of 50 mcg/kg/minute. If tachycardia doesn't subside within 5 minutes, repeat the loading dose and follow with a maintenance infusion of 100 mcg/kg/minute. Continue titration, repeating loading infusion and increasing each maintenance infusion by 50 mcg/kg/minute. As the patient's heart rate or blood pressure reaches a safety end point, omit the loading infusion and reduce the increase in maintenance infusion from 50 to 25 mcg/kg/minute or less; also, increase the interval between titration steps from 5 to 10 minutes.
- *Action:* Esmolol selectively blocks $beta_1$-adrenergic receptors. It rapidly decreases blood pressure and heart rate because of its rapid onset. It prolongs sinus node recovery time, increases sinus cycle length, and slows conduction in the AV node.

Contraindications and cautions
- Because the drug may worsen cardiac depression, don't give it to patients with cardiac failure, cardiogenic shock, second- or third-degree AV block, or sinus bradycardia.
- Use esmolol, like all beta blockers, with caution in atopic patients and patients with bronchial asthma, emphysema, or bronchitis because it may precipitate bronchospasm.
- Use cautiously in diabetes because esmolol may mask tachycardia associated with hypoglycemia.
- Use cautiously in elderly patients.
- Pregnancy risk category C

Life-threatening adverse reactions
- CHF
- Bronchospasm
- Seizures

Common adverse reactions
- Hypotension (20% to 50%) with 12% of it symptomatic and dose related
- Nausea
- Local induration or inflammation at infusion site
- Pain, fever

Infrequent adverse reactions
- Peripheral ischemia, pallor, flushing, diaphoresis, bradycardia, chest pain, syncope, pulmonary edema, heart block
- Breathing difficulty, wheezing
- Speech disorders, dizziness, somnolence, confusion, paresthesia, headache, agitation, fatigue, depression, anxiety
- Vomiting, anorexia
- Urine retention
- Nasal congestion
- Local edema, local erythema

Interactions
- *Antihypertensives:* Concomitant use may potentiate the hypotensive effects of antihypertensives and require dosage adjustments based on blood pressure measurements.
- *Digoxin:* Esmolol may increase serum digoxin levels by 10% to 20%.
- *Insulin or oral antidiabetic agents:* Concurrent use with esmolol may mask symptoms of developing hypoglycemia, such as rising pulse rate and blood pressure.

- *Morphine:* May increase esmolol blood levels by up to 50%. Titrate esmolol carefully.
- *Nondepolarizing neuromuscular blocking agents such as gallamine, metocurine, pancuronium, or tubocurarine; succinylcholine:* Esmolol may potentiate and prolong neuromuscular blockade.
- *Sympathomimetic amines having beta-adrenergic stimulant activity:* Concurrent use with esmolol may cause mutual inhibition.
- *Xanthines, especially aminophylline or theophylline:* Use with esmolol may cause mutual inhibition of therapeutic effects and (except for dyphylline) decrease theophylline clearance, especially in patients with increased theophylline clearance induced by smoking. Concurrent use requires careful monitoring to prevent toxic accumulation of theophylline.

For dangerous interactions, see *Life-threatening hazards of multidrug therapy with esmolol,* page 152.

Interventions
Preparation and administration
- Dilute 10-ml ampules of esmolol for I.V. infusion. Vials containing 10 ml in a concentration of 10 mg/ml don't require dilution. To prepare esmolol injection for I.V. infusion, use a 500-ml bottle of I.V. fluid (5% dextrose injection, 5% dextrose in Ringer's injection, 5% dextrose in 0.45% NaCl injection, 5% dextrose in 0.9% NaCl injection, lactated Ringer's injection, 0.45% NaCl injection, or 0.9% NaCl injection). Add 5 g of esmolol injection (two 10-ml ampules containing 250 mg/ml each) to the bottle to

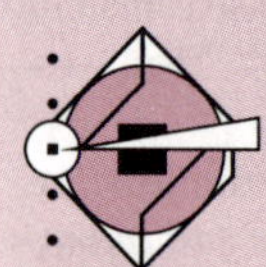

Interactions alert

Life-threatening hazards of multidrug therapy with esmolol

Interacting drug	Effects
Reserpine (rauwolfia alkaloid)	May result in bradycardia and hypotension
Verapamil (calcium channel blocker)	May result in severe cardiac depression or arrest

produce a solution containing approximately 10 mg/ml of esmolol.
• Be aware that esmolol isn't compatible with 5% sodium bicarbonate injection and certain drugs. (See *Esmolol combinations to avoid*.)
• Know that diluted solutions of esmolol hydrochloride are stable for at least 24 hours at room temperature.
• Don't give esmolol by I.V. push; use a controlled infusion device. Use of butterfly needles for I.V. administration of esmolol isn't recommended.
Safety tip. Concentrations that exceed 10 mg/ml of esmolol may produce irritation. If irritation occurs at the infusion site, stop the infusion and resume it at another site.

Monitoring and supportive care
• Be aware that esmolol has an extremely short duration of action and can be accurately titrated, making it superior to other beta blockers in treating cardiac arrhythmias.
• Know that many of the drug interactions associated with other beta blockers don't apply to esmolol

because of its short duration of action and the short periods of time over which it's used.
• Monitor the patient's ECG and blood pressure continuously during infusion, especially if the patient's pretreatment blood pressure was low.
• Hypotension is common and can usually be reversed by decreasing or stopping the infusion.
• Esmolol shouldn't be administered for longer than 48 hours.
• When the patient's heart rate stabilizes, esmolol will be replaced by longer-acting antiarrhythmics, such as propranolol, digoxin, or verapamil. As the replacement drug is started, you will gradually reduce the esmolol infusion over 1 hour, cutting it by 50% 30 minutes after you have administered the first dose of the alternative agent. Discontinue esmolol if the second dose of the alternative agent maintains a satisfactory response during the first hour.

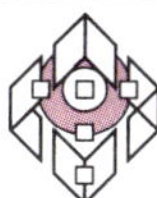 **MedTest**

1. To achieve an antiarrhythmic effect, administer esmolol:
   a. P.O.
   b. S.C.
   c. I.M.
   d. I.V.

2. During treatment with esmolol, monitor the patient's:
   a. ABGs and oxygen saturation.
   b. ECG and blood pressure.
   c. apical pulse rate and hourly urine output.
   d. PAWP and cardiac output.

3. Following the initial loading dose and maintenance therapy, tachycardia should subside within:
   a. 5 minutes.
   b. 15 minutes.
   c. 30 minutes.
   d. 1 hour.

Ethacrynate sodium and ethacrynic acid

Also known by the brand names Edecrin, Edecrin Sodium, and (in Australia) Edecril, ethacrynic acid is a loop diuretic. It's available in 25- and 50-mg tablets, and in a 50-mg vial for injection.

Pharmacokinetics

• *Absorption:* Tablets absorbed rapidly from GI tract; diuresis occurs in 30

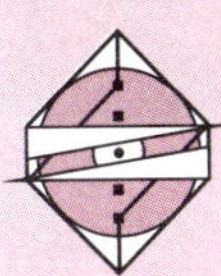

Esmolol can be incompatible with 5% sodium bicarbonate injection; deterioration can occur, but with no precipitation. Esmolol is incompatible with furosemide (with visible precipitation) as well as with diazepam and thiopental sodium (with visible changes).

minutes and peaks in 2 hours. After I.V. administration of ethacrynate sodium, diuresis occurs in 5 minutes and peaks in 15 to 30 minutes.

• *Distribution:* In animal studies, drug accumulates in the liver. It doesn't enter the CSF, and its distribution into breast milk or the placenta is unknown.

• *Metabolism:* In animals, metabolized by the liver to a potentially active metabolite.

• *Excretion:* Animal studies show that 30% to 65% of ethacrynate sodium is excreted in urine and 35% to 40% is excreted in bile as metabolite. Duration of action is 6 to 8 hours after oral administration and about 2 hours after I.V. administration.

Indications, dosage, and action

Acute pulmonary edema

• *Adult dosage:* 50 to 100 mg of ethacrynate sodium I.V. slowly over several minutes.

Edema
• *Adult dosage:* 50 to 200 mg P.O. daily. Refractory cases may require up to 200 mg b.i.d.
• *Pediatric dosage:* Initially, 25 mg P.O., given cautiously and increased in 25-mg increments daily until desired effect is achieved.
• *Dosage for neonates and infants:* 0.5 to 1 mg/kg (not approved).
• *Action:* Ethacrynic acid inhibits sodium and chloride reabsorption in the proximal part of the ascending loop of Henle, promoting the excretion of sodium, water, chloride, and potassium.

Contraindications and cautions
• Avoid use in patients with anuria, hypotension, dehydration with low serum sodium levels, or metabolic alkalosis with hypokalemia because the drug may exacerbate these conditions.
• Use cautiously in patients with cirrhosis, especially those with a history of previous electrolyte imbalance or hepatic encephalopathy.
• Use carefully in diabetes because the drug may alter carbohydrate metabolism.
• Use with caution in patients with increasing azotemia or oliguria because hearing impairment has occurred in these patients.
• Give cautiously to patients receiving digitalis glycosides because ethacrynic acid–induced hypokalemia may predispose such patients to digitalis toxicity.
• Know that the drug may need to be discontinued if excessive diuresis, electrolyte imbalances, increasing azotemia, oliguria, hematuria, bloody stools, or severe or watery diarrhea occurs.
• Closely observe elderly and debilitated patients, who are more susceptible to drug-induced diuresis. Reduced dosages may be indicated.
• Avoid use in breast-feeding women.
• Pregnancy risk category B

Life-threatening adverse reactions
• Hepatic coma in patients with liver disease
• Renal failure
• Agranulocytosis, thrombotic episodes due to hemoconcentrations of plasma
• Dehydration, electrolyte imbalance

Common adverse reactions
None noted

Infrequent adverse reactions
• Orthostatic hypotension, volume depletion and dehydration
• Headache, fatigue, apprehension, confusion
• Abdominal discomfort and pain, diarrhea, acute pancreatitis, GI bleeding, anorexia, vomiting
• Transient or permanent deafness (especially with I.V. injection or high-dose oral therapy), tinnitus, vertigo
• Hematuria, agranulocytosis, neutropenia, thrombocytopenia
• Hypochloremic alkalosis; asymptomatic hyperuricemia; fluid and electrolyte imbalances, including hypokalemia, hypocalcemia, hypomagnesemia, and hyponatremia; hyper-

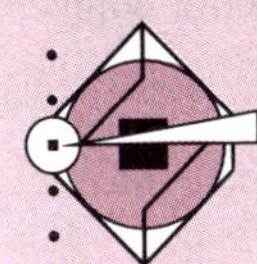

Hazards of multidrug therapy with ethacrynic acid

Interacting drug	Effects
Amphotericin B (antifungal agent)	May cause severe potassium loss
Antihypertensives (such as carteolol)	May potentiate the hypotensive effects of antihypertensives
Corticosteroids (such as prednisone)	May cause severe potassium loss
Digoxin	May deplete potassium, potentially leading to digoxin toxicity

glycemia and impairment of glucose tolerance
- Dermatitis
- Fever, chills

Interactions
- *Aminoglycoside antibiotics:* Potentiated ototoxic adverse effects for both ethacrynic acid and aminoglycosides. Use together cautiously.
- *Diuretics:* Concomitant use of ethacrynic acid with other diuretics may enhance the diuretic effect of other drugs; reduce dosage when adding ethacrynic acid to a diuretic regimen.
- *Insulin or oral antidiabetic agents:* Diabetic patients may need increased dosages when taking ethacrynic acid.
- *Lithium:* Ethacrynic acid may reduce renal clearance of lithium, elevating serum lithium levels. Monitor lithium levels.
- *NSAIDs:* Decreased diuretic effectiveness. Use together cautiously.
- *Potassium-sparing diuretics:* Concomitant use with these agents (spironolactone, triamterene, amiloride) may decrease the potassium loss induced by ethacrynic acid and may be a therapeutic advantage.
- *Warfarin:* Potentiated anticoagulant effect. Use together cautiously.

For dangerous interactions, see *Hazards of multidrug therapy with ethacrynic acid.*

Interventions
Preparation and administration
- Give P.O. doses in the morning to prevent nocturia.
- Tell the patient that he may take the medicine on an empty stomach. However, if the drug upsets his stomach, he may take it with milk or meals. (See *Taking loop diuretics at home,* page 98.)
- Don't give ethacrynate sodium I.M. or S.C. because it may cause severe local pain and irritation. When giving I.V., check infusion site frequently

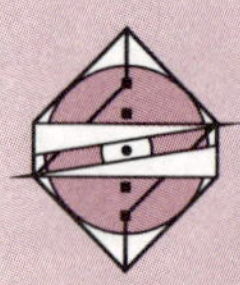

Incompatibility warning

Ethacrynate combinations to avoid

Because hemolysis may occur, don't mix ethacrynate sodium with whole blood or blood products. Ethacrynate is also incompatible with balanced electrolyte maintenance solutions, although a mixture of the two may be accompanied by no visible changes. It's also incompatible with solutions of hydralazine HCl, procainamide HCl, or tolazoline HCl; decomposition may occur, but with no visible change.

for infiltration (edema or skin blanching).

• For I.V. use, reconstitute the vacuum vial with 50 ml of D_5W or 0.9% NaCl solution. Discard unused solution after 24 hours. Don't use cloudy or opaque solutions.

• Give ethacrynate sodium slowly over 20 to 30 minutes by I.V. infusion, or by direct I.V. injection over a period of several minutes. Rapid injection may cause hypotension.

• Don't administer ethacrynate sodium simultaneously with whole blood or blood products. (See *Ethacrynate combinations to avoid*.)

Monitoring and supportive care

• This drug is a very potent diuretic. Monitor the patient's fluid intake and output, weight, blood pressure, and serum electrolyte levels.

• Watch for signs of hypokalemia (for example, muscle weakness and cramps). Potassium chloride supplements may be needed.

• Consult with the doctor and dietitian to provide a high-potassium diet if indicated. Foods rich in potassium include citrus fruits, tomatoes, bananas, dates, and apricots.

• Periodic assessment of the patient's hearing should be performed, especially in patients receiving high-dose therapy.

• Observe for diarrhea or runny stools. Severe diarrhea may necessitate discontinuing the drug.

• Monitor serum uric acid levels, especially in patients with a history of gout.

• Be aware that ethacrynic acid therapy alters electrolyte balances and liver and renal function tests.

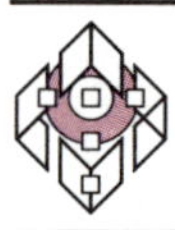

MedTest

1. Ethacrynic acid's diuretic action in the proximal part of the ascending loop of Henle promotes excretion of:

    a. water.

    b. sodium and water.

    c. sodium, water, chloride, and potassium.

    d. potassium and water.

2. When assessing patients taking ethacrynic acid, be particularly alert for:

    a. weight loss.

    b. electrolyte imbalances.

    c. orthostatic hypotension.

    d. hearing loss.

3. The proper diluent for reconstituting ethacrynic acid is:

   a. D_5W or 0.9% NaCl solution.

   b. bacteriostatic water for injection.

   c. 0.45% NaCl solution.

   d. the special diluent supplied with the vacuum vial.

Flecainide acetate

Also known by the brand name Tambocor, flecainide is a benzamide-derivative, local anesthetic (amide) that's classified therapeutically as a ventricular antiarrhythmic agent. It's available in 50-, 100-, and 150-mg tablets.

Pharmacokinetics

• *Absorption:* Rapidly and almost completely from GI tract; bioavailability of tablets is 85% to 90%. Peak plasma levels usually occur within 3 hours.

• *Distribution:* About 40% bound to plasma proteins. Trough serum levels ranging from 0.2 to 1 mcg/ml provide the greatest therapeutic benefit. Trough serum levels higher than 0.7 mcg/ml are associated with adverse effects.

• *Metabolism:* In the liver to active and inactive metabolites. About 30% of an oral dose is excreted in urine unchanged.

• *Excretion:* Elimination half-life averages about 20 hours. Plasma half-life may be longer in CHF and renal disease.

Indications, dosage, and action
Life-threatening sustained VT

• *Adult dosage:* 100 mg P.O. q 12 hours; may be increased in increments of 50 mg b.i.d. every 4 days until efficacy is achieved. Maximum dosage is 400 mg daily for most patients with VT.

Paroxysmal atrial flutter and PSVT in the absence of structural heart defects

• *Regular adult dosage:* 50 mg q 12 hours; may be increased in increments of 50 mg b.i.d. every 4 days until efficacy is achieved. Maximum daily dosage for most patients with paroxysmal atrial flutter or PSVT is 300 mg. In patients with CHF or myocardial dysfunction, initial dosage shouldn't exceed 100 mg q 12 hours; common initial dosage is 50 mg q 12 hours.

• *Dosage in renal failure:* In patients with a creatinine clearance below 35 ml/minute, therapy should begin at 50 mg b.i.d.; dosage should be increased cautiously at intervals longer than 4 days.

• *Action:* A class Ic antiarrhythmic agent, flecainide suppresses SA node automaticity and prolongs conduction in the atria, AV node, ventricles, accessory pathways, and His-Purkinje system. It has the most pronounced effect on the His-Purkinje system, as shown by QRS-complex widening, leading to a prolonged QT interval. The drug has relatively little effect on action potential duration except in Purkinje's fibers, where it shortens the duration. An arrhythmogenic action may result from the drug's potent effects on the conduction system. Effects on the sinus node are strongest in patients with sinus node disease. Flecainide also exerts a moderate negative inotropic effect. All class I drugs have membrane-stabilizing effects.

Contraindications and cautions

- Don't use in patients with significant conduction delay, including second- or third-degree AV block, SSS, and right bundle-branch heart block with bifascicular block (unless a pacemaker is in place) because it may further depress cardiac conduction.
- Don't use in cardiogenic shock because of the drug's mild negative inotropic and arrhythmogenic effects.
- Use with caution in patients with preexisting sinus node dysfunction because it may cause marked effects on the sinus node.
- Use carefully in patients with permanent artificial pacemakers or temporary pacing electrodes because the drug may increase pacing thresholds and suppress ventricular escape rhythms.
- Use with caution in preexisting left ventricular dysfunction or sustained VT because the drug may cause arrhythmogenic effects.
- Use cautiously in hepatic or renal dysfunction because these conditions can cause increased drug levels and subsequent toxicity. Dosage reduction may be necessary and patients should be monitored for signs of toxicity. Serum levels also must be monitored.
- The drug should be discontinued if CHF worsens; if QT is prolonged 25% over baseline; or if unexplained jaundice, signs of hepatic dysfunction, or blood dyscrasias develop.
- Because elderly patients are more susceptible to adverse reactions, monitor them carefully.
- Flecainide is excreted in breast milk; avoid its use in breast-feeding women.
- Pregnancy risk category C

Life-threatening adverse reactions

- Cardiac arrest, new or worsened arrhythmias, CHF

Common adverse reactions

- Dyspnea
- Dizziness (19%), headache, fatigue
- Palpitations (with dosage of 400 mg/day)
- Nausea
- Blurred vision and other visual disturbances (16%)

Infrequent adverse reactions

- Edema, chest pain, tachycardia, palpitations (decreased incidence with 200 to 300 mg/day)
- Dyspnea (4% incidence with doses of 400 mg/day)
- Fatigue, malaise, asthenia, tremor
- Constipation, abdominal pain
- Fever

Interactions

- *Amiodarone:* May increase serum flecainide levels. Monitor for toxicity.
- *Beta-adrenergic blockers, propranolol:* Increase of 20% to 30% in both flecainide and propranolol plasma levels; may cause additive negative inotropic effects.
- *Cimetidine:* May decrease both the renal and nonrenal clearance of flecainide. Monitor for toxicity.

• *Digitalis glycosides:* Flecainide may increase plasma digoxin levels by 15% to 25%. Monitor for digoxin toxicity.

• *Disopyramide:* May cause an additive negative inotropic effect.

• *Urine acidifying and alkalinizing agents, such as ammonium chloride, high-dose antacids, carbonic anhydrase inhibitors, or sodium bicarbonate:* Extremes of urine pH may substantially alter excretion of flecainide (alkalinization decreases renal flecainide excretion, and acidification increases it). Monitor for possible subtherapeutic or toxic levels and effects.

• *Verapamil:* May have an additive negative inotropic effect and may exacerbate AV node dysfunction.

Interventions

Preparation and administration

• You may administer flecainide without regard to food. (See *Taking antiarrhythmics at home*, page 74.)

• Loading doses shouldn't be given because they may exacerbate arrhythmias. Dosage should be adjusted at intervals of at least 4 days because of this drug's long half-life.

• You can give most patients the drug on a q 12 hour dosage schedule, but you may need to give the drug to some q 8 hours.

Monitoring and supportive care

• Hypokalemia or hyperkalemia may alter drug effects and should be corrected before beginning drug therapy.

• Flecainide therapy should be started in the hospital with careful monitoring of patients with symptomatic CHF, sinus node dysfunction, sus-

tained VT, or underlying structural heart disease.

• Also monitor patients changing from another antiarrhythmic if discontinuation of that antiarrhythmic is likely to cause life-threatening arrhythmias.

Safety tip. Monitor patients for increasing signs and symptoms of CHF (dyspnea, fatigue, fluid retention), and monitor the ECG for worsening or development of arrhythmias.

• You may need to administer I.V. lidocaine for the first 3 to 5 days of therapy because this drug's full therapeutic effect may not be evident for that duration.

Safety tip. Periodically monitor serum flecainide levels, especially in patients with renal failure or CHF.

• For patients with artificial pacemakers, the patient's pacing threshold should be determined before administering the drug, after 1 week of therapy, and regularly thereafter. The drug shouldn't be given to patients with preexisting poor thresholds or nonprogrammable artificial pacemakers unless pacing rescue is available.

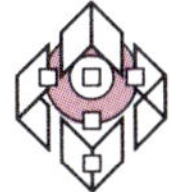 **MedTest**

---

1. When initiating therapy with flecainide, closely monitor the patient's:

   a. heart rate and rhythm.

   b. CVP.

   c. blood pressure.

   d. PAWP.

2. Dosage increases of 50 mg should occur q:
    a. 12 hours.
    b. 24 hours.
    c. 72 hours.
    d. 4 days.

3. While awaiting full therapeutic effect, the patient may be maintained on I.V.:
    a. propranolol.
    b. procainamide.
    c. lidocaine.
    d. amrinone.

Fosinopril sodium

Also known by the brand name Monopril, fosinopril is an ACE inhibitor that's classified therapeutically as an antihypertensive agent. It's available in 10- and 20-mg tablets.

Pharmacokinetics

• *Absorption:* About 36% slowly through GI tract.
• *Distribution:* More than 95% protein-bound. Peak concentrations occur in about 3 hours.
• *Metabolism:* Hydrolyzed mainly in the liver and intestinal wall by esterases to its active metabolite fosinoprilat, which has a half-life of about 12 hours.
• *Excretion:* Half excreted in urine, half in feces.

Indications, dosage, and action
Hypertension
• *Adult dosage:* Initially, 10 mg P.O. daily; dosage should be adjusted based on blood pressure response at peak and trough levels. Usual daily dosage is 20 to 40 mg up to a maximum of 80 mg. Dosage may be divided.
• *Action:* Fosinopril lowers blood pressure by inhibiting ACE, which prevents conversion of angiotensin I to angiotensin II. Reduced formation of angiotensin II decreases peripheral arterial resistance, which results in decreased aldosterone secretion. This reduces sodium and water retention and lowers blood pressure.

Contraindications and cautions
• Use with caution in patients taking potassium-containing salts or sodium substitutes, in those with impaired liver function, and in those undergoing surgery.
• Don't use in children.
• Avoid use in breast-feeding women; significant levels have been detected in breast milk.
• Pregnancy risk category D

Life-threatening adverse reactions
• MI, hypertensive crisis
• Bronchospasm
• Neutropenia, agranulocytosis
• Angioedema of tongue, glottis, or larynx
• Fetal or neonatal mortality when administered to pregnant women

Common adverse reactions
• None noted

Infrequent adverse reactions
• Chest pain, angina, rhythm disturbances, palpitations, hypotension, flushing, claudication, orthostatic hypotension

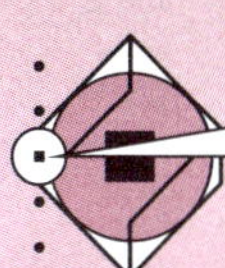

Interactions alert

Hazards of multidrug therapy with fosinopril

Interacting drug	Effects
Diuretics (such as hydrochlorothiazide)	Cause excessive hypotension, especially if patient is volume depleted
Lithium	May increase lithium levels and cause symptoms of lithium toxicity
Potassium-sparing diuretics (such as spironolactone)	May cause hyperkalemia
Potassium supplements (such as potassium chloride)	May cause hyperkalemia

- Cough, pharyngitis, laryngitis, hoarseness
- CVA
- Headache, dizziness, fatigue, lightheadedness, syncope, memory disturbances, mood change, paresthesia, sleep disturbance, drowsiness, weakness
- Nausea and vomiting, diarrhea, pancreatitis, hepatitis, dysphagia, abdominal distention, abdominal pain, flatulence, constipation, heartburn, appetite change, weight change, dry mouth, jaundice
- Sexual dysfunction, decreased libido, urinary frequency, renal insufficiency, acute renal failure
- Tinnitus, vision disturbances, eye irritation, epistaxis, sinusitis, rhinitis
- Lymphadenopathy, neutropenia, agranulocytosis, pancytopenia, anemia, thrombocytopenia
- Hyperkalemia, hypernatremia
- Urticaria, rash, photosensitivity, pruritus
- Angioedema, fever, musculoskeletal pain, gout

Interactions
- *Antacids:* May impair absorption. Separate administration times by at least 2 hours.
- *Sodium substitutes containing potassium:* Risk of hyperkalemia. Avoid concomitant use. Monitor potassium levels.

For dangerous interactions, see *Hazards of multidrug therapy with fosinopril.*

Interventions
Preparation and administration
- You may give fosinopril with or without food. (See *Taking ACE inhibitors at home,* page 87.)
- Give antacids 2 hours before or after fosinopril.

Monitoring and supportive care
• Assess renal and hepatic function before and periodically throughout therapy.
• Diuretic therapy should be discontinued 2 to 3 days before the start of ACE-inhibitor therapy to reduce the risk of hypotension. If fosinopril doesn't adequately control blood pressure, a diuretic may be reinstituted with care.

Safety tip. Monitor potassium levels to reduce the risk of hyperkalemia.

Safety tip. Monitor blood pressure daily at first and then periodically. Blood pressure generally decreases within 1 hour of a dose, with peak reductions occurring within 2 to 6 hours. The antihypertensive effect lasts 24 hours.
• Be aware that inadequate fluid intake, vomiting, diarrhea, and excessive perspiration can lead to lightheadedness and syncope. However, the incidence of orthostatic hypotension is low.
• Other ACE inhibitors have been associated with agranulocytosis and neutropenia. Monitor for signs of infection (sore throat and fever), and check the patient's CBC with differential count periodically as indicated.
• Tell the patient that, like other ACE inhibitors, this drug may cause dry, persistent, tickling, nonproductive cough that's reversible when therapy is discontinued.
• Know that the effectiveness of fosinopril is unaffected by age, sex, or weight.
• Be aware that transient elevations of BUN and serum creatinine levels, liver function tests, and decreases in hematocrit or hemoglobin levels, may also occur.

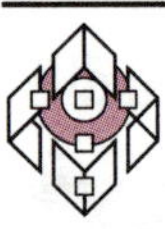 **MedTest**

1. Administration of which drug should be separated by 2 hours from fosinopril?
   a. Metoprolol
   b. Furosemide
   c. An antacid
   d. Nitrates

2. How long does the antihypertensive effect of fosinopril usually last?
   a. 6 hours
   b. 12 hours
   c. 24 hours
   d. 48 hours

3. Adjust the dosage of fosinopril based on:
   a. supine, sitting, and standing blood pressures.
   b. peak and trough blood pressures.
   c. early morning blood pressures.
   d. late evening and bedtime blood pressures.

Furosemide

Also called frusemide, furosemide is known by the brand names Lasix, Furomide M.D., and Myrosemide. In Canada, the drug is also known as Apo-Furosemide, Furoside, Lasix Special, Novosemide, and Uritol. A loop diuretic, furosemide is classified therapeutically as an antihypertensive agent. It's available in 20-, 40-, 80-, and (in Canada) 500-mg tablets; in an oral solution in concentrations of 8 mg/ml, 10 mg/ml, and (in Canada) 50 mg/ml and 40 mg/5 ml; and for injection in 10-mg/ml vials, ampules, and prefilled syringes.

Pharmacokinetics

• *Absorption:* About 60% of oral dose absorbed from GI tract. Food delays oral absorption but doesn't alter diuretic response. Diuresis begins in 30 to 60 minutes; peak diuresis occurs 1 to 2 hours after oral administration. Diuresis follows I.V. administration within 5 minutes and peaks in 20 to 60 minutes.

• *Distribution:* 95% plasma protein–bound. Drug crosses placenta and is excreted in breast milk.

• *Metabolism:* Slightly by the liver.

• *Excretion:* 50% to 80% excreted in urine; its plasma half-life is about 30 minutes. Duration of action is 6 to 8 hours after oral administration and about 2 hours after I.V. administration.

Indications, dosage, and action

Acute pulmonary edema

• *Adult dosage:* Initially, 40 mg I.V. injected slowly; then 80 mg I.V. within 60 to 90 minutes if needed.

• *Pediatric dosage:* 1 mg/kg I.M. or I.V. q 2 hours until response is achieved; maximum dosage is 6 mg/kg/day.

Edema

• *Adult dosage:* 20 to 80 mg P.O. daily in morning, with second dose given in 6 to 8 hours, titrated up to 600 mg daily if needed; or 20 to 40 mg I.M. or I.V. Increase by 20 mg q 2 hours until desired response is achieved. Give I.V. dosage slowly over 1 to 2 minutes.

• *Pediatric dosage:* 2 mg/kg/day, increased by 1 to 2 mg/kg in 6 to 8 hours if needed, carefully titrated not to exceed 6 mg/kg/day.

• *Action:* Inhibits sodium and chloride reabsorption in the proximal part of the ascending loop of Henle, promoting the excretion of sodium, water, chloride, and potassium.

Hypertension

• *Adult dosage:* 10 to 20 mg P.O. b.i.d. Dosage may be adjusted according to the patient's response.

• *Pediatric dosage:* 2 mg/kg P.O. daily; increase dose by 1 to 2 mg/kg in 6 to 8 hours if needed. May be carefully titrated up to 6 mg/kg daily if needed.

Hypertensive crisis

• *Adult dosage:* 100 to 200 mg I.V. over 1 to 2 minutes.

• *Action:* Antihypertensive effect may be due to renal and peripheral vasodilatation, a temporary rise in glomerular filtration rate, reduced peripheral vascular resistance, and plasma volume reduction.

Contraindications and cautions

• Don't use in anuria, hepatic coma, oliguria, or electrolyte depletion, or when BUN and serum creatinine levels rise, even though furosemide is used to produce diuresis in patients with renal impairment. Rapid fluid and electrolyte changes can exacerbate these conditions.

• Use with caution in patients who are hypersensitive to sulfonamides.
• Use carefully in hepatic cirrhosis and ascites because changes in electrolyte balance may precipitate hepatic encephalopathy.
• Use cautiously in patients receiving digitalis glycosides because furosemide-induced hypokalemia may predispose them to digitalis toxicity.
• The drug should be discontinued or the dosage reduced if dehydration or hypotension occurs or if BUN and serum creatinine levels rise.
• Know that rapid I.V. administration of furosemide increases the risk of ototoxicity.
• Closely observe elderly and debilitated patients who are more susceptible to drug-induced diuresis. Reduced dosages may be indicated.
• Use caution in neonates. The usual pediatric dosage can be used, but dosing intervals should be extended.
• Avoid use in breast-feeding women.
• Be aware that diuretics are usually contraindicated during pregnancy.
• Pregnancy risk category C

Life-threatening adverse reactions

• Agranulocytosis
• Dehydration, electrolyte imbalances

Common adverse reactions

• Hypotension, especially with I.V. doses
• Dehydration, decreased potassium level

Infrequent adverse reactions

• Abdominal discomfort and pain, diarrhea (with oral solution)

• Transient or permanent deafness, especially with rapid I.V. injection or high doses, though not necessarily dose related
• Transient leukopenia, thrombocytopenia
• Hypochloremic alkalosis; asymptomatic hyperuricemia; fluid and electrolyte imbalances, including hypocalcemia, hypokalemia, hypomagnesemia, and hyponatremia; hyperglycemia and impairment of glucose tolerance
• Dermatitis, photosensitivity, pain at injection site

Interactions

• *Antihypertensive agents:* Increased risk of hypotension. Use together cautiously.
• *Lithium:* Furosemide may reduce renal clearance of lithium and increase lithium levels; lithium dosage may require adjustment.
• *Nephrotoxic or ototoxic drugs:* Concomitant administration with furosemide may increase toxicity.
• *NSAIDs:* Inhibited diuretic response. Use cautiously.
• *Other diuretics:* Potentiated diuretic and hypotensive actions. Use cautiously together.
• *Potassium-sparing diuretics:* Concomitant use with potassium-sparing diuretics (spironolactone, triamterene, and amiloride) may decrease furosemide-induced potassium loss.

For dangerous interactions, see *Hazards of multidrug therapy with furosemide.*

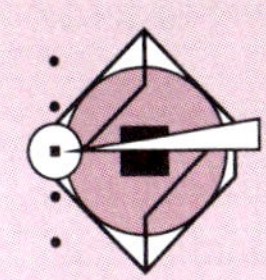

Interactions alert

Hazards of multidrug therapy with furosemide

Interacting drug	Effects
Amphotericin B	May cause severe potassium loss
Corticosteroids (such as prednisone)	May cause severe potassium loss
Digoxin	May lead to digoxin toxicity because of potassium depletion caused by furosemide
Ticarcillin	May cause severe potassium loss

Interventions

Preparation and administration

• Give I.V. furosemide slowly at a rate not to exceed 4 mg/minute; for I.V. infusion, dilute furosemide in D_5W, 0.9% NaCl solution, or lactated Ringer's solution, and use within 24 hours.

Safety tip. Don't use discolored (yellow) injectable preparation.

• Give the first dose in the morning and the second dose in the early afternoon to prevent nocturia. Tell the patient he may take the drug without regard to meals. (See *Taking loop diuretics at home,* page 98.)

Monitoring and supportive care

• Furosemide can lead to profound water and electrolyte loss. Monitor blood pressure, pulse rate, serum potassium and other electrolytes, and BUN levels during rapid diuresis and with chronic use.

• You may need to stop the drug if oliguria or azotemia appear or worsen.

Safety tip. Watch for signs of hypokalemia (muscle weakness, cramps, and ventricular arrhythmias).

• Consult with the doctor and dietitian to provide a high-potassium diet if indicated. Foods rich in potassium include citrus fruits, tomatoes, bananas, dates, and apricots.

• Be aware that the sorbitol content of oral liquid preparations may cause diarrhea, especially at high dosages.

• Monitor blood glucose levels in patients with diabetes. Severe hyperglycemia may be treated with oral antidiabetic agents as needed.

• Monitor serum uric acid levels, especially in patients with a history of gout.

• Furosemide has been used to treat hypercalcemia at dosages of 80 to 100 mg I.V., given q 1 to 2 hours.

• Be aware that furosemide alters liver and renal function tests.

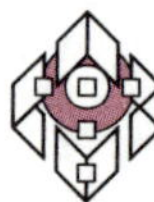 **MedTest**

1. Following oral administration of furosemide, expect diuresis to begin within:
   a. 10 to 20 minutes.
   b. 30 to 60 minutes.
   c. 1 to 2 hours.
   d. 2 to 4 hours.

2. Furosemide is contraindicated in patients with:
   a. renal impairment.
   b. oliguria or anuria.
   c. hypersensitivity to sulfonamides.
   d. hepatic cirrhosis and ascites.

3. Which of the following adverse reactions may occur with rapid I.V. administration of furosemide?
   a. Dizziness
   b. Photosensitivity
   c. Hypokalemia
   d. Transient or permanent deafness

Gemfibrozil

Also known by the brand name Lopid, gemfibrozil is a fibric acid derivative that's classified therapeutically as an antilipemic agent. It's available in 600-mg tablets and (in Canada) in 300-mg capsules.

Pharmacokinetics
- *Absorption:* Well absorbed from GI tract; peak plasma levels occur 1 to 2 hours after an oral dose.
- *Distribution:* 95% plasma protein–bound. Drug crosses placenta.
- *Metabolism:* By the liver to active metabolites.
- *Excretion:* Gemfibrozil and its metabolites eliminated mostly in urine, but some in feces. Elimination half-life is 1½ hours. Plasma levels of VLDLs decrease in 2 to 5 days; peak clinical effect occurs in 4 weeks. Further decreases in plasma VLDL levels occur over several months.

Indications, dosage, and action
Type IV hyperlipidemia and severe hypercholesterolemia unresponsive to diet and other drugs; reducing risk of CAD untreatable with bile acid sequestrants or niacin
- *Adult dosage:* 1,200 mg P.O. administered in two divided doses 30 minutes before morning and evening meals. Usual dosage range is 900 to 1,500 mg daily. If no beneficial effect is seen after 3 months of therapy, drug should be discontinued.
- *Action:* Gemfibrozil increases levels of serum HDL cholesterol, inhibits lipolysis in adipose tissue, and reduces hepatic triglyceride synthesis. The drug is closely related to clofibrate.

Contraindications and cautions
- Don't use in patients with gallbladder disease, because the drug may cause cholelithiasis.
- Don't use in patients with hepatic dysfunction (including primary biliary cirrhosis) or severe renal dysfunction. The drug may cause a paradoxical increase in serum cholesterol levels in patients with primary biliary cirrhosis. Hepatic or severe renal disease may increase the possibility of adverse reactions.

• This drug should be discontinued if liver function test results rise significantly or show worsening abnormalities, if gallstones are found, or if the clinical response is inadequate after 3 months of treatment.
• Pregnancy risk category C

Life-threatening adverse reactions
None noted

Common adverse reactions
• Abdominal and epigastric pain, dry mouth, dyspepsia (20%), anorexia, diarrhea

Infrequent adverse reactions
• Headache, dizziness, fatigue, depression
• Nausea and vomiting, constipation, acute appendicitis, flatulence, elevated hepatic enzyme levels, cholestatic jaundice
• Blurred vision
• Anemia, leukopenia
• Rash, dermatitis (eczema)
• Painful extremities, flulike symptoms

Interactions
• *Lovastatin and similar cholesterol-lowering drugs (such as pravastatin and simvastatin):* Myopathy with rhabdomyolysis may occur with use of gemfibrozil. Use together with caution.
• *Oral anticoagulants:* Increased risk of bleeding. Monitor PT closely and adjust anticoagulant dosage as prescribed.

Interventions
Preparation and administration
• For best absorption, administer the drug 30 minutes before breakfast and dinner. (See *Taking gemfibrozil at home,* page 168.)
• If the patient experiences GI discomfort, give the drug with food.

Monitoring and supportive care
• Because gemfibrozil is pharmacologically related to clofibrate, adverse reactions associated with clofibrate may also occur with gemfibrozil. Some studies suggest clofibrate increases the risk of death from cancer, heart disease, postcholecystectomy complications, and pancreatitis. These hazards haven't been studied in gemfibrozil but are theoretically possible. This drug shouldn't be used indiscriminately.
• Monitor CBC and liver function test results periodically during the first 12 months of therapy.
• Observe bowel movements for evidence of steatorrhea or other signs of bile duct obstruction.
• Be aware that gemfibrozil therapy may elevate serum CK, ALP, ALT, AST, and LD levels. It may decrease serum potassium, hematocrit, and hemoglobin levels, and leukocyte counts.

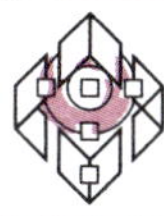 **MedTest**

---

1. For optimal absorption, the patient should take gemfibrozil:
   a. 30 minutes before breakfast and dinner.
   b. with food.
   c. 1 hour after breakfast and dinner.
   d. on arising and h.s.

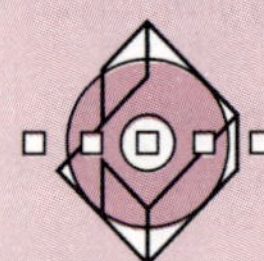

Patient-teaching checklist

Taking gemfibrozil at home

In addition to explaining the drug's action and dosage, teach the patient who will continue gemfibrozil therapy after discharge to follow these important guidelines.

Take your medication correctly
☐ Take gemfibrozil 30 minutes before breakfast and dinner.
☐ If you experience stomach discomfort, take gemfibrozil with food.
☐ Take gemfibrozil as prescribed even when you're feeling well. Be aware that the drug may take up to 4 weeks to produce optimal effects. Don't take more than the prescribed dose.

Watch for adverse effects
☐ Continue taking the drug even if unpleasant adverse reactions occur because when you stop taking it, your blood cholesterol levels may increase again. But make sure you discuss any adverse reactions with your doctor.
☐ Remember to promptly report flulike symptoms or severe stomach pain with nausea and vomiting to your doctor.

☐ Look at your bowel movements, and report any changes in their appearance, especially bulky, fatty-looking stools.
☐ Avoid driving or operating machinery until you've adjusted to the drug's effects.

Modify your lifestyle
☐ Take steps to correct any cardiac risk factors that you may have, such as obesity (lose weight), smoking (enroll in a stop-smoking program), and a sedentary lifestyle (start exercising moderately under a doctor's supervision). These risk factors not only may shorten your life, but also may make the drug less effective.
☐ Adhere to a low-fat, low-cholesterol diet because gemfibrozil is most effective when used in conjunction with dietary restrictions.

2. Advise the patient taking gemfibrozil to examine his bowel movements and to report changes, especially:
  a. dry, constipated stools.
  b. soft or liquid stools.
  c. mucus in the stools.
  d. bulky, fatty stools.

3. Because of the special risks that this drug poses, which studies should be monitored periodically during the first 12 months of therapy?
  a. ALP and CK
  b. ALT and AST
  c. LD
  d. CBC and liver function tests

Heparin calcium, heparin sodium

Classified therapeutically as an anticoagulant, heparin calcium is derived from porcine intestinal mucosa, and heparin sodium is derived from beef lung or porcine intestinal mucosa. Usually given as the sodium salt, heparin is equally effective in calcium form. Heparin calcium is known by the brand names Calciparine, Calcilean (in Canada), and Caprin and Uniparin-Ca (in Australia). Heparin sodium is known by the brand names Liquaemin Sodium, Hepalean (in Canada), and Uniparin (in Australia). All forms are measured in USP units and given by injection.

Heparin calcium is available in a syringe containing 5,000 units/0.2 ml and (in Canada) in ampules containing 12,500 units/0.5 ml and 20,000 units/0.8 ml.

Heparin sodium is available in vials, unit-dose ampules, and disposable syringes of 1,000 units/ml, 5,000 units/ml, and 10,000 units/ml in a variety of dilutions.

Heparin sodium also is available in prefilled cartridges of 5,000 units/ml and in premixed I.V. solutions.

Heparin sodium flush, known by the brand names Hep Lock and Hep Lock U/P, is available in vials containing 10 units/ml and 100 units/ml and in disposable syringes containing 10 units/ml, 25 units/2.5 ml, and 2,500 units/2.5 ml.

Pharmacokinetics
- *Absorption:* Must be given parenterally. After I.V. use, onset is almost immediate; after S.C. injection, onset takes 20 to 60 minutes.
- *Distribution:* Extensively bound to lipoproteins, globulins, and fibrinogen; it doesn't cross the placenta.
- *Metabolism:* Apparently removed by the reticuloendothelial system, with some liver metabolism.
- *Excretion:* A small fraction is excreted in urine as unchanged drug. Plasma half-life is between 1 and 2 hours.

Indications, dosage, and action
Deep vein thrombosis, pulmonary embolism, acute stroke, unstable angina, MI
- *Adult dosage:* Initially, 5,000 to 7,500 units by I.V. push; then 4,000 to 5,000 units I.V. q 4 hours. Or 5,000 to 7,500 units by I.V. bolus; then 1,000 units hourly by I.V. infusion pump. Wait 6 hours after bolus dose, and adjust dosage according to PTT. Or, 10,000 to 15,000 units S.C. q 8 hours. Dosages adjusted according to PTT.
- *Pediatric dosage:* Initially, 50 to 100 units/kg by I.V. drip. Maintenance dosage is 50 to 100 units/kg by I.V. drip q 4 hours or 10 to 15 units/kg/hour by continuous I.V. infusion. Alternatively, continuous infusion of 20,000 units/m^2 daily. Dosages adjusted according to PTT.

Embolism prophylaxis
- *Adult dosage:* 5,000 units S.C. q 8 to 12 hours.

Open-heart surgery
• *Adult dosage:* 150 to 300 units/kg continuous I.V infusion for total body perfusion.

Disseminated intravascular coagulation
• *Adult dosage:* 50 to 100 units/kg I.V. q 4 hours as a single injection or continuous infusion. Discontinue if no improvement in 4 to 8 hours.
• *Pediatric dosage:* 25 to 50 units/kg I.V. q 4 hours, as a single injection or continuous infusion. Discontinue if no improvement in 4 to 8 hours.
• *Anticoagulant action:* Heparin binds to and activates antithrombin III. This antithrombin III–heparin complex inactivates factors Xa, IIc, IX, XI, and XII. It also inactivates thrombin and prevents conversion of fibrinogen to fibrin.

Contraindications and cautions
• Typically, avoid giving heparin in active bleeding and in patients with blood dyscrasias or bleeding tendencies, such as hemophilia, thrombocytopenia, or hypoprothrombinemia; intracranial hemorrhage; suppurative thrombophlebitis; inaccessible ulcerative lesions (especially GI); open ulcers; extensive denudation of skin; conditions causing capillary permeability; during or after brain, eye, or spinal surgery; during continuous GI tube drainage; and in patients with subacute bacterial endocarditis, shock, advanced renal disease, threatened abortion, or severe hypertension.
• Use heparin cautiously during menstruation and the postpartum period.

• Give the drug carefully to elderly patients; patients with hepatic or renal disease, GI ulcers, or alcoholism; and patients who are at risk for physical injury.
• Exercise caution in patients with a history of allergy or asthma because the drug is potentially allergenic.
• Use cautiously in breast-feeding women because osteoporosis can develop after 2 to 4 weeks of therapy. Heparin isn't excreted into breast milk.
• Discontinue the drug if signs of hemorrhage or new thrombosis occur.
• Pregnancy risk category C

Life-threatening adverse reactions
• Hemorrhage with excessive dosage, thrombocytopenia
• "White clot" syndrome (a type of arterial thrombosis caused by heparin-induced thrombocytopenia)

Common adverse reactions
• Overly prolonged PTT
• Mild thrombocytopenia (up to 30%)

Infrequent adverse reactions
• Local tissue irritation, mild pain, pruritus, ecchymosis, hematoma, ulceration, local necrosis, hypersensitivity reactions, arthralgia, urticaria, osteoporosis (after long-term use with large doses)

Interactions
• *Oral anticoagulants, NSAIDs, salicylates:* Increased risk of bleeding. Monitor carefully.
• *Vitamin C:* Large doses of vitamin C may antagonize the effects of heparin.

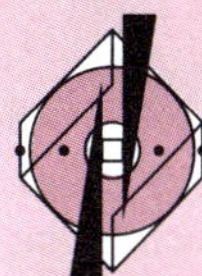

Administration guidelines

Giving heparin I.V. or S.C.

The preferred route of administration for heparin is I.V. However, the drug also can be given S.C.

I.V. administration
The three basic methods of I.V. heparin infusion are direct injection, intermittent infusion, and continuous infusion.
• For *direct injection,* give the drug diluted or undiluted through an intermittent infusion device or through an I.V. line containing a free-flowing compatible solution.
• For *intermittent infusion,* dilute ordered dose in 50 to 100 ml of 0.9% NaCl solution. Administer through a peripheral or central venous line over the prescribed duration using an infusion pump.
• For *continuous infusion,* use an infusion pump and give the diluted solution at the prescribed rate over 24 hours or as specified.

S.C. administration
• Administer a low-dose injection sequentially between iliac crests and at least 2″ (5 cm) from the umbilicus, in the lower abdomen deep into subcutaneous fat. Leave the needle in place for 10 seconds after injection; then withdraw it.
• Alternate sites. If administering the drug q 12 hours, inject it into the patient's right side in the morning and left side in the evening. Record the site used. Don't massage the injection site.
• Check the site for bleeding.

Interventions
Preparation and administration
• Be aware that the heparin dosage is highly individualized, depending on the patient's disease state, age, and renal and hepatic status.
• I.V. administration is preferred because dosage titration is difficult with S.C. injection.

Safety tip. Use an infusion pump when giving the drug I.V.
• Never mix any drug with heparin in a syringe when bolus therapy is used.
• I.V. heparin should be given on time; try not to skip a dose or "catch up" with an I.V. line containing heparin.
• For S.C. injection, use one needle to withdraw solution from the vial and another to inject the drug.

Safety tip. Don't massage the injection site after S.C. injection; watch for local bleeding, hematoma, or inflammation. (See *Giving heparin I.V. or S.C.*)
• Avoid I.M. injection of other drugs to prevent or minimize hematomas.
• Check compatibility before administering heparin with another drug. (See *Heparin combinations to avoid,* page 172.)

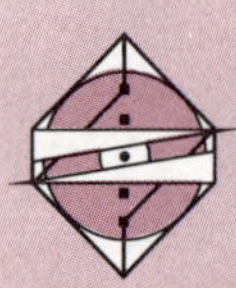

Incompatibility warning

Heparin combinations to avoid

Heparin is incompatible with well over 100 drugs. So make sure you check the compatibility of any planned admixture before administering it concomitantly through the same I.V. site. Consult an incompatibility chart, a specialized text, or a pharmacist.

Safety tip. Heparin is available in various concentrations, so check the order and vial carefully.

Monitoring and supportive care

• Check the baseline platelet count and PTT; monitor PTT results at least daily. Dosage is adjusted to maintain PTT values at 1½ to 2½ times the control values.

• Monitor the platelet count every 3 days. Heparin should be discontinued if the count falls below 50,000/mm³; if the count is below 100,000/mm³, the patient should be tested for the presence of heparin-associated antiplatelet antibodies and discontinuation of the drug should be considered.

Safety tip. Check the patient for bleeding gums, arm or leg bruises, petechiae, nosebleeds, melena, tarry stools, hematuria, or hematemesis. (See *Taking heparin at home.*)

• Draw blood 30 minutes before the next scheduled dose when administering heparin intermittently to avoid a falsely prolonged PTT. You can draw blood for PTT any time after 6 hours of continuous I.V. heparin therapy.

• Don't draw blood from the infusion tubing or the vein used for infusion. Always draw blood from the other arm.

• Don't piggyback other drugs into the infusion line unless these drugs are known to be compatible; many drugs, including antibiotics, inactivate heparin.

• Remember that heparin concentrations greater than 100 units/ml can irritate blood vessels.

Safety tip. Place a notice above the patient's bed to inform the I.V. team or lab personnel to apply pressure dressings after drawing blood.

• Full-dose heparin therapy is usually followed by oral anticoagulants.

• Severe hemorrhage may require treatment with protamine sulfate. Usually, 1 mg of protamine sulfate will neutralize 90 units of bovine heparin or 115 units of porcine heparin.

• Give protamine as a 25- to 50-mg loading dose, followed by a constant infusion of the rest of the calculated dose over 8 to 16 hours. Protamine dosage depends on the heparin dose, administration route, and time elapsed since heparin was given.

• Give protamine slowly — not more than 50 mg in any 10-minute period.

• Transfusions may be required for severe bleeding.

• Be aware that heparin prolongs PT, may falsely elevate ALT and AST levels, and causes false elevations in serum thyroxine tests.

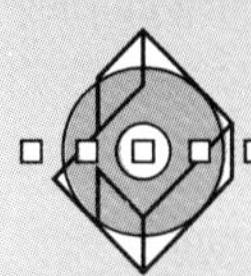

Patient-teaching checklist

Taking heparin at home

In addition to explaining the drug's action and dosage, teach the patient who will continue heparin therapy after discharge to follow these important guidelines.

Take your medication correctly

☐ Inject heparin into your abdomen between the bony prominences of your hip bones and at least 2″ (5 cm) from your navel, deep into the fatty tissue under the skin. Your doctor or nurse will provide you with more detailed instructions.

☐ Always double-check the dosage to be sure you are taking the right amount of heparin and following the prescribed schedule.

☐ If you miss a dose of heparin, take it as soon as possible. However, if it's almost time for your next dose, skip the missed dose and don't double the next one. Doubling the dose may cause bleeding. Continue your regular dosing schedule.

☐ Keep a record of each dose and where you injected it to avoid mistakes.

☐ Take heparin exactly as prescribed, even when you're feeling well.

Know when to call your doctor

☐ Tell your doctor immediately if you experience signs of bleeding, such as bleeding gums, bruises on your arms or legs, nosebleeds, tarry stools, or blood in your urine or vomitus.

☐ Avoid OTC medications containing aspirin because the interaction may cause excessive bleeding. Also check with your doctor or pharmacist before taking any other OTC medications.

☐ Keep scheduled follow-up visits with your doctor, who will determine how well heparin is working and detect any adverse reactions promptly.

Other instructions

☐ Have blood tests drawn as scheduled to monitor heparin's effect on your blood's clotting ability.

☐ Avoid sports and other activities that may cause you to be injured. Also report any falls, blows to the body or head, or other injuries because serious bleeding inside your body may occur without your knowing about it.

☐ Take special care in brushing your teeth and in shaving. Use a soft toothbrush or sponge stick and floss gently. Use an electric shaver, not a razor.

☐ Tell all doctors and dentists that you visit that you're using heparin.

☐ Carry medical identification stating that you're using heparin.

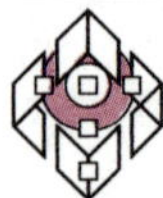 **MedTest**

1. When administering heparin S.C.:
   a. aspirate before injecting the drug to make sure you're not in a blood vessel.
   b. inject slowly, deep into S.C. fat.
   c. leave the needle in place for 30 seconds after injecting.
   d. alternate left to right abdominal sites daily.

2. Which of the following values should you monitor to avoid "white clot" syndrome?
   a. PTT at least daily
   b. Lee-White coagulation time 30 minutes prior to next scheduled dose
   c. PT 12 to 24 hours after S.C. dose
   d. Platelet count every 3 days

3. If severe hemorrhaging occurs, treat the patient, as prescribed, with:
   a. protamine sulfate.
   b. phentolamine mesylate.
   c. penbutolol sulfate.
   d. procainamide hydrochloride.

Hydralazine hydrochloride

Also known by the brand names Alazine Tabs, Apresoline, Novo-Hylazin (in Canada), and Supres (in Australia), hydralazine HCl is a peripheral vasodilator that's classified therapeutically as an antihypertensive agent. It's available in 10-, 25-, 50-, and 100-mg tablets and in 20-mg/ml vials for injection.

Pharmacokinetics

- *Absorption:* Absorbed rapidly from the GI tract; food enhances absorption. Peak plasma levels occur in 1 hour. Onset occurs 20 to 30 minutes after oral dose, 5 minutes after I.V. dose, and 10 to 30 minutes after I.M. dose.
- *Distribution:* About 88% to 90% of the drug is protein-bound.
- *Metabolism:* Metabolized extensively in the GI mucosa and the liver to inactive metabolites.
- *Excretion:* Excreted in urine, primarily as metabolites; about 10% of an oral dose is excreted in feces.

Indications, dosage, and action
Moderate to severe hypertension
- *Regular adult dosage:* Initially, 10 mg P.O. q.i.d. for 2 to 4 days; then increased to 25 mg q.i.d. for the remainder of the week. If necessary, increase dosage to 50 mg q.i.d. Maximum recommended dosage is 200 mg daily, but some patients may require 300 to 400 mg daily.
- *Dosage for severe hypertension:* 10 to 50 mg I.M. or 10 to 20 mg given slowly I.V. and repeated as necessary, generally q 4 to 6 hours. Switch to oral antihypertensives as soon as possible.
- *Dosage for hypertensive crisis associated with pregnancy:* Initially, 5 mg I.V., followed by 5 to 10 mg I.V. q 20 to 30 minutes until adequate reduction in blood pressure is achieved (usual range is 5 to 20 mg).

• *Regular pediatric dosage:* Initially, 0.75 mg/kg P.O. daily in four divided doses (25 mg/m^2 daily); may increase gradually to 7.5 mg/kg daily.
• *I.M. or I.V. pediatric dosage:* 1.7 to 3.5 mg/kg daily or 50 to 100 mg/m^2 daily in four to six divided doses.
• *Antihypertensive action:* Has a direct vasodilating effect on vascular smooth muscle, thus lowering blood pressure. Drug's effect on resistance vessels (arterioles and arteries) is greater than that on capacitance vessels (venules and veins). Its antihypertensive effect persists 2 to 4 hours after an oral dose and 2 to 6 hours after I.V. or I.M. administration.

Short-term management of severe CHF (unlabeled use)
• *Adult dosage:* Initially, 50 to 75 mg P.O., then adjusted according to patient response. Most patients respond to 200 to 600 mg daily, divided every 6 to 12 hours, but dosages as high as 3 g daily have been used.
• *Action:* Causes a reduction in afterload, thereby improving cardiac function and increasing cardiac output.

Contraindications and cautions
• Use with caution in patients with mitral valve disorders, rheumatic heart disease, history of stroke, or severe renal damage because these conditions may be exacerbated by hypotension.
• Discontinue if the patient develops lupus-like syndrome or blood dyscrasias, a positive antinuclear antibody (ANA) titer, or positive lupus erythematosus (LE) cell preparation.

• Be aware that elderly patients may be more sensitive to drug's antihypertensive effects.
• Use in children only if potential benefit outweighs risk.
• Avoid use in breast-feeding women.
• Pregnancy risk category C

Life-threatening adverse reactions
• MI

Common adverse reactions
• Tachycardia, angina, palpitations
• Headache
• Anorexia, nausea, vomiting, diarrhea
• Weight gain

Infrequent adverse reactions
• Orthostatic hypotension, arrhythmias, edema
• Dyspnea
• Peripheral neuritis, dizziness, paresthesia, tremors, depression, disorientation, anxiety
• Constipation, paralytic ileus, difficulty urinating
• Nasal congestion, lacrimation, conjunctivitis
• Reduced hemoglobin and RBC count, neutropenia, leukopenia, lymphadenopathy, splenomegaly
• Rash, urticaria, pruritus, flushing
• Lupus-like syndrome (with dosages greater than 200 mg/day), muscle cramps

Interactions
• *Diuretics, MAO inhibitors, other antihypertensives:* Risk of hypotension. Monitor patient closely.

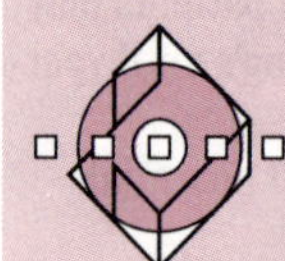

Taking hydralazine at home

In addition to explaining the drug's action and dosage, teach the patient who will continue hydralazine therapy after discharge to follow these important guidelines.

Take your medication correctly
□ Take hydralazine with meals to increase absorption and help minimize gastric irritation.
□ Take the drug at the same time every day. If possible, take your blood pressure before each dose of hydralazine. Check your blood pressure frequently. Notify the doctor of any significant changes.
□ Take hydralazine as prescribed even when you're feeling well.
□ Continue taking the drug even if unpleasant adverse reactions occur.

Watch for adverse reactions
□ Be aware that headache and palpitations may occur 2 to 4 hours after the first dose but should subside spontaneously.
□ Report sore throat, fever, muscle and joint aches, a rash, and any other adverse reactions to your doctor immediately.

□ Remember to change positions slowly (especially from lying flat or sitting down to sitting upright) and to dangle your legs over the bedside for a few minutes before standing. These measures will minimize the potential for light-headedness. Lie down immediately if dizziness occurs.
□ Avoid driving or operating machinery until you've adjusted to the drug's effects.

Other instructions
□ Limit your fluid and salt intake to minimize fluid retention.
□ Weigh yourself at least weekly at the same time of day and in the same type of clothing. Report a weight gain that exceeds 5 lb (2 kg) per week.
□ Check with your doctor or pharmacist before drinking alcohol or taking OTC medications, especially cold or allergy remedies.

• *Epinephrine:* Decreased pressor response to epinephrine.

Interventions
Preparation and administration
• Be aware that food enhances oral absorption and helps minimize gastric irritation. (See *Taking hydralazine at home.*)

• Administer I.V. doses slowly, monitoring blood pressure every 5 minutes until stable, then every 15 minutes. Too-rapid reduction in blood pressure can cause mental changes.
 Safety tip. Put the patient in Trendelenburg's position if he's faint or dizzy.

Monitoring and supportive care
• CBC, LE cell preparation, and ANA titer studies should be performed before therapy and at regular intervals during long-term therapy. Hydralazine may cause a positive ANA titer; a positive LE cell preparation; blood dyscrasias, including leukopenia and agranulocytosis; and a decreased hemoglobin level or RBC count.
• Monitor the patient's blood pressure and pulse rate frequently.
• Watch the patient closely for signs of lupus-like syndrome. Call the doctor immediately if any of these develops.
• Keep in mind that the incidence of hydralazine-induced lupus-like syndrome is greatest in patients receiving more than 200 mg/day for prolonged periods.
• Sodium retention can occur with long-term use. Know that some clinicians combine hydralazine therapy with diuretics.
• Hydralazine also may be combined with beta-adrenergic blockers to prevent headaches, tachycardia, and anginal attacks.
• Some preparations contain tartrazine, which may precipitate allergic reactions, especially in aspirin-sensitive patients.
• Remember that patients with renal impairment may respond to lower maintenance doses of hydralazine.
• Know that use in CHF is limited because tolerance may develop with prolonged use.
• Hydralazine has been prescribed during pregnancy for treatment of eclampsia.

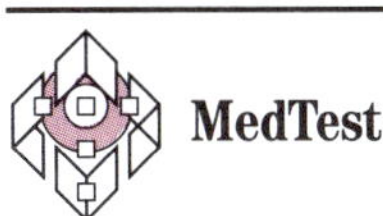

MedTest

1. Hydralazine's antihypertensive action occurs primarily because of its direct vasodilating action on:
   a. arteries and veins.
   b. coronary vasculature.
   c. arteries and arterioles.
   d. veins and venules.

2. A common adverse effect of hydralazine is:
   a. constipation.
   b. leukopenia.
   c. orthostatic hypotension.
   d. headache.

3. You should teach patients to take their hydralazine:
   a. without regard to meals.
   b. 30 to 60 minutes a.c. to enhance absorption.
   c. with food to enhance absorption and minimize gastric irritation.
   d. 1 to 2 hours p.c. to help minimize gastric irritation.

Hydrochlorothiazide

Also known by the brand names Aprozide, Chlorzide, Diaqua, Esidrix, HydroDIURIL, Hyperetic, and Oretic, and (in Canada) Apo-Hydro, Novohydrazide, and Urozide, hydrochlorothiazide is a thiazide diuretic that's classified therapeutically as a diuretic and an antihypertensive agent. It's available in 25-, 50-, and 100-mg tablets and as an oral solution containing 50 mg/ 5 ml.

Pharmacokinetics
• *Absorption:* The rate and extent of absorption haven't been well defined.
• *Distribution:* Unknown.
• *Metabolism:* None.
• *Excretion:* Excreted unchanged in urine within 24 hours.

Indications, dosage, and action
Edema
• *Adult dosage:* Initially, 25 to 100 mg P.O. daily or intermittently for maintenance.
• *Pediatric dosage:* Ages 6 months and older, give 2 to 2.2 mg/kg P.O. daily divided b.i.d. Ages younger than 6 months, give up to 3.3 mg/kg P.O. daily divided b.i.d.
• *Diuretic action:* Increases urinary excretion of sodium and water by inhibiting sodium reabsorption in the cortical diluting tubule of the nephron, thus relieving edema.

Hypertension
• *Adult dosage:* 12.5 to 50 mg P.O. once daily or in divided doses. Daily dosage increased or decreased according to blood pressure. Full antihypertensive effect may take up to 12 weeks to achieve.
• *Antihypertensive action:* Blocks sodium and water reabsorption by the kidneys, causing diuresis and reducing circulating blood volume.

Contraindications and cautions
• Don't use in patients with anuria or hypersensitivity to sulfonamide derivatives.
• Use cautiously in elderly patients, in patients with severe renal disease because the drug may cause azotemia, and in patients with liver disease because the drug may cause hepatic coma.
• Know that hydrochlorothiazide-induced hypokalemia may predispose patients to digitalis toxicity.
• Use cautiously in breast-feeding women.
• Pregnancy risk category B

Life-threatening adverse reactions
• Aplastic anemia, agranulocytosis

Common adverse reactions
• Fluid and electrolyte imbalances, including hyponatremia, hypochloremia, hypercalcemia, and hypokalemia

Infrequent adverse reactions
• Orthostatic hypotension, hypercholesterolemia, hypertriglyceridemia
• Vertigo, dizziness, headache, transient blurred vision, paresthesia, weakness, restlessness
• Anorexia, nausea, vomiting, cramping, diarrhea, constipation, gastric irritation, pancreatitis, jaundice, hepatic encephalopathy
• Leukopenia, thrombocytopenia
• Asymptomatic hyperuricemia, gout, hyperglycemia and impaired glucose tolerance, metabolic alkalosis
• Dermatitis, photosensitivity, rash, urticaria, purpura
• Muscle spasm, hypersensitivity reactions, such as pneumonitis and vasculitis

Interactions
• *Amphetamines, quinidine:* Decreased excretion and enhanced toxicity.

• *Antidiabetic agents:* Dosage adjustments may be necessary. Monitor blood glucose levels.
• *Cholestyramine, colestipol:* Decreased absorption of thiazides. Keep doses as separate as possible.
• *Digitalis glycosides:* Increased risk of toxicity in patients with thiazide-induced hypokalemia.
• *Lithium:* Reduced renal clearance of lithium. May necessitate reduction in lithium dosage by 50%.
• *Methenamine compounds:* Decreased effectiveness.
• *NSAIDs:* Decreased diuretic effectiveness. Avoid concomitant use.
• *Other antihypertensives:* increased risk of hypotension. Use together cautiously.

Interventions
Preparation and administration
• Give the drug in the morning to prevent nocturia. Studies have shown that the drug is as effective when administered once daily as it is when given more frequently. (See *Taking hydrochlorothiazide at home*, page 180.)

Monitoring and supportive care
• Monitor intake and output, weight, blood pressure, and serum electrolyte levels.
• If needed, give the patient foods rich in potassium, including citrus fruits, tomatoes, bananas, dates, and apricots, as well as salt substitutes. Also, know that reducing sodium intake increases renal conservation of potassium.

• Discuss discontinuing the drug with the doctor if signs of renal failure develop.
• Monitor serum creatinine and BUN levels regularly. The drug is not as effective if these levels are more than twice the normal levels.
• Monitor serum cholesterol and triglyceride levels and reinforce a low-cholesterol, low-fat diet.
• Monitor blood uric acid levels, especially in patients with a history of gout.
• Be aware that hydrochlorothiazide therapy may interfere with tests for parathyroid function and should be discontinued before such tests.

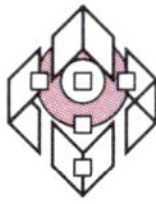 **MedTest**

1. You should discuss with the doctor discontinuing hydrochlorothiazide if the patient develops signs of:
   a. renal failure.
   b. hypokalemia.
   c. orthostatic hypotension.
   d. hyperglycemia.

2. Hydrochlorothiazide is most effective and causes the patient less lifestyle disruption when administered:
   a. h.s.
   b. with meals.
   c. on an empty stomach.
   d. first thing in the morning.

3. Hydrochlorothiazide shouldn't be used for patients with known hypersensitivity to:
   a. penicillins.

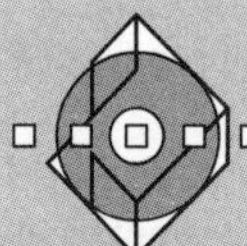

Taking hydrochlorothiazide at home

In addition to explaining the drug's action and dosage, teach the patient who will continue hydrochlorothiazide therapy after discharge to follow these important guidelines.

Take your medication correctly

☐ Take hydrochlorothiazide in the morning to prevent the need to urinate during the night.

☐ If you are taking the liquid form of hydrochlorothiazide, you must measure your dose with the specially marked dropper that comes with the drug to ensure accuracy.

☐ Take hydrochlorothiazide as prescribed even when you're feeling well. Be aware that the drug may take several days to weeks to produce optimal effects.

☐ Continue taking the drug even if unpleasant adverse reactions occur. Make sure you discuss any adverse reactions with your doctor as soon as possible.

☐ If so advised, monitor your fluid intake and output daily.

☐ Weigh yourself daily at the same time of day wearing the same type of clothing.

Watch for adverse reactions

☐ Report any evidence of fluid retention (swollen hands, feet, or ankles; tight rings or shoes), a weight gain or loss of more than 2 lb (1 kg) per day, or excessive urination. Be aware that urine volume should decrease as the body's fluid balance normalizes.

☐ Avoid high-sodium foods to minimize fluid retention. Also incorporate high-potassium foods into your daily diet if so instructed by your doctor. This is important because hydrochlorothiazide causes loss of potassium in your urine.

☐ Elevate your legs when possible to help relieve foot or ankle swelling.

☐ Remember to change positions slowly (especially from lying flat to sitting upright) and dangle your legs over the bedside for a few minutes before standing. This will help to minimize the potential for drug-induced dizziness and light-headedness.

Other instructions

☐ Avoid direct sun exposure as much as possible because this drug may cause a photosensitivity reaction. When you must be in the sun, take proper sun precautions (wear sunscreen, a hat, a long-sleeved shirt, and gloves), especially if prolonged exposure is anticipated.

☐ Monitor your blood glucose levels closely if you have diabetes because you may require a dosage adjustment in your insulin or other antidiabetic drug.

☐ Check with your doctor or pharmacist before taking OTC medications.

b. sulfonamides.
c. aminoglycosides.
d. cephalosporins.

Isoproterenol

Also known by the brand name Isuprel, isoproterenol is an adrenergic that's classified therapeutically as a bronchodilator and a cardiac stimulant. As a cardiac stimulant, isoproterenol is available in 10- and 15-mg sublingual tablets and in 20- and 200-mcg/ml ampules for injection.

Pharmacokinetics
• *Absorption:* Absorbed rapidly after injection; after sublingual administration, absorption is variable and often unreliable. Effects persist for a few minutes after I.V. injection, up to 2 hours after S.C. or sublingual administration, and up to 4 hours after rectal administration of sublingual tablet.
• *Distribution:* Drug is distributed widely throughout the body.
• *Metabolism:* Metabolized primarily by tissue uptake and by enzymes in the GI tract, liver, lungs, and other tissues.
• *Excretion:* Excreted in urine as unchanged drug and metabolites.

Indications, dosage, and action
Complete AV block
• *Adult dosage:* 0.04 to 0.06 mg of isoproterenol HCl (2 to 3 ml of a 1:50,000 dilution) as I.V. bolus.

• *Pediatric dosage:* 0.01 to 0.03 mg of isoproterenol HCl (0.5 to 1.5 ml of a 1:50,000 dilution) as I.V. bolus.

Prevention of transient AV block, Stokes-Adams attacks
• *Adult dosage:* 10 to 30 mg of isoproterenol HCl sublingually 4 to 6 times daily.

Cardiac arrest
• *Adult dosage:* Initially, 0.02 to 0.06 mg of isoproterenol HCl as an I.V. bolus. Subsequent I.V. doses of 0.01 to 0.2 mg. Alternatively, 5 mcg/minute titrated to patient's response. Range is 2 to 20 mcg/minute. Alternatively, 0.2 mg I.M. or S.C.; subsequent doses of 0.02 to 1 mg I.M. or 0.15 to 0.2 mg S.C. In extreme cases, 0.02 mg (0.1 ml of 200 mcg/ml) intracardiac injection.
• *Pediatric dosage:* May give one-half of initial adult dose.

Temporary control of symptomatic bradycardia
• *Adult dosage:* 2 to 10 mcg/minute of isoproterenol HCl by I.V. infusion titrated to patient's response.
• *Pediatric dosage:* 0.1 mcg/kg/minute of isoproterenol HCl titrated to patient's response. Maximum rate is 1 mcg/kg/minute.

Adjunctive treatment of shock
• *Adult and pediatric dosage:* 0.5 to 5 mcg/minute of isoproterenol HCl by continuous infusion titrated to patient's response.
• *Cardiac stimulant action:* Isoproterenol acts on beta$_1$- and beta$_2$-adren-

ergic receptors. Beta$_1$-receptors in the heart produce a positive chronotropic and inotropic effect, thus increasing cardiac output. In patients with AV block, isoproterenol decreases AV node refractory time, shortens conduction time, and increases heart rate. Beta$_2$-receptors in the respiratory tract cause bronchodilation; in the peripheral vasculature, they mediate vasodilation.

Contraindications and cautions

• Avoid use in patients with cardiac arrhythmias, especially ventricular arrhythmias and tachycardia, because of the drug's cardiac stimulant effects.
• Don't use in patients who are hypersensitive to sympathomimetics.
• Administer cautiously to elderly patients, children, diabetic patients, and those with renal or cardiovascular disease or hyperthyroidism because the drug may worsen these conditions.
• Administer cautiously to sulfite-sensitive patients because some formulations contain sulfite preservatives.
• Discontinue the drug if precordial distress, angina, ventricular arrhythmias, swelling of the parotid glands, or airway resistance develops.
• Use with caution in breast-feeding women because it's unknown whether the drug is excreted in breast milk.
• Pregnancy risk category C

Life-threatening adverse reactions

• Arrhythmias, hypotension
• Bronchial inflammation and edema, paradoxical bronchospasm
• Anaphylaxis

Common adverse reactions

• Palpitations, tachycardia, angina, changes in blood pressure, arrhythmias, precordial discomfort
• Bronchial irritation
• Headache

Infrequent adverse reactions

• Restlessness, insomnia, anxiety, tension, fear, excitement, weakness, dizziness, mild tremor, light-headedness
• Nausea, vomiting
• Tinnitus
• Hyperglycemia
• Sweating, flushing of face or skin

Interactions

• *Digitalis glycosides, potassium-depleting drugs:* Arrhythmias may occur more readily when drug is administered to patients receiving digitalis glycosides, potassium-depleting drugs, or other drugs that affect cardiac rhythm. Monitor for arrhythmias during initial therapy.
• *Ergot alkaloids:* Concomitant use may raise blood pressure. Monitor patient's blood pressure.

For dangerous interactions, see *Life-threatening hazards of multidrug therapy with isoproterenol.*

Interventions

Preparation and administration
• Don't inject solutions intended for oral inhalation.
• Expect to titrate dosage based upon patient response.

Safety tip. Because of the danger of precipitating arrhythmias, decrease the rate of infusion if

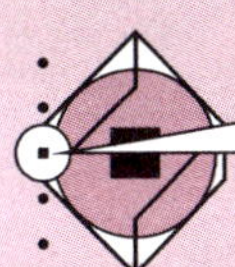

Interactions alert

Life-threatening hazards of multidrug therapy with isoproterenol

Interacting drug	Effects
Beta blockers (such as propranolol)	May antagonize isoproterenol's cardiac-stimulating, bronchodilating, and vasodilating effects but can be lifesaving during an emergency
Cyclopropane (general anesthetic)	Increases risk of life-threatening arrhythmias
Halogenated hydrocarbon general anesthetics (such as halothane)	Increase risk of life-threatening arrhythmias resulting from combined drug effects
Sympathomimetic agents (such as epinephrine)	Increase risk of additive CV reactions and cardiotoxicity

the patient's heart rate exceeds 110 beats/minute. Doses sufficient to increase the heart rate to more than 130 beats/minute may induce ventricular arrhythmias.

Safety tip. Use an infusion pump to regulate infusion flow rate.

• Don't give sublingual doses more frequently than q 3 to 4 hours or more often than t.i.d. (See *Taking isoproterenol at home*, page 184.)

• You may give sublingual tablets rectally, if indicated.

• If possible, don't give dose h.s. because it interrupts sleep patterns.

Monitoring and supportive care

• Be aware that this drug may cause a slight rise in systolic blood pressure and a slight-to-marked drop in diastolic blood pressure.

• Continuously monitor ECG during I.V. administration.

Safety tip. If precordial distress or anginal pain occurs, stop the drug immediately.

• Hypovolemia must be corrected before isoproterenol is administered.

Safety tip. When administering I.V. isoproterenol for shock, closely monitor blood pressure, CVP, ECG, ABG measurements, and urine output.

• Keep in mind that oral and sublingual tablets are poorly absorbed.

• If three to five treatments within 6 to 12 hours provide minimal or no relief, reevaluate therapy.

• Know that isoproterenol may reduce the sensitivity of spirometry in the diagnosis of asthma.

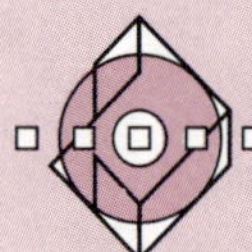

Patient-teaching checklist

Taking isoproterenol at home

In addition to explaining the drug's action and dosage, teach the patient who will continue isoproterenol therapy after discharge to follow these important guidelines.

Take your medication correctly

☐ If you're taking isoproterenol sublingually, don't suck it; hold the tablet under your tongue until it dissolves and is absorbed. Don't swallow saliva until that time because it may cause epigastric pain.

☐ Measure your pulse rate before and after each dose of oral isoproterenol, and notify your doctor if it increases more than 20 beats per minute.

☐ Discuss when you should take the last daily dose of isoproterenol with your doctor because if it's taken too close to bedtime, the effects of the drug may interrupt your sleep pattern.

☐ Take isoproterenol as prescribed even when you're feeling well. Don't increase the dose or frequency of administration because serious cardiac adverse reactions may occur. If the prescribed dosage doesn't relieve your symptoms or if your condition worsens, notify your doctor. Never take sublingual doses more frequently than every 3 to 4 hours.

Know when to call your doctor

☐ Stop the drug and notify your doctor immediately if you develop a fluttering sensation in the heart, rapid heartbeat, shortness of breath or dyspnea, or chest pain or tightness. Continue taking the drug if other unpleasant adverse reactions occur. However, make sure you discuss them with your doctor.

Other instructions

☐ Be aware that prolonged use of sublingual isoproterenol tablets can cause tooth decay. Rinse your mouth with water after taking your dose, and see your dentist regularly.

☐ Rinse your mouth with water between drug doses to prevent drug-induced mouth dryness.

☐ Reduce your intake of foods containing caffeine, such as coffee, colas, and chocolates, because their stimulating effects can increase your heart rate and cause fluttering or palpitations.

☐ Check with your doctor or pharmacist before taking OTC medications.

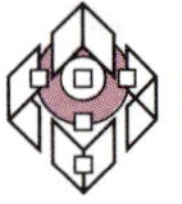

MedTest

1. What should you do if patient's heart rate exceeds 110 beats/minute while receiving I.V. isoproterenol?

a. Continue to monitor closely for increases to 130 beats/minute.
b. Report increase appropriately.
c. Stop administering the drug.
d. Decrease the infusion rate.

2. A common CNS adverse effect of isoproterenol that you would warn the patient about is:
  a. headache.
  b. nervousness.
  c. dizziness.
  d. tremor.

3. The primary cardiac use of isoproterenol is management of:
  a. heart failure.
  b. ventricular arrhythmias.
  c. AV block.
  d. angina pectoris.

Isosorbide dinitrate, isosorbide mononitrate

Isosorbide dinitrate is known by the brand names Dilatrate-SR, Iso-Bid, Isonate, Isorbid, Isordil, Sorbitrate, and Sorbitrate SA; Apo-ISDN, Cedocard-SR, Coronex, and Novosorbide (in Canada); and Nitro-Spray (in Australia). Brand names of isosorbide mononitrate include Monoket and Ismo.

This drug is classified therapeutically as a vasodilator. It's available in 5-, 10-, 20-, 30-, and 40-mg tablets; 5- and 10-mg chewable tablets; 2.5-, 5-, and 10-mg sublingual tablets; 40-mg sustained-release tablets; 40-mg capsules; 40-mg sustained-release capsules; and 20-mg tablets and 60-mg sustained-release tablets (isosorbide mononitrate).

Pharmacokinetics

• *Absorption:* Absorbed rapidly after oral administration. With dinitrate forms, action begins within 5 minutes after administration of sublingual or chewable forms, 30 minutes after regular-release forms, and 1 hour after sustained-release forms. With mononitrate, onset of action is within 1 hour.

• *Distribution:* Distributed to total body water. Duration of action for dinitrate forms is as follows: sublingual, 2 hours; chewable, $1\frac{1}{2}$ to 2 hours; oral, 5 to 6 hours; and sustained-release, 6 to 8 hours. For mononitrate, duration with oral tablets is up to 12 hours; with sustained-release, up to 24 hours.

• *Metabolism:* Isosorbide dinitrate is metabolized to isosorbide mononitrate, the active metabolite. Isosorbide mononitrate has almost 100% bioavailability. It's cleared from the serum by denitrification, glucuronidation, and hydration.

• *Excretion:* Metabolites and a small percentage of isosorbide mononitrate are eliminated in the urine, with a half-life of about 5 hours.

Indications, dosage, and action

Treatment or prophylaxis of acute angina; chronic ischemic heart disease

• *Adult dosage:* Sublingual form — 2.5 to 10 mg under the tongue for prompt relief of anginal pain, repeated q 5 to 10 minutes (maximum of three doses per 30-minute period). For prophylaxis, repeat q 2 to 3 hours.

Chewable form — 5 to 10 mg p.r.n. for acute attack or q 2 to 3 hours for prophylaxis but only after initial test dose of 5 mg to determine risk of severe hypotension.

Oral form (for prophylaxis only) — 5 to 30 mg isosorbide dinitrate P.O. q.i.d. or 40 mg P.O. of sustained-release form q 6 to 12 hours. Alternatively, give 10 to 20 mg isosorbide mononitrate P.O. b.i.d., usually 7 hours apart (the first dose upon awakening), or 30 to 60 mg of sustained-release form P.O. daily.

Adjunctive treatment of severe chronic CHF

• *Adult dosage:* 20 to 40 mg of oral or chewable forms q 4 to 12 hours.

• *Vasodilator action:* Nitrates relax vascular smooth muscle with greater dilation of veins and venules (capacitance vessels) than of arteries and arterioles (resistance vessels). Venous dilation decreases venous return to the heart, which decreases preload. Arteriolar relaxation decreases systemic vascular resistance, mean arterial pressure, and afterload. Cardiac oxygen demand is reduced. Dilation of coronary arteries and enhanced collateral coronary circulation also occur.

Contraindications and cautions

• Avoid use in patients with anuria, severe dehydration, acute pulmonary edema, or severe cardiac decompensation because the osmotic effects of the drug may worsen the symptoms or disorders.

• Don't use in patients with hypersensitivity to nitrates.

• Don't use in patients with head trauma, cerebral hemorrhage, or severe anemia.

• Use cautiously in elderly patients and in patients with hypotension.

• Give repeated doses with caution in patients with diseases associated with sodium retention.

• Discontinue the drug if fluid or electrolyte imbalances occur or if urine output decreases drastically.

• Use caution when administering to breast-feeding women because it's unknown whether the drug is excreted in breast milk.

• Pregnancy risk category C

Life-threatening adverse reactions

• Severe hypotension

Common adverse reactions

• Symptomatic hypotension (up to 36%)

• Headache, sometimes with throbbing (mononitrate form, 19%; dinitrate form, 25%); dizziness (dinitrate form, up to 36%)

• Sublingual burning or tingling (locally)

Infrequent adverse reactions

• Orthostatic hypotension, tachycardia, palpitations, arrhythmias, ankle edema, angina

• Dizziness, light-headedness, fainting, confusion, disorientation, irritability, lethargy

• Nausea, vomiting, GI discomfort, thirst, hiccups, diarrhea, anorexia

• Cutaneous vasodilation, flushing, rash, pruritus

• Hypersensitivity reactions

Interactions

For dangerous interactions, see *Hazards of multidrug therapy with*

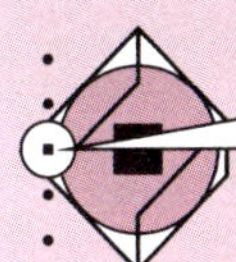

Hazards of multidrug therapy with isosorbide dinitrate and mononitrate

Interacting drug	Effects
Alcohol (CNS depressant)	May cause serious hypotension
Antihypertensive agents (such as fosinopril)	May cause serious hypotension
Beta blockers (such as propranolol)	May cause serious hypotension
Other nitrates	May cause serious hypotension
Phenothiazines (such as chlorpromazine)	May cause serious hypotension

isosorbide dinitrate and mononitrate.

Interventions

Preparation and administration
• Teach the patient how to take the drug. (See *Taking isosorbide dinitrate or mononitrate at home*, page 188.)

Safety tip. Administer doses on a schedule that provides a nitrate-free interval of 8 to 12 hours per day to decrease the incidence of tolerance.

Monitoring and supportive care
• Monitor blood pressure and intensity and duration of response to the drug.
• Monitor the patient for 5 to 10 minutes after administration of sublingual or chewable forms.
• The drug should not be discontinued abruptly because coronary vasospasm may occur.

• Don't confuse isosorbide dinitrate or mononitrate with isosorbide, an osmotic diuretic used to treat glaucoma.

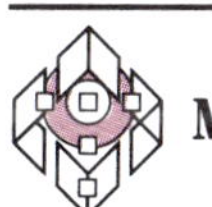 **MedTest**

1. The onset of action of chewable isosorbide dinitrate is:
    a. less than 5 minutes.
    b. 10 to 15 minutes.
    c. 30 minutes.
    d. 1 hour.

2. Isosorbide's vasodilator action occurs primarily in:
    a. coronary arteries.
    b. collateral coronary circulation.
    c. resistance vessels (arteries and arterioles).
    d. capacitance vessels (veins and venules).

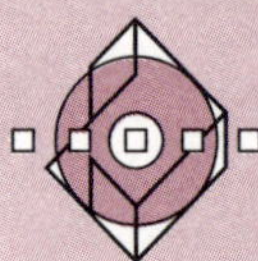

Taking isosorbide dinitrate or mononitrate at home

In addition to explaining the drug's action and dosage, teach the patient who will continue isosorbide dinitrate or mononitrate therapy after discharge to follow these important guidelines.

Take your medication correctly

☐ Chew chewable tablets thoroughly before swallowing.

☐ To take a sublingual tablet, wet the tablet with saliva, then place it under your tongue until it's completely absorbed. You may also hold the tablet in the side of your mouth.

☐ Repeat sublingual dose every 5 to 10 minutes, as needed, up to a maximum of three doses within 30 minutes. If no relief is obtained, call your doctor immediately or have someone take you to the hospital emergency department.

☐ Take the oral tablet or capsule form with a full (8-oz) glass of water either 30 minutes before or 1 to 2 hours after meals. Swallow the tablet or capsule whole. Don't break, crush, or chew these forms.

☐ If you miss a scheduled dose, take it as soon as possible. However, if the next scheduled dose is within 2 hours (or within 6 hours for a sustained-release form), skip the missed dose and go back to your regular dosing schedule. Don't double doses.

Know when to call your doctor

☐ Don't stop taking this drug suddenly (even if unpleasant adverse reactions occur). Discuss any adverse reactions with your doctor.

☐ Call your doctor if you experience no change or an increase in your anginal attacks because your medication may not be effective.

☐ Be aware that these drugs may cause headaches, especially at first. To relieve headaches, take acetaminophen or aspirin. Notify your doctor if headaches persist or become worse.

Other instructions

☐ Avoid alcoholic beverages, prolonged standing, excessive exercise, and hot weather when possible.

☐ Remember to change positions slowly (especially from lying flat to sitting upright) and to dangle your legs over the bedside for a few minutes before standing to minimize light-headedness. Lie down immediately if dizziness occurs.

☐ If you're taking antihypertensive medications and experience increased fatigue or dizziness, space your medicines 1 to 2 hours apart.

☐ If you're taking the sustained-release form of these drugs, be alert for partially dissolved tablets in your stools. If you discover such pieces, notify your doctor because the drug must be properly digested to provide the correct dose.

☐ Check with your doctor or pharmacist before taking OTC medications.

3. You should advise your patient that he may initially experience which adverse reaction:

   a. dizziness.
   b. headache.
   c. orthostatic hypotension.
   d. nausea and vomiting.

Labetalol hydrochloride

Also known by the brand names Normodyne, Trandate, and (in Australia) Presolol, labetalol is an alpha- and beta-adrenergic blocking agent that's classified therapeutically as an antihypertensive. It's available in 100-, 200-, and 300-mg tablets and in 20- and 40-ml vials for injection as 5 mg/ml.

Pharmacokinetics

• *Absorption:* Labetalol undergoes extensive first-pass metabolism in the liver and only about 25% of an oral dose reaches the systemic circulation. Onset occurs in 20 minutes to 2 hours, with peak effect in 1 to 4 hours. After I.V. administration, onset occurs in 2 to 5 minutes, with peak effect in 5 to 15 minutes.
• *Distribution:* Approximately 50% protein-bound.
• *Metabolism:* Metabolized extensively in the liver and possibly in GI mucosa to inactive metabolites.
• *Excretion:* About 5% is excreted unchanged in urine; the remainder is excreted as metabolites in urine and feces. Elimination half-life is 6 to 8 hours.

Indications, dosage, and action
Hypertension

• *Adult dosage:* 100 mg P.O. b.i.d. Increase by 100 mg b.i.d. daily every 2 or 4 days until optimum response is reached. Usual maintenance dosage is 200 to 400 mg b.i.d.

Severe hypertension, hypertensive crisis, clonidine-withdrawal hypertension
• *Adult dosage:* Initially, 20-mg I.V. slowly over 2 minutes; if necessary, give 40 to 80 mg q 10 minutes to a maximum dosage of 300 mg.

   Alternatively, may be given by intermittent infusion, diluting 200 mg with 160 ml of D_5W and infusing at an initial rate of 2 mg/minute. Usual cumulative dosage is 50 to 200 mg. May repeat q 6 to 8 hours.
• *Antihypertensive action:* Blocks both beta-adrenergic and postsynaptic alpha-adrenergic receptor sites, and depresses renin secretion. Drug may also have a vasodilating effect. The effect of an oral dose persists for about 8 to 24 hours; after I.V. administration, it lasts 2 to 4 hours.

Contraindications and cautions

• Don't use in patients with overt cardiac failure, severe bradycardia, second- or third-degree AV block (unless a pacemaker is in place), bronchial asthma, or cardiogenic shock because the drug may worsen these conditions.
• Use with caution in patients with pheochromocytoma because paradoxical hypertensive responses have been reported.
• Use with caution in patients with diabetes mellitus or hyperthyroidism

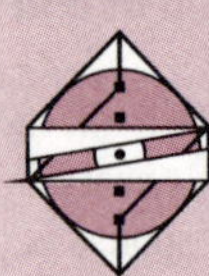

Incompatibility warning
Labetalol combinations to avoid

Be aware that labetalol is incompatible with 5% sodium bicarbonate injection because it forms a white precipitate within 6 hours after mixing. The precipitate results because the mixture has a pH of 7.6 to 8. (Labetalol is most stable in acidic solutions with a pH of 2 to 4.)

because labetalol may mask tachycardia (but not sweating or dizziness) caused by hypoglycemia or hyperthyroidism.
- Use cautiously in elderly patients and in patients with impaired hepatic function (lower dosage may be necessary).
- Use in children only if potential benefit outweighs risk.
- Use cautiously in breast-feeding women because the drug is excreted into breast milk.
- Pregnancy risk category C

Life-threatening adverse reactions
- Severe hypotension, CHF
- Severe hepatocellular injury

Common adverse reactions
- Dizziness, fatigue
- Nausea

Infrequent adverse reactions
- Orthostatic hypotension, peripheral vascular insufficiency, bradycardia

- Dyspnea, increased airway resistance
- Headache, vivid dreams
- Vomiting, dyspepsia, diarrhea, elevated liver function test results, hepatitis, jaundice
- Sexual dysfunction, urine retention
- Nasal stuffiness
- Rash, tingling scalp

Interactions
- *Beta-adrenergic agonists:* Labetalol may antagonize bronchodilation produced by beta-adrenergic agonists.
- *Cimetidine:* May decrease labetalol metabolism, causing accumulation. Give together cautiously.
- *Diuretics, other antihypertensive agents:* May cause additive hypotension. Use together cautiously.
- *Inhaled anesthetics such as halothane:* Increased risk of arrhythmias or hypotension.
- *Insulin, oral antidiabetic drugs:* Can alter dosage requirements in previously stabilized diabetics. Observe patient carefully.

Interventions
Preparation and administration
- For I.V. use, administer labetalol with an infusion pump.

Safety tip. Monitor blood pressure closely: q 5 minutes for 30 minutes, then q 30 minutes for 2 hours, and then hourly for 6 hours. Keep the patient supine for 3 hours after infusion. (See *Labetalol combinations to avoid.*)

Monitoring and supportive care
- Monitor the patient's blood pressure frequently. (See *Taking labetalol at home.*)

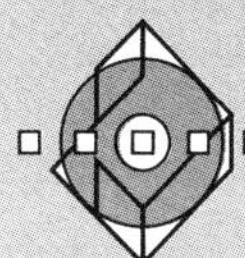

Patient-teaching checklist

Taking labetalol at home

In addition to explaining the drug's action and dosage, teach the patient who will continue labetalol therapy after discharge to follow these important guidelines.

Take your medication correctly

☐ You may take labetalol with or without food.

☐ Take labetalol as prescribed even when you're feeling well. Be aware that dosage changes are common at the beginning of therapy and that it may take days for the drug to produce optimal effects.

Know when to call your doctor

☐ Continue taking the drug even if unpleasant adverse reactions occur because abrupt discontinuation can exacerbate angina and MI. But be sure to discuss adverse reactions with your doctor.

☐ Take your blood pressure frequently when taking labetalol, and notify the doctor of any significant changes.

☐ Report new or increasing fatigue. If you take labetalol with other antihypertensive medications, discuss spacing out your medications to minimize excessive fatigue.

Watch for adverse reactions

☐ Remember to change positions slowly (especially from lying flat to sitting upright) and to dangle your legs over the bedside for a few minutes before standing to minimize the potential for drug-induced lightheadedness.

☐ Lie down immediately if dizziness or faintness occurs.

☐ During labetalol therapy, avoid drinking alcoholic beverages, prolonged standing, and excessive exercising, especially in hot weather, because these activities can increase your risk of fainting or developing dizziness or light-headedness.

☐ Avoid driving or operating machinery if dizziness occurs.

☐ Be aware that transient scalp tingling sometimes occurs at the beginning of therapy, but this usually subsides quickly.

Other instructions

☐ Schedule frequent rest periods throughout the day if fatigue occurs as a result of labetalol use.

☐ Monitor your blood glucose level closely if you have diabetes and take medication to control your blood glucose level because labetalol may alter your dosage requirements. Be prepared to treat labetalol-induced hypoglycemia immediately and notify your doctor if hypoglycemic episodes are severe or recur frequently.

☐ Check with your doctor or pharmacist before taking OTC medications.

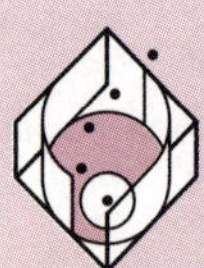

Compliance builder

Changing labetalol dosage

To increase compliance with oral labetalol therapy in the patient experiencing dizziness, ask the doctor if the patient can take one dose h.s. or take smaller doses t.i.d. These dosage changes can help minimize this adverse reaction.

• To minimize dizziness, have the patient rise slowly and avoid sudden position changes. Taking a dose at bedtime or taking smaller doses t.i.d. will also help the patient deal with this common reaction.

Safety tip. Discuss changes in the medication schedule with the doctor. (See *Changing labetalol dosage*.)

• Tell the patient that although transient scalp tingling occurs occasionally at the beginning of labetalol therapy, it usually subsides quickly.

• Titration of hospitalized patients from parenteral to oral labetalol should begin with 200 mg and then proceed to 200 to 400 mg P.O. 6 to 12 hours later. Thereafter, the same total daily dosage should be given orally that the patient received I.V., except divided t.i.d.

• Know that this drug masks common signs of shock and hypoglycemia.

Safety tip. Assess for CNS signs of hypoglycemia, such as changes in mental status, restlessness, and irritability. Monitor blood glucose levels as necessary.

• Be aware that labetalol therapy may cause a false-positive increase in urine free and total catecholamine levels when measured by a nonspecific fluorometric method.

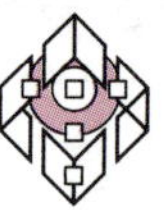

MedTest

1. When labetalol is first administered I.V., you should:
   a. give it by slow push, over a 5-minute period.
   b. monitor cardiac rate and rhythm.
   c. observe the patient closely for bronchospasm.
   d. monitor blood pressure closely (q 5 minutes for 30 minutes).

2. The most troublesome adverse effect of labetalol is:
   a. dizziness.
   b. sexual dysfunction.
   c. dyspnea.
   d. scalp tingling.

3. Which of the following signs of hypoglycemia would not be evident in the diabetic patient taking labetalol?
   a. Restlessness
   b. Tachycardia
   c. Dizziness
   d. Mental status changes

Lidocaine hydrochloride

Also known by the brand names Alphacaine, Anestacon, L-caine, Lidoject, LidoPen Auto-Injector,

Xylocaine, and (in Canada and Australia) Xylocard, lidocaine is an amide derivative that's classified therapeutically as a ventricular anti-arrhythmic. It's available for injection — for direct I.V. use in syringes containing 50 mg/5 ml, 100 mg/10 ml, and in vials, syringes, and ampules containing 100 mg/5 ml; for I.M. use in 300 mg/3 ml automatic injection device or 500 mg/5 ml ampules; for I.V. admixture in vials containing 1 g/10 ml and in vials and syringes containing 1 g/5 ml, 1 g/25 ml, 2 g/10 ml, and 2 g/50 ml. It's also available for infusion, premixed with D_5W as 2-, 4-, and 8-mg/ml solutions.

Pharmacokinetics

• *Absorption:* A significant first-pass effect by the liver prevents oral administration.

• *Distribution:* After I.V. bolus administration, there is an early, rapid decline in drug concentration in the plasma. This is due primarily to the distribution of the drug into highly perfused tissues, such as the kidneys, lungs, and heart. This is followed by metabolism and redistribution of the drug into skeletal muscle and adipose tissue. Lidocaine has a high affinity for adipose tissue. As the concentration of the drug in the plasma falls, lidocaine diffuses from the highly perfused tissues and adipose tissue back into the blood. Distribution volume declines in patients with CHF, resulting in potentially toxic concentrations with usual doses. About 60% to 80% of circulating drug is bound to plasma proteins. Usual

therapeutic drug level is 1.5 to 5 mcg/ml.

• *Metabolism:* Metabolized in the liver to two active metabolites. Less than 10% of a parenteral dose reaches the kidneys unchanged. Metabolism is affected by hepatic blood flow, which may decrease after MI and with CHF or pretreatment with beta blockers. Liver disease also may limit metabolism.

• *Excretion:* The half-life of the initial phase is 7 to 30 minutes; terminal elimination half-life is 1½ to 2 hours. Hepatic disease, CHF, or continuous infusions longer than 24 hours may cause an increase in half-life.

Indications, dosage, and action

Ventricular arrhythmias from MI or myocardial ischemia, cardiac manipulation, or digitalis toxicity

• *Adult dosage:* ACLS dosage is 1.5 mg/kg by I.V. bolus at 25 to 50 mg/minute, followed by an additional 1.5 mg/kg in 10 to 20 minutes to a maximum of 3 mg/kg. Additional bolus doses may be given q 3 to 5 minutes until arrhythmia subsides, but no more than 300 mg total bolus during a 1-hour period. Give one-half this amount to elderly or light-weight patients and to those with CHF.

In circumstances not requiring ACLS, give 1 mg/kg by I.V. bolus, followed by 0.5 mg/kg in 10 to 20 minutes. Simultaneously start an infusion at 2 mg/minute to maintain therapeutic serum level. After 24 hours, decrease infusion rate by one-half.

I.M. administration — 200 to 300 mg in deltoid muscle in early stages of acute MI.
• *Pediatric dosage:* 1 mg/kg by I.V. bolus, followed by infusion of 30 mcg/kg/minute.
• *Antiarrhythmic action:* A local anesthetic that acts as a class Ib antiarrhythmic, lidocaine suppresses automaticity and shortens the effective refractory period and action potential duration of His-Purkinje fibers; it also suppresses spontaneous ventricular depolarization during diastole. Therapeutic concentrations do not significantly affect conductive atrial tissue and AV conduction. The drug seems to act preferentially on diseased myocardial tissue.

Contraindications and cautions
• Avoid use in patients with Stokes-Adams syndrome or severe SA, AV, or intraventricular heart block who don't have an artificial pacemaker because the drug may worsen these conditions.
• Don't use in patients with hypersensitivity to amide-type anesthetic agents.
• Avoid use in patients with inflammation or infection in a puncture region, septicemia, severe hypertension, spinal deformities, and neurologic disorders.
• Use cautiously in debilitated, acutely ill, or obstetric patients.
• Use with caution in patients with severe shock, first- or second-degree AV block, general drug allergies, and paracervical block.

• Use cautiously in patients with WPW syndrome, bradycardia, incomplete heart block, or atrial fibrillation because the drug may exacerbate these conditions and precipitate other arrhythmias.
• Use cautiously in elderly patients and in patients with CHF, renal or hepatic disease, or those who weigh less than 110 lb (50 kg). These patients will need a reduced dosage.
• Use cautiously in breast-feeding women because it is not known whether this drug is excreted in breast milk.
• Pregnancy risk category B

Life-threatening adverse reactions
• Cardiac arrest, new or worsened arrhythmias
• Seizures
• Anaphylaxis

Common adverse reactions
None at prescribed dosage

Infrequent adverse reactions
• Myocardial depression, hypotension, bradycardia, edema
• Anxiety, apprehension, nervousness, seizures followed by drowsiness, unconsciousness, respiratory arrest, confusion, tremors, lethargy, somnolence, stupor, restlessness, slurred speech, euphoria, depression, light-headedness, paresthesia, muscle twitching
• Nausea, vomiting
• Tinnitus, blurred or double vision
• Dermatologic reactions (local sensitization, rash)

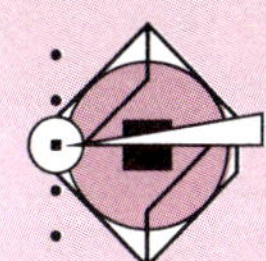

Interactions alert

Life-threatening hazards of multidrug therapy with lidocaine

Interacting drug	Effects
Antiarrhythmic agents (such as procainamide and quinidine)	Predispose patient to proarrhythmia
Beta blockers (such as propranolol)	May cause antagonistic effects as well as lidocaine toxicity
Cimetidine (antiulcer agent)	May cause lidocaine toxicity
Phenytoin (anticonvulsant agent)	May cause additive or antagonist effects as well as lidocaine toxicity

• Soreness at injection site, cold sensation, diaphoresis, hypersensitivity reactions

Interactions

• *Hepatic enzyme inducers (barbiturates, phenytoin, rifampin):* Enhanced lidocaine metabolism. Dosage adjustments may be needed.
• *Succinylcholine:* Concomitant use may increase succinylcholine's neuromuscular effects.

For dangerous interactions, see *Life-threatening hazards of multidrug therapy with lidocaine.*

Interventions

Preparation and administration

• Patients receiving I.V. lidocaine infusion should be placed on a cardiac monitor at all times. (See *Giving I.V. lidocaine safely*, page 196.)

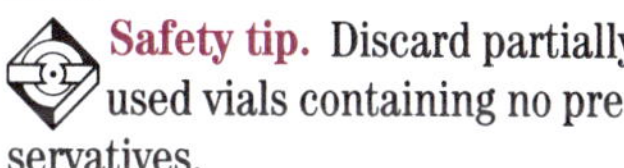
Safety tip. Don't exceed an infusion rate of 4 mg/minute. A faster rate greatly increases the risk of toxicity.

Safety tip. Don't administer lidocaine with epinephrine (for local anesthesia) to treat arrhythmias.

Safety tip. Discard partially used vials containing no preservatives.

Monitoring and supportive care

• Monitor the patient's response, vital signs, and serum electrolyte, BUN, and creatinine levels.
• Know that seizures may be the first sign of toxicity. However, severe reactions are usually preceded by somnolence, confusion, and paresthesia. Regard all signs and symptoms of toxicity as serious, and promptly reduce the dosage or discontinue therapy.
• Know that lidocaine therapy may increase CK levels. Isoenzyme tests should be performed for differential diagnosis of acute MI.

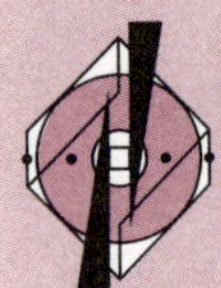

Administration guidelines

Giving I.V. lidocaine safely

To ensure your patient's safety during I.V. lidocaine therapy, follow these guidelines.

Starting therapy
• Be prepared to administer lidocaine as an I.V. bolus first. Administer the bolus dose slowly (no faster than 50 mg/minute).
• Expect to repeat the bolus in 10 to 20 minutes or to give the drug by I.V. push every 3 to 5 minutes until the patient's arrhythmia has disappeared, a maximum of 300 mg has been given, or adverse reactions (such as CNS disturbances, bradycardia, hypotension, or other arrhythmias) develop. Be aware that a bolus *not* followed by an infusion will have only a transient effect.

Administering continuous infusion
• Following bolus administration, administer by continuous infusion at the rate prescribed. Take care not to exceed 4 mg/minute because a faster rate increases the risk of toxicity.
• Use an infusion pump to administer the prescribed dosage precisely.
• Throughout lidocaine administration, observe the patient closely and monitor his cardiac rate and rhythm.

Stopping therapy
• Discontinue lidocaine by shutting off the infusion. The drug weans itself; you don't need to wean the patient over a period of hours or days.

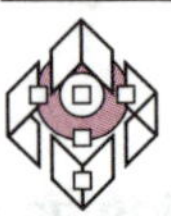

MedTest

1. Your 165-lb (75-kg) male patient is in ventricular fibrillation. According to current ACLS criteria, you would administer a lidocaine bolus of:
   a. 75 mg.
   b. 100 mg.
   c. 112.5 mg.
   d. 363 mg.

2. You would administer this bolus at the rate of:
   a. 10 to 25 mg/minute.
   b. 25 to 50 mg/minute.
   c. 50 to 100 mg/minute.
   d. more than 100 mg/minute (as rapidly as possible).

3. Your patient has been receiving lidocaine by continuous infusion at a rate of 2 mg/minute, and it's to be discontinued. You should:
   a. slow to 1 mg/minute for the next 24 hours, then 0.5 mg/minute for 24 hours, and then discontinue.
   b. slow to 1 mg/minute for 12 hours, then 0.5 mg/minute for 12 hours, and then discontinue.
   c. slow to 1 mg/minute for 6 hours and then discontinue.
   d. shut off the lidocaine infusion.

Lisinopril

Also known by the brand names Prinivil and Zestril, lisinopril is an ACE inhibitor that's classified therapeutically as an antihypertensive

Two alternatives: Quinapril and ramipril

In addition to lisinopril, a number of other ACE inhibitors are available today. Two of the more recently approved ones are quinapril hydrochloride and ramipril.

Similarities and differences

All three of these drugs are relatively equal in their antihypertensive effectiveness. But quinapril and ramipril differ significantly from lisinopril in their pharmacokinetics.

Quinapril and ramipril are "prodrugs" — inactive compounds that are metabolized in the body into pharmacologically active components: in this case, quinaprilat and ramiprilat. Lisinopril, by contrast, is a lysine analog of enalaprilat (the activated form of enalapril) and doesn't require activation.

All three of these drugs are long-acting and need to be given only once a day. Consequently, patients are more likely to comply with their drug therapy.

Unlike many other ACE inhibitors, quinapril and ramipril do not contain sulfhydryl groups — chemical structures that researchers have linked to various adverse reactions, including rash, leukopenia, and dysgeusia.

Quinapril hydrochloride

Known by the brand name Accupril, quinapril produces the greatest decrease in peripheral vascular resistance of all currently available ACE inhibitors. Quinapril is available in 5-, 10-, 20-, and 40-mg tablets. The usual adult dosage is 10 mg P.O. daily. Dosage should be adjusted based on the patient's response after about 2 weeks. Most patients are controlled at 20, 40, or 80 mg daily as a single dose or in two divided doses.

Ramipril

Known by the brand name Altace, ramipril is available in 1.25-, 2.5-, 5-, and 10-mg capsules. The usual adult dosage is 2.5 mg P.O. daily. Dosage is adjusted based on the patient's response after about 2 weeks. The usual maintenance dosage is 2.5 to 20 mg daily as a single dose or in two equal doses.

---

agent. It's available in 5-, 10-, and 20-mg tablets. (See *Two alternatives: Quinapril and ramipril*.)

Pharmacokinetics

• *Absorption:* Only about 25% of an oral dose is absorbed. Peak serum levels occur in about 7 hours. Onset of antihypertensive activity occurs in about 1 hour, with peak effect in about 6 hours.

• *Distribution:* Plasma protein–binding appears to be insignificant. Minimal amounts enter the brain; drug crosses the placenta.

• *Metabolism:* Not metabolized.

• *Excretion:* Excreted unchanged in the urine.

Indications, dosage, and action
Mild to severe hypertension
• *Adult dosage:* Initially, 10 mg P.O. daily. Most patients are well controlled on 20 to 40 mg daily as a single dose.
• *Antihypertensive action:* Inhibits ACE, preventing pulmonary conversion of angiotensin I to angiotensin II, a potent vasoconstrictor. Reduced formation of angiotensin II decreases peripheral arterial resistance and aldosterone secretion, thereby reducing sodium and water retention and blood pressure.

Contraindications and cautions
• Don't give to patients hypersensitive to ACE inhibitors.
• Use with caution in elderly patients and in patients with impaired renal function because the drug may worsen oliguria or progressive azotemia.
• Use with caution in patients with severe CHF.
• Use in children only if potential benefits outweigh risks.
• Use cautiously in breast-feeding women because the drug may be distributed into breast milk.
• Pregnancy risk category C (D in second and third trimesters)

Life-threatening adverse reactions
• Angioedema

Common adverse reactions
• Dizziness, headache

Infrequent adverse reactions
• Hypotension, orthostatic hypotension, chest pain

• Upper respiratory symptoms, cough
• Fatigue, depression, somnolence, paresthesia
• Diarrhea, nausea, vomiting, dyspepsia, loss of taste
• Impotence, decreased libido
• Nasal congestion
• Neutropenia
• Hyperkalemia
• Rash
• Muscle cramps

Interactions
• *Indomethacin, NSAIDs:* Attenuated antihypertensive effect. Monitor patient closely.
• *Insulin, oral antidiabetic agents:* Risk of hypoglycemia, especially at initiation of lisinopril therapy. Monitor closely.
  For dangerous interactions, see *Life-threatening hazards of multidrug therapy with lisinopril.*

Interventions
Preparation and administration
• Know that lisinopril absorption is unaffected by food. (See *Taking ACE inhibitors at home*, page 87.)

Monitoring and supportive care
• Lisinopril enhances the antihypertensive effect of diuretics. Diuretics should be discontinued 2 to 3 days before starting lisinopril.
• Diuretics should be added cautiously to the patient's regimen if lisinopril doesn't adequately control blood pressure.
• Review WBC and differential counts before treatment and periodically thereafter.

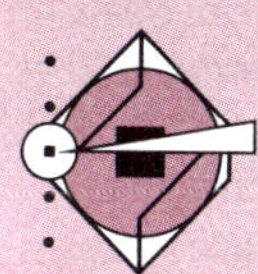

Life-threatening hazards of multidrug therapy with lisinopril

Interacting drug	Effects
Diuretics (such as hydrochlorothiazide)	May cause excessive hypotension
Potassium-containing salt substitutes (such as Co-salt and Chlor-3 condiment)	May result in hyperkalemia
Potassium-sparing diuretics (such as spironolactone)	May result in hyperkalemia
Potassium supplements (such as potassium chloride)	May result in hyperkalemia

• Remember that the drug's physiologic effects may lead to elevations of serum potassium, serum creatinine, BUN, and serum bilirubin levels; minor reductions of hemoglobin and hematocrit levels; and changes in liver enzyme tests.

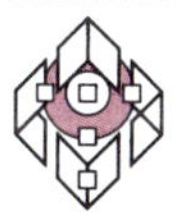

MedTest

1. Which of the following medications should be discontinued before starting lisinopril therapy?
  a. Diuretics
  b. Digitalis glycosides
  c. Anticonvulsants
  d. Anticoagulants

2. Common adverse effects of lisinopril include:
  a. upper respiratory symptoms.
  b. angioedema.
  c. nausea and vomiting.
  d. headache or dizziness.

3. Which of the following ACE inhibitors produces the greatest decrease in peripheral vascular resistance?
  a. Lisinopril
  b. Ramipril
  c. Quinapril
  d. Fosinopril

Lovastatin

Also known by the brand name Mevacor, lovastatin is a lactone that's classified therapeutically as a cholesterol-lowering agent. It's available in 20- and 40-mg tablets.

Pharmacokinetics

• *Absorption:* About 30% of an oral dose is absorbed. Administration of the drug with food increases plasma levels of active drug by about 30%.

Onset occurs in 3 days, with peak effect seen in 4 to 6 weeks.
• *Distribution:* Less than 5% of an oral dose reaches the systemic circulation because of extensive first-pass hepatic metabolism; the liver is the drug's principal site of action. Both the parent compound and its metabolite are highly bound (more than 95%) to plasma proteins. Lovastatin can cross the placenta and the blood-brain barrier.
• *Metabolism:* Lovastatin is converted to the active beta-hydroxy acid form in the liver. Other metabolites include the 6′ hydroxy derivative and two unidentified compounds.
• *Excretion:* Mostly excreted in the feces with a small amount (about 10%) excreted in urine.

Indications, dosage, and action
Reduction of LDL and total cholesterol in primary hypercholesterolemia (types IIa and IIb)
• *Adult dosage:* Initially, 20 mg P.O. once daily with the evening meal. For patients with severely elevated cholesterol levels (over 300 mg/dl), the initial dose should be 40 mg. The recommended range is 20 to 80 mg P.O. in single or divided doses.
• *Antilipemic action:* Lovastatin's active metabolite inhibits 3-hydroxy-3-methylglutaryl-coenzyme A reductase (HMG-CoA reductase). This enzyme is an early (and rate-limiting) step in the synthetic pathway of cholesterol.

Contraindications and cautions
• Don't use in patients with evidence of liver disease because the drug may be hepatotoxic.
• Avoid use in breast-feeding women because it's not known whether the drug is excreted in breast milk.
• This drug is contraindicated in women of childbearing age unless there's no risk of pregnancy.
• Marked persistent elevations in serum levels of ALT and AST have been noted. It's recommended that liver function tests be performed q 4 to 6 weeks during the first few months of therapy and periodically thereafter.
• Use cautiously in patients with a history of liver disease and in those who consume substantial quantities of alcohol.
• Use cautiously in patients at risk for developing renal failure secondary to rhabdomyolysis, such as trauma patients and patients undergoing major surgery, and in patients with severe acute infection, hypotension, uncontrolled seizures, or severe metabolic, endocrine, or electrolyte disorders.
• Pregnancy risk category X

Life-threatening adverse reactions
• Rhabdomyolysis

Common adverse reactions
• Headache
• Diarrhea, flatus, abdominal pain or cramps
• Rash, pruritus

Infrequent adverse reactions
• Dizziness
• Constipation, dyspepsia, heartburn, nausea
• Blurred vision, dysgeusia

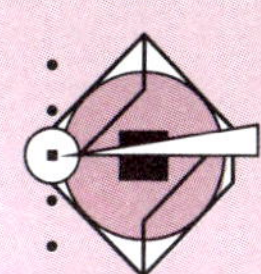

Life-threatening hazards of multidrug therapy with lovastatin

Interacting drug	Effects
Cyclosporine (immunosuppressant)	Increases risk of severe myopathy or rhabdomyolysis
Erythromycin (antibiotic)	Increases risk of severe myopathy or rhabdomyolysis
Gemfibrozil (antilipemic)	Increases risk of severe myopathy or rhabdomyolysis
Niacin (B-complex vitamin)	Increases risk of severe myopathy or rhabdomyolysis
Warfarin (oral anticoagulant)	Increases risk of bleeding

- Elevated serum AST and ALT levels, abnormal liver test results
- Muscle cramps, myalgia, myositis, peripheral neuropathy

Interactions

For dangerous interactions, see *Life-threatening hazards of multidrug therapy with lovastatin*.

Interventions

Preparation and administration

- Give lovastatin with the evening meal; absorption is enhanced and cholesterol biosynthesis is greater in the evening. (See *Taking lovastatin at home,* page 202.)

Monitoring and supportive care

- Lovastatin should be initiated only after diet and other nonpharmacologic therapies have proved ineffective. Continue a low-cholesterol diet throughout therapy.

- Monitor for signs of myositis; have the patient report any muscle aches and pains.
- Periodically monitor CK and liver enzyme levels.

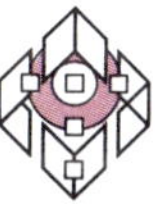

MedTest

1. Lovastatin produces its antilipemic effect by:

  a. reducing triglyceride synthesis in the liver.

  b. inhibiting an enzyme that's an early step in synthesizing cholesterol.

  c. accelerating hepatic catabolism of cholesterol.

  d. combining with bile acid to form an insoluble compound that's excreted.

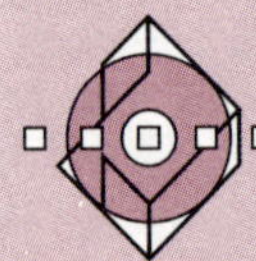

Patient-teaching checklist

Taking lovastatin at home

In addition to explaining the drug's action and dosage, teach the patient who will continue lovastatin therapy after discharge to follow these important guidelines.

Take your medication correctly

☐ Take lovastatin with your evening meal because absorption of this drug is enhanced by food.

☐ Take lovastatin as prescribed even when feeling well. Be aware that the drug may take up to 6 weeks to produce optimal effects.

☐ Continue taking the drug even if unpleasant reactions occur. Make sure you discuss any adverse reactions (especially muscle aches and pain) with your doctor.

☐ Adhere to your prescribed diet restricting total fat and cholesterol intake as well as caloric intake if you are overweight.

Other instructions

☐ Incorporate a regular exercise program into your lifestyle after obtaining approval by your doctor. Regular exercise, along with a low-fat, low-cholesterol diet, will help lovastatin lower your serum lipid levels.

☐ Remember to report for regular blood tests, which are used to measure drug effectiveness and toxicity.

☐ Restrict alcohol intake because alcohol can adversely affect your cholesterol profile. It can also damage the liver.

☐ Avoid driving or operating machinery if dizziness or blurred vision occurs.

---

2. A life-threatening adverse effect of lovastatin is:

    a. status asthmaticus.
    b. anaphylaxis.
    c. rhabdomyolysis.
    d. status epilepticus.

3. The patient should take lovastatin once daily:

    a. on an empty stomach.
    b. with breakfast.
    c. with dinner.
    d. h.s.

Metaraminol bitartrate

Also known by the brand name Aramine, metaraminol is an adrenergic agent that's classified therapeutically as a vasopressor. It's available for injection in 10-mg/ml ampules.

Pharmacokinetics

• *Absorption:* Onset after I.M. injection occurs within 10 minutes; after I.V. injection, within 1 to 2 minutes; after S.C. injection, within 5 to 20

minutes. Pressor effects may persist 20 to 90 minutes.
- *Distribution:* Not completely known.
- *Metabolism:* Not metabolized. Effects are terminated by uptake of drug into tissues and by urine excretion.
- *Excretion:* Excreted in urine; excretion may be accelerated by acidifying urine.

Indications, dosage, and action
Hypotension
- *Adult dosage:* 2 to 10 mg I.M. or S.C. Wait at least 10 minutes before administering additional doses so that the effects of the first dose may be evaluated. Subsequent doses are determined by the pressor response.
- *Pediatric dosage:* 0.1 mg/kg or 3 mg/m^2 S.C. or I.M. Wait at least 10 minutes before administering additional doses so that the effects of the first dose may be evaluated. Subsequent doses are determined by the pressor response.

Hypotension in severe shock
- *Adult dosage:* 0.5 to 5 mg direct I.V. followed by I.V. infusion. If necessary, mix 15 to 100 mg in 500 ml of 0.9% NaCl solution or D$_5$W; titrate infusion based on response.
- *Pediatric dosage:* 0.01 mg/kg or 0.03 mg/m^2 direct I.V. followed by I.V. infusion, if necessary, of 0.4 mg/kg or 12 mg/m^2 diluted and titrated to maintain desired blood pressure.
- *Vasopressor action:* Metaraminol acts predominantly by direct stimulation of alpha-adrenergic receptors, which constrict both capacitance and resistance blood vessels, resulting in increased total peripheral resistance and increased systolic and diastolic blood pressure. It also has a direct stimulating effect on beta$_1$ receptors of the heart, producing a positive inotropic response, and an indirect effect, releasing norepinephrine from its storage sites, which, with repeated use, may result in tachyphylaxis.

Contraindications and cautions
- Don't use metaraminol in patients with peripheral or mesenteric vascular thrombosis because it may increase ischemia and extend the area of infarction.
- Don't use in patients with pulmonary edema or those with metabolic or respiratory acidosis.
- Administer cautiously to hypertensive or hyperthyroid patients because the drug can increase adverse reactions.
- Use with caution in elderly patients and patients with diabetes, heart disease, cirrhosis, Buerger's disease, peripheral vascular disease, acidosis, or history of malaria (relapse may occur).
- Administer cautiously to patients with known sensitivity to sulfites because commercially available formulations contain sulfites.
- Prepare I.V. infusion solutions by diluting 1 mg of metaraminol per 25 ml of diluent. Use D$_5$W or 0.9% NaCl.
- Pregnancy risk category C

Life-threatening adverse reactions
- Severe hypertension, arrhythmias (including VT)
- Respiratory distress

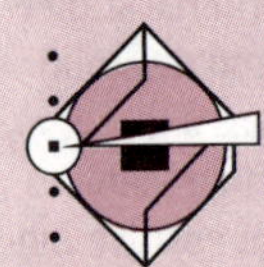

Life-threatening hazards of multidrug therapy with metaraminol

Interacting drug	Effects
Beta blockers (such as propranolol)	Block cardiac-stimulating effects of metaraminol, increasing potential for excessive bradycardia with possible AV block
MAO inhibitors (such as isocarboxazid)	May prolong and intensify cardiac-stimulating and vasopressor effects of MAO inhibitors, resulting in hypertensive crisis if metaraminol is given within 14 days of last MAO inhibitor dose

- Seizures (with excessive use)
- Metabolic acidosis in hypovolemia

Common adverse reactions
None noted

Infrequent adverse reactions
- Precordial pain, palpitations, arrhythmias, sinus or ventricular tachycardia, bradycardia, AV dissociation, hypotension, hypertension
- Apprehension, anxiety, tremor, restlessness, weakness, faintness, dizziness, headache
- Nausea, vomiting
- Decreased urine output
- Hyperglycemia
- Pallor, sweating, fever; local abscess, necrosis, and sloughing upon extravasation

Interactions
- *Alpha-adrenergic blocking agents:* Pressor effects of metaraminol may be decreased, but not completely blocked. Monitor patient response.
- *Antihypertensive agents:* Metaraminol may decrease antihypertensive effects.
- *Atropine:* Reflex bradycardia caused by metaraminol is blocked and pressor effect is enhanced. Monitor patient response.
- *Digitalis glycosides, general anesthetics, inhaled hydrocarbon, levodopa, maprotiline, other sympathomimetics, thyroid hormones:* Increased risk of adverse cardiac effects. Monitor closely.
- *Doxapram, ergot alkaloids, mazindol, methylphenidate, trimethaphan:* Pressor effects of metaraminol may be increased. Monitor patient response.

For dangerous interactions, see *Life-threatening hazards of multidrug therapy with metaraminol.*

Interventions

Preparation and administration

• Keep solution in light-resistant container away from heat.

• Check compatibility before mixing with other drugs. (See *Metaraminol combinations to avoid*.)

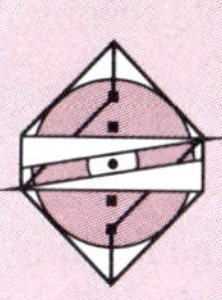 **Safety tip.** Ask the patient about allergy to sulfites before administering.

• For I.V. administration, use a central venous catheter or a large vein, such as one in the antecubital fossa, to minimize the risk of extravasation. Use an infusion pump to regulate the flow rate and a piggyback setup to allow continuation of the infusion if this drug is stopped.

Safety tip. Watch the infusion site carefully for signs of extravasation. If it occurs, stop the infusion immediately and call the doctor.

• Allow at least 10 minutes to elapse before administering additional doses because the maximum effect is not immediately apparent.

Monitoring and supportive care

• Blood volume depletion should be corrected before metaraminol administration. This drug is not a substitute for blood, plasma, fluids, or electrolyte replacement.

• During infusion, check blood pressure every 5 minutes until the patient is stabilized; then recheck every 15 minutes.

• Also monitor ECG, cardiac output, CVP, PAWP, pulse rate, urine output, and extremity color and temperature often during infusion. Titrate the in-

Metaraminol combinations to avoid

Be aware that metaraminol is incompatible with drugs that dissolve poorly in acid solutions, such as sulfonamides. When the two are mixed, a precipitate may form. Similarly, metaraminol shouldn't be mixed with acid-sensitive drugs, such as penicillins or erythromycins, because it may cause them to precipitate and increase the rate of their decomposition.

Because compatibility of metaraminol with other drugs may depend on several factors (such as concentration of the drugs, specific diluents used, resulting pH, and temperature), you should check with your pharmacist before administering metaraminol with any other drug.

fusion rate according to these findings, as ordered.

• Generally, blood pressure should be raised to slightly less than the patient's normal level.

• Remember that headache may be a symptom of hypertension. A rapidly induced hypertensive response can cause acute pulmonary edema, arrhythmias, and cardiac arrest.

• Withdraw the drug gradually; recurrent hypotension may follow abrupt withdrawal.

Safety tip. After metaraminol is withdrawn, continue to monitor blood pressure and heart rate and rhythm until the patient is sta-

ble, watching for a possible severe drop in blood pressure.
• Know that tachyphylaxis is possible with prolonged use.
• Urine output may decline initially and then increase as blood pressure reaches normal level.

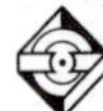 **Safety tip.** Report persistently decreased urine output.

• To treat extravasation, use a fine needle to infiltrate the site promptly with 10 to 15 ml of 0.9% NaCl solution containing 5 to 10 mg of phentolamine.
• Closely monitor fluid and electrolyte status.

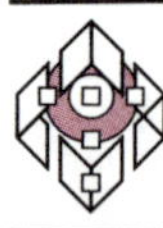 **MedTest**

1. Before administering metaraminol, you should ask the patient if he's allergic to:
   a. iodine or other radiopaque agents.
   b. insect stings.
   c. antibiotics.
   d. sulfites.

2. While administering metaraminol, you should closely monitor the patient's blood pressure and watch for:
   a. respiratory distress.
   b. extravasation at the infusion site.
   c. coolness and pallor of the extremities.
   d. dizziness.

3. A symptom that would alert you to an excessive metaraminol response (hypertension) is:
   a. increased urine output.

   b. a rapid pulse rate.
   c. headache.
   d. dizziness.

Methyldopa

Also known by the brand names Aldomet; Apo-Methyldopa and Novomedopa (in Canada); and Hydopa (in Australia), methyldopa is a centrally acting antiadrenergic agent that's classified therapeutically as an antihypertensive. It's available in 125-, 250-, and 500-mg tablets; as an oral suspension containing 250 mg/5 ml; and in 5-ml vials for injection (as methyldopate HCl) in a 250 mg/5-ml concentration.

Pharmacokinetics

• *Absorption:* About 50% of an oral dose is absorbed. After oral administration, maximal decline in blood pressure occurs in 3 to 6 hours; however, full effect is not evident for 2 to 3 days. No correlation exists between plasma concentration and antihypertensive effect. After I.V. administration, blood pressure usually begins to fall in 4 to 6 hours.
• *Distribution:* Bound weakly to plasma proteins.
• *Metabolism:* Metabolized extensively in the liver and intestinal cells to its active metabolite, alpha-methylnorepinephrine. Some inactive metabolites are also formed.
• *Excretion:* Methyldopa and its metabolites are excreted in urine; the unabsorbed drug is excreted unchanged in feces. Elimination half-life is approximately 2 hours.

Indications, dosage, and action
Moderate to severe hypertension

• *Adult dosage:* Initially, 250 mg P.O. b.i.d. to t.i.d. for first 48 hours, then increased or decreased p.r.n. q 2 days. Entire daily dose may be given in the evening or h.s. Dosage may need adjustment if other antihypertensive drugs are added to or deleted from therapy. Maintenance dosage is 500 mg to 2 g daily in two to four divided doses. Maximum recommended daily dosage is 3 g.

For I.V. infusion, give 250 to 500 mg over 30 to 60 minutes q 6 hours. Maximum I.V. dosage is 1 g q 6 hours.

• *Pediatric dosage:* Initially, 10 mg/ kg or 300 mg/m^2 P.O. daily in two to four divided doses; or 20 to 40 mg/kg or 0.6 to 1.2 g/m^2 I.V. daily in four divided doses. Increase dosage at least every 2 days until desired response occurs. Maximum daily dosage is 65 mg/kg, 2 g/m^2, or 3 g, whichever is least.

• *Antihypertensive action:* Exact mechanism of action is unknown; it's thought to be caused by methyldopa's metabolite, alpha-methylnorepinephrine, which stimulates central inhibitory alpha-adrenergic receptors, decreasing total peripheral resistance. Drug may also act as a false neurotransmitter. Its antihypertensive effect usually persists up to 24 hours after oral administration and 10 to 16 hours after I.V. administration.

Contraindications and cautions

• Don't use in patients with active hepatic disease, such as hepatitis or cirrhosis, or in patients with a history of hepatic dysfunction, especially those who developed such dysfunction during previous methyldopa therapy.

• Also avoid use in patients with renal failure.

• The drug should be discontinued if any of the following occurs: abnormalities in liver function test results, jaundice, a positive Coombs' test, or choreoathetoid movements.

• Know that dosage reductions may be necessary in elderly patients.

• Recommend an alternative infant feeding method to breast-feeding women during therapy because the drug is distributed in breast milk.

• Pregnancy risk category B

Life-threatening adverse reactions

• Hepatic necrosis
• Hemolytic anemia

Common adverse reactions

• Orthostatic hypotension, edema, weight gain
• Sedation, decreased mental acuity
• Impotence
• Dry mouth, nasal stuffiness

Infrequent adverse reactions

• Bradycardia, aggravated angina, myocarditis
• Headache, weakness, dizziness, involuntary choreoathetoid movements, psychic disturbances, depression, nightmares
• Diarrhea, pancreatitis, hepatic necrosis, abnormal liver function test results
• Reversible granulocytopenia, thrombocytopenia

- Rash
- Gynecomastia, lactation, drug-induced fever

Interactions
- *Amphetamines, norepinephrine, phenothiazines, sympathomimetics, tricyclic antidepressants:* Possible decreased antihypertensive effects. Monitor patient response.
- *Anesthetic agents:* Patients undergoing surgery may require reduced dosages of anesthetics. Notify anesthesiologist of patient's drug regimen.
- *Haloperidol:* Concomitant use may produce dementia and sedation. Monitor patient response.
- *Levodopa:* Additive hypotension; possible increased CNS reactions. Monitor patient response.

Interventions
Preparation and administration
- Administer methyldopa HCl I.V.; I.M. or S.C. administration isn't recommended because of the drug's unpredictable absorption.
- Dilute prescribed I.V. dose in D_5W and administer over 30 to 60 minutes q 6 hours.
- Give at bedtime to minimize daytime sedation and drowsiness. (See *Taking methyldopa at home.*)

Monitoring and supportive care
- Methyldopa is dialyzable. Additional doses may be required after a dialysis session.
- At the initiation of and periodically throughout therapy, monitor hemoglobin and hematocrit levels and RBC count for hemolytic ane-

mia; also monitor liver function tests.

◆ **Safety tip.** If the patient requires a blood transfusion, make sure that both direct and indirect Coombs' tests are done to avoid crossmatching problems.

- With I.V. use, monitor for involuntary choreoathetoid movements. Report these to the doctor because the drug may need to be discontinued.
- Take blood pressure in supine, sitting, and standing positions during dosage adjustment.

◆ **Safety tip.** Take blood pressure at least q 30 minutes during I.V. infusion until the patient is stable.

- Know that sedation and drowsiness usually disappear with continued therapy.

◆ **Safety tip.** Check for orthostatic hypotension, which may indicate a need for dosage reduction.

- Know that signs of hepatotoxicity may occur 2 to 4 weeks after therapy begins.
- Monitor the patient for signs and symptoms of drug-induced depression.
- Know that methyldopa is frequently used to treat hypertension in pregnant women, apparently without ill effects to the fetus, if the patient is closely monitored. Some clinicians recommend not beginning therapy between 16 and 20 weeks' gestation if possible.
- Methyldopa alters urine uric acid, serum creatinine, and AST levels; it may also cause falsely high levels of urine catecholamines, interfering with the diagnosis of pheochromocy-

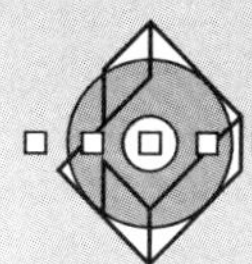

Patient-teaching checklist

Taking methyldopa at home

In addition to explaining the drug's action and dosage, teach the patient who will continue methyldopa therapy after discharge to follow these important guidelines.

Take your medication correctly

☐ Ask your doctor about taking methyldopa at bedtime until you develop tolerance to sedation, drowsiness, and other CNS reactions (usually in 2 to 3 weeks). Then take the drug during the day as prescribed, with or without food.

☐ Adhere to a consistent daily administration schedule if times other than bedtime are chosen after tolerance develops.

☐ Check your blood pressure frequently (at least once a week). Notify your doctor of any significant change.

☐ Take methyldopa as prescribed even when you're feeling well. Be aware that the drug may take up to 3 days to produce optimal effects.

Watch for adverse reactions

☐ Continue taking the drug even if unpleasant adverse reactions occur because abrupt discontinuation may worsen hypertension. However, make sure you discuss any adverse reactions (especially jerky movements or fever) with your doctor.

☐ Remember to change positions slowly (especially from lying flat to sitting upright) and to dangle your legs over the bedside for a few minutes before standing to minimize the risk of light-headedness. Lie down immediately if dizziness or faintness occurs.

☐ Avoid driving or hazardous activities until you've adjusted to the drug's effects.

☐ Relieve dry mouth caused by methyldopa with sugarless chewing gum, hard candy, or ice chips or by misting or rinsing your mouth with water.

☐ Be aware that your urine may turn dark in toilet bowls, especially if the bowl is treated with bleach.

Minimize fluid retention

☐ Restrict your salt and fluid intake to minimize fluid retention.

☐ Monitor your daily fluid intake and output if so advised.

☐ Weigh yourself daily at the same time and in the same type of clothing. Report a sudden weight gain of more than 5 lb (2.3 kg) per week to your doctor because this may indicate that you are retaining excessive fluid.

Other instructions

☐ If you feel depressed or note any changes in your sexual activity, discuss these concerns with your doctor or nurse so that drug regimen changes or other suggestions can be made to alleviate such problems.

☐ Check with the doctor or pharmacist before taking OTC medications.

☐ Store methyldopa at room temperature and protect it from moisture, direct light, and air.

toma, as well as a positive Coombs' test.

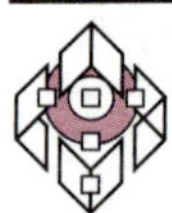 **MedTest**

1. Administer I.V. methyldopa over a period of:
  a. 1 to 2 minutes.
  b. 5 to 10 minutes.
  c. 15 to 30 minutes.
  d. 30 to 60 minutes.

2. A common distressing reaction for the patient taking methyldopa is:
  a. drug-induced fever.
  b. rash.
  c. gynecomastia.
  d. impotence.

3. Which of the following adverse reactions might signal the need to discontinue I.V. methyldopa?
  a. Sedation and drowsiness
  b. Orthostatic hypotension with dizziness
  c. Involuntary choreoathetoid movements
  d. Unexplained fever

Metolazone

A quinazoline derivative (thiazide-like) diuretic, metolazone is classified therapeutically as a diuretic and an antihypertensive agent. It's available in 2.5-, 5-, and 10-mg tablets under the names Diulo and Zaroxolyn and in 0.5-mg tablets under the name Mykrox.

Pharmacokinetics
• *Absorption:* About 65% is absorbed in healthy individuals; in cardiac patients, absorption falls to 40%. However, rate and extent of absorption vary among preparations, with Mykrox being most rapidly and completely absorbed.
• *Distribution:* 50% to 70% erythrocyte-bound and about 33% protein-bound.
• *Metabolism:* Insignificant.
• *Excretion:* About 70% to 95% of dose is excreted unchanged in urine. Elimination half-life is about 14 hours in healthy patients but may be prolonged in patients with decreased creatinine clearance.

Indications, dosage, and action
Edema in heart failure
• *Adult dosage:* 5 to 10 mg P.O. daily (when using Mykrox, 0.5 to 2 mg daily).
• *Diuretic action:* Increases urine excretion of sodium and water by inhibiting sodium reabsorption in the cortical diluting tubule of the nephron, thus relieving edema.

Hypertension
• *Adult dosage:* 2.5 to 5 mg P.O. daily (When using Mykrox tablets, give 0.5 to 1 mg daily.) Maintenance dosage determined by patient's blood pressure.
• *Antihypertensive action:* Reduces circulating blood volume and total peripheral resistance.

Contraindications and cautions
• Don't use metolazone in patients with anuria, hepatic coma, or precoma.

- Avoid use in patients with sensitivity to thiazides or other sulfonamide-derived drugs.
- Use cautiously in hyperuricemia or gout.
- Use with caution in elderly patients and patients with renal disease.
- Also use with caution in patients with liver disease because electrolyte changes may precipitate coma.
- Use cautiously in breast-feeding women.
- Pregnancy risk category D

Life-threatening adverse reactions

- Aplastic anemia, agranulocytosis
- Severe dehydration and electrolyte disturbances

Common adverse reactions

- Dizziness, light-headedness, headaches
- Muscle weakness or cramps

Infrequent adverse reactions

- Orthostatic hypotension, hypercholesterolemia, hypertriglyceridemia, chest pain (precordial discomfort)
- Fatigue
- Anorexia, nausea, pancreatitis, hepatic encephalopathy
- Leukopenia, thrombocytopenia
- Asymptomatic hyperuricemia; gout; hyperglycemia and impairment of glucose tolerance; fluid and electrolyte imbalances, including hyponatremia, hypochloremia, hypercalcemia, and hypokalemia; metabolic alkalosis
- Dermatitis, photosensitivity

- Hypersensitivity reactions, such as pneumonitis and vasculitis; joint pain and swelling

Interactions

- *Antihypertensive drugs:* Risk of hypotension. Monitor closely.
- *Cholestyramine, colestipol:* May bind to metolazone, preventing or decreasing its intestinal absorption; separate administration times as much as possible.
- *Diazoxide:* Metolazone may potentiate hyperglycemic, hypotensive, and hyperuricemic effects of diazoxide. Use together cautiously.
- *Digitalis glycosides:* Metolazone reduces serum potassium levels, leading to digoxin toxicity. Monitor closely.
- *Furosemide:* Unusually large loss of fluid and electrolytes may result when used concomitantly.
- *Lithium:* Metolazone may reduce renal clearance of lithium, elevating serum lithium levels.
- *Methenamine compounds:* Alkaline urine may decrease efficacy of methenamine compounds.
- *NSAIDs:* Decreased diuretic effect.
- *Quinidine, sympathomimetics:* Metolazone turns urine slightly alkaline and may decrease urinary excretion of some amines.

Interventions

Preparation and administration

- Mykrox tablets are more rapidly and completely absorbed than are Diulo or Zaroxolyn tablets. Mykrox absorption characteristics mimic those of an oral solution.

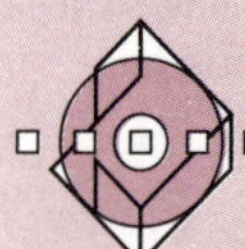

Patient-teaching checklist

Taking metolazone at home

In addition to explaining the drug's action and dosage, teach the patient who will continue metolazone therapy after discharge to follow these important guidelines.

Take your medication correctly

☐ Take metolazone in the morning to prevent nocturia.

☐ Take metolazone as prescribed even when you're feeling well. The drug may take up to several days to produce optimal effects.

☐ Continue taking the drug even if unpleasant adverse reactions occur. Make sure you discuss any adverse reaction with your doctor as soon as possible. In particular, report fatigue, confusion, nausea, vomiting, diarrhea, headache, muscle weakness and cramps, tingling, or numbness.

Watch for fluid retention

☐ If so advised, monitor your fluid intake and output daily.

☐ Weigh yourself daily at the same time of day wearing the same type of clothing. Report any signs of increased fluid retention (tight rings or shoes, puffy hands, feet, or ankles), excessive voiding, or a weight gain or loss of more than 2 lb (1 kg) per day.

☐ Avoid high-sodium foods to minimize fluid retention. Also, if indicated, incorporate high-potassium foods into your daily diet because metolazone increases potassium loss in your urine.

☐ Elevate your legs when possible to help relieve fluid retention.

Minimize other adverse reactions

☐ Remember to change positions slowly (especially from lying flat to sitting upright) and to dangle your legs over the bedside for a few minutes before standing. This will help to minimize light-headedness. Lie down immediately if dizziness or faintness occurs.

☐ Avoid direct sun exposure as much as possible because this drug may cause a photosensitivity reaction. When you must be in the sun, wear a hat, sunscreen, and a long-sleeved shirt.

☐ If you have diabetes, monitor your blood glucose levels closely. You may require an adjustment in your oral antidiabetic drug or insulin dosage.

☐ Check with your doctor or pharmacist before taking OTC medications.

Safety tip. Don't interchange Mykrox with Diulo or Zaroxolyn.

• Administer drug in the morning to prevent nocturia. (See *Taking metolazone at home.*)

Monitoring and supportive care

• Monitor fluid intake and output, daily weight, blood pressure, and serum electrolyte levels.

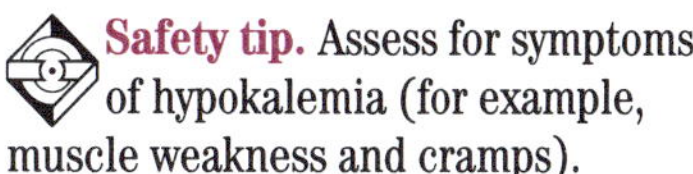 **Safety tip.** Assess for symptoms of hypokalemia (for example, muscle weakness and cramps).

• Consult with a doctor and dietitian to provide a high-potassium diet if warranted. Foods rich in potassium include bananas, citrus fruits, tomatoes, dates, and apricots.

• Remember that patients also receiving digoxin are at increased risk for digitalis toxicity from the potassium-depleting effect of this drug. You can use a potassium-sparing diuretic to prevent excessive potassium loss.

• Monitor blood uric acid levels, especially in patients with a history of gout.

• Be aware that metolazone is effective in patients with decreased renal function, unlike other thiazide and thiazide-related diuretics, and is used for edema in renal disease.

• Know that metolazone is used as an adjunct in furosemide-resistant edema.

• Discontinue thiazides and thiazide-like diuretics before performing tests for parathyroid function.

• Be aware that metolazone therapy may alter serum electrolyte levels and may increase serum urate, glucose, cholesterol, and triglyceride levels.

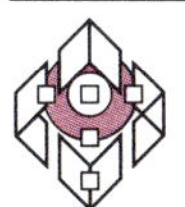 **MedTest**

1. Metolazone is contraindicated in patients with known sensitivity to:
  a. penicillins.
  b. sulfonamides.
  c. aminoglycosides.
  d. iodine preparations.

2. Metolazone should be administered:
  a. in the morning to prevent nocturia.
  b. a.c. to enhance absorption.
  c. with meals to limit gastric irritation.
  d. h.s. to reduce daytime sedation.

3. While taking metolazone, the patient may need to consume potassium-rich foods, such as:
  a. tomatoes, dates, and apricots.
  b. peaches and pears.
  c. cranberry juice, nonfat dry milk, and yogurt.
  d. fish, whole grains, and nuts.

Metoprolol tartrate

Also known by the brand names Lopressor and Toprol XL, and (in Canada) Apo-Metoprolol, Betaloc, Betaloc Durules, Lopresor, Lopresor SR, and Novometoprol, metoprolol tartrate is a beta-adrenergic blocker that's classified therapeutically as an antihypertensive and used as an adjunctive treatment in acute MI. It's available in 50- and 100-mg tablets; 50-, 100-, and 200-mg sustained-release tablets; and for injection as 5-ml ampules or prefilled syringes in concentrations of 1 mg/ml.

Pharmacokinetics

• *Absorption:* Absorbed rapidly and almost completely from the GI tract; food enhances absorption. Peak plasma concentrations occur in 90 minutes. After I.V. administration, maxi-

mum beta blockade occurs in 20 minutes.
- *Distribution:* Drug is about 12% protein-bound.
- *Metabolism:* Metabolized in the liver to inactive metabolites.
- *Excretion:* About 95% is excreted in urine as inactive metabolites; 5% is excreted unchanged. Beta blockade persists for about 24 hours after oral administration and 5 to 8 hours after I.V. administration. Maximum antihypertensive effect is seen after about 1 week of therapy.

Indications, dosage, and action
Mild to severe hypertension
- *Adult dosage:* Initially, 100 mg P.O. daily in single or divided doses. Usual maintenance dosage is 100 to 450 mg daily.
- *Antihypertensive action:* Metoprolol is a $beta_1$ antagonist that reduces blood pressure by decreasing cardiac output and sympathetic outflow from the CNS; it also suppresses renin release.

Reduction of mortality in acute MI
- *Adult dosage:* Three 5-mg I.V. boluses q 2 minutes. Then, beginning 15 minutes after last dose, 50 mg P.O. q 6 hours for 48 hours. Maintenance dosage is 100 mg P.O. b.i.d.
- *Action:* The exact mechanism by which metoprolol curbs mortality after MI is unknown.

Angina
- *Adult dosage:* 100 mg in two divided doses. Maintenance dosage is 100 to 400 mg daily.
- *Antianginal action:* Decreases heart rate, conduction velocity, myo-

cardial contractility, and cardiac output, thus reducing myocardial oxygen consumption and relieving ischemic pain.

Contraindications and cautions
- Don't give to patients with overt cardiac failure, second- or third-degree AV block (unless they have a pacemaker), or cardiogenic shock because the drug may worsen these conditions.
- Use cautiously in patients with CHF or left ventricular dysfunction because beta-adrenergic blockade may exacerbate CHF.
- Use with caution in elderly patients and in those with impaired hepatic function (dosage reduction may be necessary).
- Use cautiously in patients with diabetes mellitus or hyperthyroidism because metoprolol may mask the tachycardia associated with hypoglycemia and hyperthyroidism.
- Use with caution in patients with bronchospastic disease. Dosages higher than 100 mg/day may precipitate bronchospasm. (At lower doses, metoprolol selectively inhibits $beta_1$-receptors.)
- Use with caution in patients with sinus node dysfunction because depression of SA node automaticity may occur.
- Avoid use in breast-feeding women because metoprolol is distributed into breast milk.
- Pregnancy risk category B

Life-threatening adverse reactions
- CHF
- Bronchospasm

- Agranulocytosis

Common adverse reactions
- CHF (28%), hypotension (27% in MI), bradycardia (16%), first-degree AV block
- Fatigue, lethargy, dizziness, depression
- Diarrhea
- Pruritus or rash

Infrequent adverse interactions
- Bradycardia (in patients with hypertension or angina), second- or third-degree AV block, reduced peripheral circulation
- Dyspnea, wheezing
- Fatigue (in MI)
- Abdominal pain and nausea, vomiting, constipation, flatulence, dry mouth
- Eosinophilia, nonthrombocytopenic and thrombocytopenic purpura

Interactions
- *Barbiturates, rifampin:* Increased metabolism of metoprolol. Monitor for decreased effect.
- *Chlorpromazine, cimetidine, verapamil:* Decreased hepatic clearance. Monitor for toxicity.
- *Digitalis glycosides:* Risk of bradycardia. Monitor pulse rate, ECG, or both.
- *Diuretics, other antihypertensive agents:* May potentiate antihypertensive effects. Monitor patient response.
- *Indomethacin, NSAIDs:* Decrease in antihypertensive effect. Monitor blood pressure and adjust dosage.
- *Insulin, oral antidiabetic drugs:* Can alter dosage requirements in previously stabilized diabetics. Observe patient carefully.
- *Sympathomimetic agents:* Metoprolol may antagonize the beta-adrenergic effects of such drugs. Monitor patient response.

Interventions
Preparation and administration
If a dose is missed, give the patient only the next scheduled dose. (See *Taking beta-adrenergic blockers at home*, page 63.)

Safety tip. Give oral forms with meals because food enhances absorption.
- Administer I.V. boluses through a patent I.V. line.

Safety tip. Discard solution if it's discolored or contains particles.

Monitoring and supportive care
- Before initiating therapy, always check the patient's apical pulse rate. If it's less than 50 beats/minute, hold the dose and notify the doctor.
- Monitor the patient's blood pressure frequently.
- Know that this drug masks common signs of shock and hypoglycemia.

Safety tip. Although metoprolol masks tachycardia associated with acute hypoglycemia, it doesn't mask CNS symptoms (such as dizziness, headache, or mental status changes), so monitor for these symptoms. Also monitor blood glucose levels.
- Discontinue metoprolol by slowly tapering the dose over 3 to 14 days. Stopping abruptly can exacerbate angina and MI.

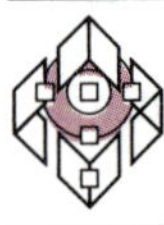

Safety tip. If withdrawal symptoms (angina, sweating, tremors, tachycardia, or respiratory distress) occur, ask the doctor to reinstitute the drug temporarily; then lower the dose more slowly, and monitor the patient closely.

Safety tip. If the patient is scheduled for surgery, notify the anesthesiologist that the patient is receiving this drug.
• Observe the patient for signs of mental depression.
• Be aware that metoprolol may elevate serum AST, ALT, ALP, LD, and uric acid levels.

MedTest

1. What is the maintenance dosage for oral metoprolol in hypertension?
   a. 100 mg b.i.d.
   b. 100 to 450 mg daily
   c. 150 mg t.i.d.
   d. 50 mg q 6 hours

2. To enhance absorption of oral metoprolol, you would:
   a. administer the drug h.s.
   b. give the drug 30 minutes a.c.
   c. give the drug 1 hour p.c.
   d. give the drug with meals.

3. Your diabetic patient receiving metoprolol is at risk for insulin-induced hypoglycemia, so you teach her to watch for:
   a. fatigue and lethargy.
   b. tremors.
   c. dizziness, headache, and mental status changes.
   d. tachycardia.

Mexiletine hydrochloride

Also known by the brand name Mexitil, mexiletine is a lidocaine analogue and sodium channel antagonist that's classified therapeutically as a ventricular antiarrhythmic agent. It's available in 150-, 200-, and 250-mg capsules; in 100-mg capsules (in Canada); and in 50-mg capsules (in Australia).

Pharmacokinetics
• *Absorption:* About 90% of drug is absorbed from the GI tract; peak serum levels occur in 2 to 3 hours.
• *Distribution:* Distribution volume declines in patients with hepatic disease, resulting in toxic serum drug levels with usual doses. About 50% to 60% of the circulating drug is bound to plasma proteins. Usual therapeutic drug level is 0.5 to 2 mcg/ml. Levels above 2 mcg/ml are associated with an increased incidence of adverse CNS effects.
• *Metabolism:* Metabolized in the liver to relatively inactive metabolites. Less than 10% of a parenteral dose (not yet available in the U.S.) escapes metabolism and reaches the kidneys unchanged. Metabolism is affected by hepatic blood flow, which may be reduced in patients who are recovering from MI and in those with CHF. Liver disease also limits metabolism.
• *Excretion:* Half-life is 10 to 12 hours. Elimination half-life may be prolonged in patients with CHF or liver disease. Urinary excretion in-

creases with urine acidification and slows with urine alkalinization.

Indications, dosage, and action
Refractory ventricular arrhythmias, including VT and PVCs
• *Adult dosage:* 200 to 400 mg P.O. followed by 200 mg q 8 hours. May increase dosage to 400 mg q 8 hours if satisfactory control isn't obtained. Some patients may respond well to a twice-daily schedule. May give up to 450 mg q 12 hours.

• *Antiarrhythmic action:* Mexiletine is structurally similar to lidocaine and exerts similar effects. A class Ib antiarrhythmic, it suppresses automaticity, shortens the effective refractory period and action potential duration of His-Purkinje fibers, and suppresses spontaneous ventricular depolarization during diastole. At therapeutic serum levels, the drug doesn't affect conductive atrial tissue or AV conduction.

Contraindications and cautions
• Don't use in patients with cardiogenic shock or in patients with severe degrees of SA, AV, or intraventricular block who don't have an artificial pacemaker because the drug may worsen these conditions.
• Use with caution in elderly patients and in patients with hepatic failure because the drug may accumulate and cause toxicity.
• Use cautiously in patients with seizure disorders, bradycardia, or hypotension because the drug may worsen these conditions.
• Avoid use in breast-feeding women because drug is excreted in breast milk.

• Pregnancy risk category C

Life-threatening adverse reactions
• New or worsened arrhythmias
• Seizures

Common adverse reactions
• Dizziness (19%), tremor, changes in sleep habits, blurred vision, nystagmus, diplopia, ataxia, nervousness, headache, weakness
• Nausea or vomiting (39%), diarrhea

Infrequent adverse reactions
• Hypotension, bradycardia, palpitations, arrhythmias, widened QRS complex, angina, chest pain
• Dyspnea
• Confusion, fatigue, depression, paresthesia, tinnitus
• Constipation, anorexia, abdominal discomfort, elevation of liver function test values
• Rash
• Dry mouth, arthralgia, fever

Interactions
• *Aluminum-magnesium antacids, atropine, narcotics:* Delayed mexiletine absorption. Monitor rhythm response.
• *Cimetidine:* Altered metabolism of mexiletine. Monitor carefully.
• *Metoclopramide:* Increased mexiletine absorption. Monitor response.
• *Phenobarbitol, phenytoin, rifampin:* Enhanced metabolism of mexiletine. Monitor carefully.
• *Urine acidifiers:* Concomitant use with such drugs as ammonium chloride enhances mexiletine excretion. Monitor for arrhythmias.

• *Urine alkalinizers:* Concomitant use with such drugs as high-dose antacids, carbonic anhydrase inhibitors, and sodium bicarbonate decreases mexiletine excretion. Monitor for toxicity.

Interventions
Preparation and administration
• Administer dose with food or an antacid, if possible, to minimize nausea. (See *Taking antiarrhythmics at home,* page 74.)
• Mexiletine injection is compatible with 0.9% NaCl, D_5W, 5% sodium bicarbonate, 1/6 M sodium lactate, and 10% fructose (levulose) solutions.

Monitoring and supportive care
• When changing from lidocaine to mexiletine, stop the infusion when the first mexiletine dose is given. Keep the infusion line open, however, until the arrhythmia appears to be satisfactorily controlled.
• Many patients who respond well to mexiletine can be maintained on a q-12-hour schedule. Twice-daily administration improves compliance.
• Monitor blood pressure and heart rate and rhythm. Notify the doctor of any significant change.

Safety tip. An early sign of mexiletine toxicity is a tremor, usually a fine tremor of the hands. This progresses to dizziness and later to ataxia and nystagmus as the blood level of the drug increases. Question your patient about these symptoms and report them to the doctor.
• Know that liver function test results may be altered transiently during mexiletine therapy.

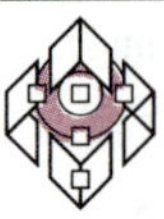 **MedTest**

1. Mexiletine is structurally similar to:
   a. metolazone.
   b. lidocaine.
   c. procainamide.
   d. simvastatin.

2. Mexiletine should be administered with food or an antacid to limit which of the following adverse reactions?
   a. Diarrhea
   b. Dizziness
   c. Nausea
   d. Anorexia

3. An early sign of mexiletine toxicity is:
   a. a fine hand tremor.
   b. dizziness.
   c. ataxia.
   d. nystagmus.

Milrinone lactate

Also known by the brand name Primacor, milrinone is a bipiridine that's classified therapeutically as an inotropic and vasodilating agent. It's available for parenteral use in concentrations of 1 mg/ml in 10- and 20-ml vials and 5-ml prefilled cartridges.

Pharmacokinetics
• *Absorption:* Drug must be administered I.V. and is absorbed almost immediately.
• *Distribution:* 70% protein-bound.

• *Metabolism:* Metabolized to inactive metabolites in the liver.
• *Excretion:* Appears in the urine mostly as unchanged drug. Elimination is rapid, with approximately 60% recovered in the first 2 hours and 90% recovered within 8 hours following administration. Elimination half-life is 2 to 3 hours.

Indications, dosage, and action
Short-term treatment of CHF
• *Adult dosage:* Initial loading dose of 50 mcg/kg I.V., slowly administered over 10 minutes, followed by continuous infusion of 0.375 to 0.75 mcg/kg/minute. Adjust infusion dose according to clinical and hemodynamic responses. Typically given with digoxin and diuretics.
• *Action:* Milrinone inhibits the breakdown of cyclic adenosine monophosphate, which alters calcium availability to cardiac and smooth muscle cells. It produces both vasodilating and positive inotropic effects. This combined effect increases myocardial contractility and decreases peripheral resistance.

Contraindications and cautions
• Avoid use in patients with severe obstructive pulmonic or aortic valve disease.
• Avoid use during an acute phase of MI.
• Use cautiously in patients with atrial fibrillation or flutter because this drug may increase ventricular response rate.
• If the patient will receive a digitalis glycoside, begin such therapy before milrinone therapy.

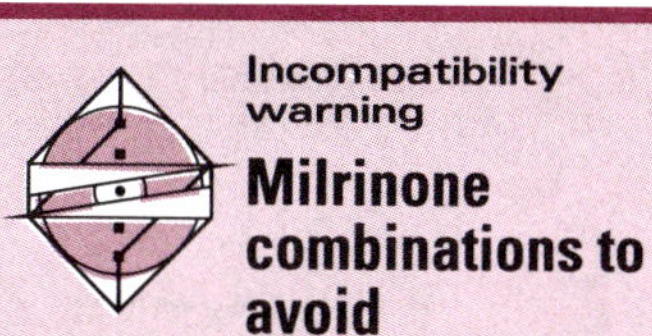

Be aware that milrinone is incompatible with furosemide. When the two drugs come in contact, precipitation occurs immediately. Administer at a different site, or flush the line completely before administering milrinone.

• Use cautiously in breast-feeding women because it's unknown whether milrinone is excreted in breast milk.
• Pregnancy risk category C

Life-threatening adverse reactions
• Sustained VT, ventricular fibrillation

Common adverse reactions
• Ventricular ectopic activity

Infrequent adverse reactions
• Supraventricular arrhythmias, non-sustained VT, hypotension, angina and chest pain
• Headache, tremor
• Thrombocytopenia
• Hypokalemia

Interactions
See *Milrinone combinations to avoid*.

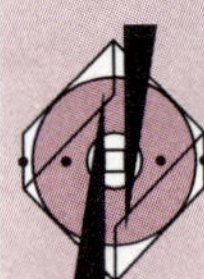

Administration guidelines

Giving I.V. milrinone safely

Follow these guidelines to ensure safe I.V. administration for patients who require milrinone therapy.

Prepararation

- Use 0.45% or 0.9% NaCl solution or D_5W to prepare milrinone for I.V. infusion.
- Inspect the product visually. Don't use if particulate matter or discoloration is present. The solution in the vial should be clear, and colorless to pale yellow.
- Prepare a 100-mcg/ml solution by adding 180 ml of diluent per 20-mg (20-ml) vial. Prepare a 150-mcg/ml solution by adding 113 ml of diluent per 20-mg (20-ml) vial. Prepare a 200-mcg/ml solution by adding 80 ml of diluent per 20-mg (20-ml) vial. Use the standard dilution determined by your hospital.

Administration

- Give the initial loading dose of 50 mcg/kg I.V. as a bolus. Administer the bolus slowly over 10 minutes.
- Follow the bolus dose of milrinone with a continuous I.V. infusion of 0.375 to 0.75 mcg/kg/minute as prescribed. Use an infusion pump to deliver the continuous infusion at the desired volume.
- Monitor the patient closely throughout milrinone use. Expect to adjust the infusion dose of milrinone according to clinical and hemodynamic responses.

Interventions

Preparation and administration

- Diluents that may be used to prepare milrinone for I.V. infusion include 0.45% NaCl, 0.9% NaCl, or D_5W solutions. (See *Giving I.V. milrinone safely.*)
- Store at room temperature.

Monitoring and supportive care

- Assess fluid and electrolyte balance, vital signs, and hemodynamic and clinical status throughout the infusion period. Improvement is evidenced by increases in cardiac output and decreases in PAWP.
- Monitor patients receiving diuretics concurrently, especially if such therapy has decreased the patient's cardiac filling pressure.
- Be aware that inotropic agents may aggravate outflow tract obstruction in patients with idiopathic hypertrophic cardiomyopathy.
- Know that patients treated with this drug have exhibited supraventricular and ventricular arrhythmias; therefore, monitor patients closely.

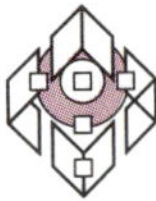

MedTest

1. A common adverse reaction to assess for when administering milrinone is:
    - **a.** ventricular fibrillation.
    - **b.** angina.
    - **c.** ventricular ectopic activity.
    - **d.** hypotension.

2. Milrinone is classified pharmacologically as:
a. an antiarrhythmic.
b. an inotropic and vasodilating agent.
c. an ACE inhibitor.
d. a diuretic and antihypertensive agent.

3. Milrinone is administered I.V. as a:
a. single bolus.
b. stat bolus followed by additional boluses q 5 minutes p.r.n.
c. bolus followed by a continuous infusion.
d. continuous infusion.

Moricizine hydrochloride

Also known by the brand name Ethmozine, moricizine is a sodium channel blocker that's classified therapeutically as an antiarrhythmic agent. It's available in 200-, 250-, and 300-mg tablets.

Pharmacokinetics

• *Absorption:* Moricizine undergoes significant first-pass metabolism, which limits bioavailability. Peak plasma concentrations are usually reached within 30 minutes to 2 hours. Administration within 30 minutes of mealtime delays absorption and lowers peak plasma levels, but has no effect on extent of absorption.
• *Distribution:* 95% plasma protein–bound.

• *Metabolism:* Metabolized in the liver. At least 26 metabolites, both active and inactive, have been identified. No single one represents at least 1% of the administered dose. Moricizine has been shown to induce its own metabolism.
• *Excretion:* 56% is excreted in feces; 39%, in urine; some is also recycled through enterohepatic circulation. Elimination half-life is $1\frac{1}{2}$ to $3\frac{1}{2}$ hours.

Indications, dosage, and action
Life-threatening ventricular arrhythmias

• *Adult dosage:* Dosage must be individualized. Usual range is 600 to 900 mg daily given q 8 hours in equally divided doses. Dosage may be adjusted within this range in increments of 150 mg daily at 3-day intervals until desired effect is obtained. Hospitalization is recommended for initiation of therapy because patient will be at high risk.
• *Antiarrhythmic action:* Moricizine has potent local anesthetic activity and myocardial membrane–stabilizing effects. A class I antiarrhythmic agent, it reduces the fast inward current carried by sodium ions. In patients with VT, moricizine prolongs AV conduction but has no significant effect on ventricular repolarization. Atrial conduction or effective refractory periods aren't consistently affected, and moricizine has minimal effect on sinus cycle length and sinus node recovery time. This may be significant in patients with sinus node dysfunction.

In patients with impaired left ventricular function, moricizine has minimal effects on measurements of cardiac performance. Small but consistent increases in resting blood pressure and heart rate are seen. Moricizine has no effect on exercise tolerance in patients with ventricular arrhythmias, CHF, or angina pectoris.

Contraindications and cautions
• Don't use in patients with preexisting second- or third-degree AV block, those with right bundle-branch block when associated with left hemiblock (unless a pacemaker is present), or patients in cardiogenic shock.
• Avoid use in breast-feeding women; drug is excreted in breast milk.
• Use with extreme caution in patients with SSS because the drug may cause sinus bradycardia, sinus pause, or sinus arrest.
• Use with caution in patients with hepatic or renal impairment, CHF, or preexisting conduction abnormalities and when medications that affect cardiac conduction are initiated concomitantly. Monitor all such patients carefully.
• Pregnancy risk category B

Life-threatening adverse reactions
• Proarrhythmic events, sinus arrest, sustained VT, CHF
• Apnea

Common adverse reactions
• Palpitations
• Dyspnea
• Dizziness (20% with 450-mg b.i.d. dose; 12% with 300-mg t.i.d. dose), headache, fatigue
• Nausea

Infrequent adverse reactions
• ECG abnormalities (including conduction defects, sinus bradycardia, sinus pause, junctional rhythm, or AV block), hypotension, hypertension, supraventricular arrhythmias, chest pain
• Hyperventilation, cough
• Nervousness, anxiety, sleep disorders, hypoesthesia, paresthesia, asthenia
• Vomiting, dyspepsia, abdominal pain, dry mouth, diarrhea, constipation
• Urine retention, frequency, dysuria, incontinence, impotence, decreased libido
• Sinusitis, blurred vision
• Musculoskeletal pain, drug fever, hypothermia, allergic reactions (rash, pruritus, urticaria, swelling of lips and tongue, periorbital edema)

Interactions
• *Cimetidine:* Decreased clearance of moricizine. Monitor plasma levels closely.
• *Digoxin, propranolol:* Additive prolongation of the PR interval. Monitor closely.
• *Theophylline:* Increased theophylline clearance. Monitor plasma levels; adjust theophylline dosage as needed.

Interventions
Preparation and administration
• This drug may be taken without regard to food intake. (See *Taking antiarrhythmics at home,* page 74.)

Monitoring and supportive care

• When transferring from another antiarrhythmic to moricizine, withdraw previous therapy one to two half-lives before initiating moricizine.

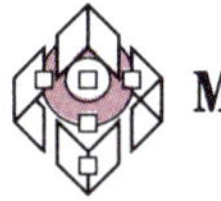 **Safety tip.** Patients who have shown a tendency to develop life-threatening arrhythmias after withdrawal of other antiarrhythmics should be hospitalized during withdrawal of these drugs and adjustment to moricizine. Moricizine therapy should begin 6 to 12 hours after the last dose of *disopyramide*; 8 to 12 hours after the last dose of *mexiletine*; 3 to 6 hours after the last dose of *procainamide*; 8 to 12 hours after the last dose of *propafenone*; 6 to 12 hours after the last dose of *quinidine*; and 8 to 12 hours after the last dose of *tocainide*.

• Know that patients with renal or hepatic impairment should be started at 600 mg daily or less and closely monitored before making dosage adjustments.

• Hypokalemia, hyperkalemia, or hypomagnesemia may alter moricizine's effects; electrolyte imbalances should be corrected before starting moricizine therapy.

MedTest

1. Moricizine is classified pharmacologically as:
   a. an ACE inhibitor.
   b. a beta blocker.
   c. a calcium channel blocker.
   d. a sodium channel blocker.

2. A common adverse effect of moricizine is:
   a. dizziness.
   b. nervousness.
   c. chest pain.
   d. abdominal pain.

3. Moricizine should be used to treat only:
   a. supraventricular tachycardias.
   b. AV block.
   c. bradyarrhythmias.
   d. life-threatening ventricular arrhythmias.

Morphine sulfate

Also known by the brand names Astramorph and Duramorph, and (in Canada) Epimorph and Statex, morphine sulfate is an opioid that's classified therapeutically as a narcotic analgesic (Controlled Substance Schedule II). It's available for injection with preservative as 1, 2, 3, 4, 5, 8, 10, and 15 mg/ml; for injection without preservative as 500 mcg/ml and 1 mg/ml; in patient-controlled analgesia (PCA) syringes of 1, 2, 3, and 4 mg/ml; and in premixed bottles of 0.2 and 1 mg/ml.

Pharmacokinetics

• *Absorption:* Onset of analgesia occurs in 15 to 60 minutes. Peak analgesic effect occurs 30 to 60 minutes after administration.

• *Distribution:* Widespread through the body.

• *Metabolism:* Metabolized primarily in the liver to inactive metabolites.

• *Excretion:* Duration of action is 3 to 7 hours. Excreted in urine and bile.

Indications, dosage, and action
Pain from acute MI
• *Adult dosage:* 8 to 15 mg I.M., S.C., or I.V. Additional, smaller doses may be given in 3- to 4-hour intervals as needed.
• *Analgesic action:* Morphine alters the patient's perception of pain. It is particularly useful in severe, acute or chronic pain. Morphine has a CNS depressant effect on respiration and on the cough reflex center. It also produces vasodilation. It's particularly helpful in treating the pain of acute MI because it produces analgesia and reduces afterload.

Contraindications and cautions
• Don't use in patients with known hypersensitivity to other opioids.
• Administer morphine with extreme caution to patients with supraventricular arrhythmias.
• Avoid or administer with extreme caution to patients with head injury or increased ICP because the drug obscures neurologic signs.
• Administer morphine cautiously to debilitated or elderly patients and to patients with renal or hepatic dysfunction because drug accumulation may occur.
• Use cautiously in COPD patients because the drug depresses respirations and suppresses the cough reflex.
• Use with caution in patients with biliary disorders or those undergoing biliary tract surgery because drug may cause biliary spasm.
• Use with caution in patients prone to physical or psychological addiction because of the high risk of addiction to this drug.
• Use cautiously in breast-feeding women because the drug is excreted in breast milk.
• Avoid or administer with extreme caution during pregnancy and labor because the drug readily crosses the placenta (premature infants are especially sensitive to respiratory and CNS depressant effects).
• Pregnancy risk category C

Life-threatening adverse reactions
• Respiratory arrest

Common adverse reactions
• Hypotension
• Sedation, somnolence, clouded sensorium, euphoria; nightmares (with long-acting dosage form)
• Nausea, vomiting, constipation
• Urinary hesitancy or urine retention
• Flushing (with epidural use)
• Physical dependence

Infrequent adverse reactions
• Tachycardia, asystole, bradycardia, palpitations, chest wall rigidity, hypertension, syncope, edema
• Respiratory depression
• Insomnia, agitation, confusion, headache, tremor, miosis, seizures, psychological dependence
• Dry mouth, anorexia, biliary spasms (colic), ileus

- Decreased libido
- Rash, pruritus, pain at injection site

Interactions
- *Anticholinergics:* Combined use with anticholinergics may cause paralytic ileus.
- *Cimetidine, CNS depressants:* Additive CNS depression, sedation, hypotension, and respiratory depressive effects. Use together cautiously.
- *Narcotic antagonists:* Patients who become physically dependent on this drug may experience acute withdrawal syndrome if given a narcotic antagonist.

Interventions
Preparation and administration
- Be aware that in cardiac patients, morphine is almost always administered I.V.

Monitoring and supportive care
- Know that morphine is the drug of choice in relieving pain of MI. It may cause a transient decrease in blood pressure.
- Monitor circulatory, respiratory, bladder, and bowel functions carefully. The drug may cause respiratory depression, hypotension, urine retention, nausea, vomiting, ileus, or altered level of consciousness without regard to route of administration. Hold a dose if respiratory rate falls below 8 breaths/minute.
- **Safety tip.** Keep a narcotic antagonist (naloxone) and resuscitation equipment available.
- Adhere to regimented scheduling (around the clock) in severe, chronic pain.

- **Safety tip.** Constipation is often severe. Make sure a stool softener or laxative is ordered.
- Remember that oral solutions are available in various concentrations.
- Be aware that preservative-free preparations are available for epidural and intrathecal administration. The use of the epidural route is increasing.
- Know that morphine may worsen or mask gallbladder pain.
- Keep in mind that morphine increases serum amylase levels.

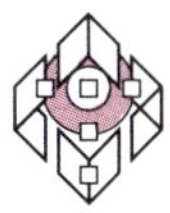 **MedTest**

1. Morphine proves effective in treating pain from acute MI because it produces analgesia and:
    a. lowers the respiratory rate.
    b. increases afterload.
    c. causes physical dependence.
    d. reduces afterload.

2. A common adverse reaction to assess for when administering morphine is:
    a. hyperventilation.
    b. blurred vision.
    c. hypotension.
    d. hypokalemia.

3. How long after administration does morphine achieve its peak analgesic effect?
    a. 3 to 5 minutes
    b. 5 to 15 minutes
    c. 15 to 30 minutes
    d. 30 to 60 minutes

Nadolol

Also known by the brand name Corgard, nadolol is a noncardioselective beta-adrenergic blocker that's classified therapeutically as an antihypertensive and antianginal agent. It's available in 20-, 40-, 80-, 120-, and 160-mg tablets.

Pharmacokinetics
• *Absorption:* 30% to 40% absorbed from the GI tract; peak plasma concentrations occur in 2 to 4 hours. Food doesn't affect absorption.
• *Distribution:* Distributed throughout the body; about 30% protein-bound.
• *Metabolism:* None.
• *Excretion:* Most of given dose excreted unchanged in urine; the remainder in feces. Plasma half-life is 10 to 24 hours; effects persist for about 24 hours.

Indications, dosage, and action
Hypertension
• *Adult dosage:* Initially, 40 mg P.O. once daily. Dosage may be increased in 40- to 80-mg increments until optimum response occurs. Usual maintenance dosage range is 40 to 240 mg once daily.
• *Action:* Blocks beta-adrenergic receptors, thus decreasing cardiac output. May also act by decreasing sympathetic outflow from the CNS or by suppressing renin release.

Chronic stable angina
• *Adult dosage:* Initially, 40 mg P.O. once daily. Dosage may be increased in 40- to 80-mg increments until optimum response occurs. Usual mainte-

nance dosage is 40 or 80 mg once daily. Dosages of up to 240 mg daily may be needed.
• *Antianginal action:* Decreases cardiac output and heart rate, thereby reducing myocardial oxygen consumption.

Contraindications and caution
• Don't use in sinus bradycardia, overt cardiac failure, second- or third-degree AV block (unless the patient has an artificial pacemaker), heart failure, or bronchial asthma because the drug may worsen these conditions.
• Use cautiously and adjust dosage in impaired renal function.
• Use with caution in diabetes mellitus and hyperthyroidism because the drug may mask tachycardia (but not sweating and dizziness) caused by hypoglycemia.
• Discontinue the drug if the patient develops signs of heart failure.
• Be aware that elderly patients may require lower dosages.
• Recommend an alternative feeding method for breast-feeding mothers during therapy. Nadolol is distributed into breast milk.
• Pregnancy risk category C

Life-threatening adverse reactions
• CHF
• Bronchospasm

Common adverse reactions
None noted at usual dosages

Infrequent adverse reactions
• Hypotension, bradycardia, rhythm disturbances, peripheral vascular insufficiency

- Increased airway resistance
- Dizziness, fatigue, sedation, behavioral changes, paresthesia, headache, reversible mental depression with catatonia, visual disturbances, nightmares
- Nausea, vomiting, diarrhea, constipation, indigestion, anorexia, bloating, flatulence, abdominal discomfort
- Decreased libido
- Dry mouth, cough, nasal stuffiness, tinnitus
- Rash, pruritus, reversible alopecia

Interactions
- *Antiarrhythmic agents:* May cause additive antagonistic cardiac effects.
- *Antihypertensive agents:* May cause hypotension.
- *Atropine:* Antimuscarinic agents may antagonize nadolol-induced bradycardia.
- *Beta-adrenergic agonists:* May cause mutual antagonism.
- *Epinephrine:* May cause severe vasoconstriction, hypertension, and reflex bradycardia with first- or second-degree AV block.
- *Insulin, oral antidiabetic drugs:* Can alter dosage requirements in previously stabilized diabetic patients. Observe patient carefully.
- *Neuromuscular blocking agents:* At high doses, nadolol may potentiate effects of tubocurarine and related agents.

Interventions
Preparation and administration
- Give nadolol with or without food. (See *Taking beta-adrenergic blockers at home,* page 63.)

Monitoring and supportive care
- Always check the patient's apical pulse before giving this drug. If it's slower than 55 beats/minute, withhold the drug and call the doctor. (For some patients, 50 may be the acceptable low rate.)
- Monitor blood pressure frequently.
- Don't discontinue drug abruptly; sudden discontinuation can exacerbate angina and cause MI. Gradually reduce dosage over 1 to 2 weeks.
- Know that this drug masks common signs of shock, hyperthyroidism, and hypoglycemia.

Safety tip. To detect shock, hyperthyroidism, and hypoglycemia, monitor for CNS signs, rather than CV signs. Observe for changes in mental status, restlessness, and dizziness.
- You may need to adjust dosage in patients with renal impairment.

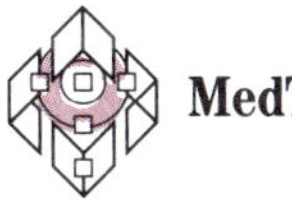 **MedTest**

1. Which of the following is a life-threatening adverse effect of nadolol?
    a. Ventricular arrhythmias
    b. Bronchospasm
    c. Seizures
    d. Agranulocytosis

2. Reduced dosage of nadolol may be required in patients with:
    a. CHF.
    b. hepatic impairment.
    c. heart block.
    d. renal impairment.

3. Nadolol should be administered:
   a. a.c.
   b. with food.
   c. p.c.
   d. with or without food.

Nicardipine hydrochloride

Also known by the brand names Cardene and Cardene SR, nicardipine is a calcium channel blocker that's classified therapeutically as an antianginal and antihypertensive agent. It's available in 20- and 30-mg capsules and in 30-, 45-, and 60-mg extended-release capsules.

Pharmacokinetics

• *Absorption:* Completely absorbed after oral administration. Plasma levels are detectable within 20 minutes and peak in 1 to 4 hours. Absorption may be decreased if drug is taken with food.
• *Distribution:* Over 95% bound to plasma proteins.
• *Metabolism:* Substantial first-pass effect reduces absolute bioavailability to about 35%. Extensively metabolized in the liver to inactive metabolites. Increased dosage yields nonlinear increases in plasma levels.
• *Excretion:* Inactive metabolites eliminated in urine, feces, and bile. Elimination half-life is about 9 hours after steady state is reached.

Indications, dosage, and action
Chronic stable angina
• *Adult dosage:* Initially, 20 mg P.O. t.i.d. (immediate-release only). Titrate dosage according to patient response. Usual dosage range is 20 to 40 mg t.i.d.
• *Antianginal action:* Inhibits calcium ion influx across cardiac and smooth muscle cells, thus decreasing myocardial contractility and oxygen demand; also dilates coronary arteries and arterioles.

Hypertension
• *Adult dosage:* Initially, 20 to 40 mg P.O. t.i.d. (immediate-release) or 30 mg b.i.d. (extended-release). Increase dosage according to patient response.
• *Antihypertensive action:* Appears to act specifically on vascular muscle and may cause a smaller decrease in cardiac output than other calcium channel blockers because of its vasodilating effect.

Contraindications and cautions
• Don't use in advanced aortic stenosis because the decrease in afterload produced by the drug may upset myocardial oxygen balance.
• Use cautiously in cardiac conduction disturbances and hypotension. Monitor blood pressure carefully.
• Recommend against breast-feeding during therapy. Substantial levels of nicardipine have been found in the milk of animals given this drug.
• Pregnancy risk category C

Life-threatening adverse reactions
• Sustained VT

Common adverse reactions
• Peripheral edema, angina

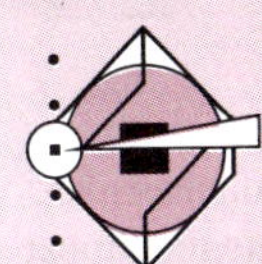

Life-threatening hazards of multidrug therapy with nicardipine

Interacting drug	Effects
Antihypertensive agents (such as prazosin)	May cause profound hypotension
Beta blockers (such as propranolol)	May increase cardiac depressant effects, possibly causing CHF
Cyclosporine (immunosuppressant)	May increase risk of cyclosporine toxicity, resulting in tremors, seizures, or renal failure

• Dizziness (in angina), headache, asthenia (in angina), flushing

Infrequent adverse reactions
• Palpitations, tachycardia
• Dyspnea
• Dizziness (in hypertension), paresthesia, somnolence, asthenia (in hypertension)
• Nausea, dyspepsia, dry mouth, constipation
• Rash
• Myalgia

Interactions
• *Cimetidine:* May decrease metabolism of calcium channel blocking agents. Monitor for increased pharmacologic effect.
• *Digoxin:* May increase plasma digoxin. Monitor levels closely.
• *Fentanyl anesthesia:* Severe hypotension has been reported.

For dangerous interactions, see *Life-threatening hazards of multidrug therapy with nicardipine.*

Interventions
Preparation and administration
• Administer this drug on an empty stomach because food may interfere with absorption. (See *Taking calcium channel blockers at home,* page 77.)

Monitoring and supportive care
• Measure blood pressure frequently during initial therapy. Maximum antihypertensive response occurs about 1 hour after administering the immediate-release form and 2 to 4 hours after giving the extended-release form. Because large swings in blood pressure may occur based on blood levels of the drug, assess adequacy of antihypertensive effect 8 hours after administration.

Safety tip. Check for orthostatic hypotension and take appropriate measures to prevent falls or injuries.
• Be aware that some patients may experience increased frequency, severity, or duration of chest pain at

the beginning of therapy or during dosage adjustments. The mechanism for this adverse reaction is not known. Assess for and advise the patient to report chest discomfort immediately.
• Patients with renal impairment require slow titration to optimal response. Therapy begins with 20 mg P.O. t.i.d.
• Patients with hepatic impairment require lower initial dosages (20 mg P.O. b.i.d.) and then careful titration to optimal response.
• Allow at least 3 days between dosage adjustments to achieve steady plasma levels.

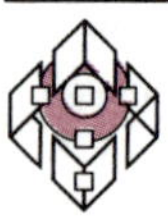 **MedTest**

1. Nicardipine is classified pharmacologically as:
    a. an ACE inhibitor.
    b. a beta blocker.
    c. a calcium channel blocker.
    d. a nitrate.

2. Nicardipine dosage should be reduced in patients with:
    a. aortic stenosis.
    b. CHF or hypotension.
    c. AV block.
    d. hepatic impairment.

3. When using the immediate-release form of nicardipine, the maximum antihypertensive effect will occur in about:
    a. 1 hour.
    b. 2 hours.
    c. 4 hours.
    d. 8 hours.

Nifedipine

Also known by the brand names Adalat, Apo-Nifed, Novo-Nifedin, Procardia, Procardia XL and, in Canada, Adalat P.A., nifedipine is a calcium channel blocker that's classified therapeutically as an antianginal agent. It's available in 10- and 20-mg capsules and in 30-, 60-, and 90-mg sustained-release tablets. (See *Other dihydropyridines: Felodipine and isradipine.*)

Pharmacokinetics
• *Absorption:* About 90% of dose is absorbed rapidly from GI tract after oral administration, but only about 65% to 70% reaches systemic circulation because of significant first-pass effect in the liver. After sublingual administration, less than 20% of dose reaches systemic circulation. With capsules, peak serum levels occur in 30 minutes to 2 hours; with sustained-release forms, 6 hours. (See *Giving nifedipine capsules,* page 232.)
• *Distribution:* 92% to 98% of circulating nifedipine is bound to plasma proteins.
• *Metabolism:* Metabolized in the liver to inactive metabolites.
• *Excretion:* Excreted in urine and feces as inactive metabolites. Elimination half-life is 2 to 5 hours. Duration of effect ranges from 4 to 12 hours.

Indications, dosage, and action
Prinzmetal's (or variant) angina or chronic stable angina
• *Adult dosage:* Starting dosage is 10 mg P.O. t.i.d. Usual effective dosage range is 10 to 20 mg t.i.d. Some pa-

Other dihydropyridines: Felodipine and isradipine

Along with nicardipine and nifedipine, felodipine and isradipine are calcium channel blockers that belong to the chemical group known as dihydropyridines. Unlike other calcium channel blockers, dihydropyridines are selective for smooth muscle found on blood vessels. Most dihydropyridines have negligible effects on the heart and its structures.

Dihydropyridines lower blood pressure by causing vasodilation, which reduces peripheral resistance. Most dihydropyridines are also effective antianginals. Dilation of peripheral blood vessels reduces cardiac afterload (the force against which the heart must pump), lessening myocardial wall tension, cardiac workload, and oxygen requirements of myocardial tissues.

Felodipine
Known by the brand name Plendil, felodipine is available in 5- or 10-mg extended-release tablets. The usual initial dosage of 5 mg P.O. once daily is adjusted according to patient response at 2-week intervals. Most patients respond to 5 or 10 mg daily; the maximum recommended dosage is 20 mg/day.

Isradipine
Known by the brand name DynaCirc, isradipine is available in 2.5- or 5-mg tablets. The usual initial dosage of 2.5 mg P.O. b.i.d. is adjusted according to patient response at 2- to 4-week intervals. Although the maximum recommended dosage is 20 mg/day, dosages above 10 mg/day have resulted in a higher incidence of adverse effects without an increase in response.

tients may require up to 30 mg q.i.d. Maximum daily dosage is 120 mg. Common dosage of sustained-release form is 30 mg once daily. Effective dosage range is 30 to 60 mg daily, with maximum daily dosage of 90 mg.
- *Antianginal action:* Causes arterial dilation, decreasing total peripheral resistance, afterload, myocardial workload, and myocardial oxygen consumption. Also dilates coronary arteries and inhibits coronary artery spasm.

Hypertension
- *Adult dosage:* Initially, 30 to 60 mg P.O. once daily (sustained-release tablets); or capsules can be given t.i.d. to provide same total daily dosage. Adjust dosage at 7- to 14-day intervals according to patient tolerance and response. Maximum dosage is 120 mg daily.
- *Antihypertensive action:* Dilates systemic arteries, resulting in decreased total peripheral resistance.

Contraindications and cautions
- Use with caution in CHF or aortic stenosis, especially if patients are receiving concomitant beta blockers. In these patients, the drug may precipitate or worsen heart failure and cause excessive hypotension because

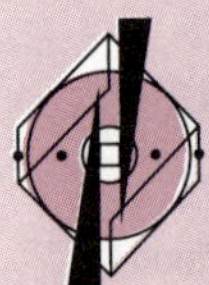

Administration guidelines

Giving nifedipine capsules

Sublingual nifedipine has routinely been used to produce a rapid onset of antihypertensive effect. Because a sublingual preparation isn't available, nurses often puncture the liquid-filled capsules and expel the contents under the patient's tongue.

But recent studies show that a better way to administer nifedipine capsules is to have the patient bite the capsule before swallowing. Not only is this more effective, producing peak drug levels in a shorter amount of time, but it's also easier for the patient and the nurse.

of its peripheral vasodilating effects. It may exacerbate angina symptoms when therapy begins or dosage is increased.

• Use cautiously in elderly patients, in whom the drug's effects may be prolonged.

• Pregnancy risk category C

Life-threatening adverse reactions
• CHF, MI

Common adverse reactions
• Peripheral edema, hypotension
• Dizziness, light-headedness, flushing, headache, weakness
• Nausea

Infrequent adverse reactions
• Palpitations, worsening angina

• Dyspnea, chest congestion
• Syncope
• Heartburn, diarrhea, constipation, cramps, flatulence
• Nasal congestion
• Muscle cramps

Interactions
• *Cimetidine, ranitidine:* Decreased nifedipine metabolism.

For dangerous interactions, see *Life-threatening hazards of multidrug therapy with nifedipine.*

Interventions
Preparation and administration
• Give with or without food. (See *Taking calcium channel blockers at home,* page 77.)

Monitoring and supportive care
• Initial doses or a dosage increase may exacerbate angina briefly. Reassure the patient that this symptom is temporary.
• Monitor blood pressure regularly.
• Patients may continue to use sublingual nitroglycerin during acute anginal attacks.
• Although a rebound effect hasn't been observed when the drug is stopped, dosage should be reduced slowly and the patient supervised.

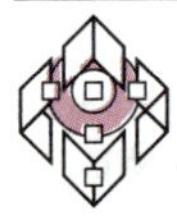

MedTest

1. If a patient develops angina during titration of his nifedipine dosage, the appropriate response should be to:

    a. discontinue his nifedipine.

    b. decrease his nifedipine dosage.

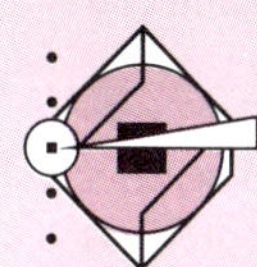

Interactions alert

Life-threatening hazards of multidrug therapy with nifedipine

Interacting drug	Effects
Antihypertensive agents (such as methyldopa)	Increase risk of severe hypotension
Beta blockers (such as propranolol)	May cause severe hypotension, exacerbation of angina, life-threatening arrhythmias, and CHF
Digitalis glycosides (such as digoxin)	Increase risk of digitalis toxicity
Fentanyl (opiate derivative)	Increases risk of severe hypotension

c. double his nifedipine dosage.
d. administer sublingual nitroglycerin.

2. One of the common adverse effects of nifedipine is:
 a. worsening of angina.
 b. palpitations.
 c. dizziness.
 d. dyspnea.

3. When nifedipine is given sublingually, how much of it reaches systemic circulation?
 a. 20% or less.
 b. 40% to 50%.
 c. 65% to 70%.
 d. 90%.

Nitroglycerin

Nitroglycerin is known by multiple brand names, depending on the type of preparation. It's available for oral use as Nitro-Bid and Nitrocap T.D. in 2.6-, 6.5-, and 9-mg sustained-release tablets and in 2.5-, 6.5- and 9-mg sustained-release capsules; for sublingual use as Nitrostat in 0.15-, 0.3-, 0.4-, and 0.6-mg tablets; for translingual use as Nitrolingual in a 0.4-mg metered spray; for I.V. use as Nitro-Bid IV, Nitrostat, and Tridil in 0.5-, 0.8-, and 5-mg/ml vials and in premixed I.V. solutions in D_5W as 100, 200, or 400 mcg/ml; for topical use as Nitrol and Nitrostat in a 2% ointment; for transdermal use as Nitrodisc, Nitro-Dur, and Transderm-Nitro in 2.5-, 5-, 7.5-, 10-, and 15-mg/24-hour systems; and for transmucosal use as Nitrogard in 1-, 2-, and 3-mg controlled-release tablets. Nitroglycerin is a nitrate that's classified therapeutically as an antianginal and a vasodilator.

Pharmacokinetics

• *Absorption:* Well absorbed from GI tract. However, because it undergoes first-pass metabolism in the liver,

bioavailability is low after oral administration. Onset of action for oral preparations is slow. After sublingual or translingual administration, absorption from the oral mucosa is relatively complete and onset of action is less than 3 minutes. Nitroglycerin also is well absorbed after topical administration as an ointment or transdermal system, and onset of action occurs in 20 to 60 minutes.
• *Distribution:* About 60% of circulating drug is bound to plasma proteins.
• *Metabolism:* Metabolized in the liver and serum to metabolites that have a slight vasodilating effect.
• *Excretion:* Metabolites excreted in urine; elimination half-life about 1 to 4 minutes. Duration of effect for various preparations is as follows: I.V. or sublingual, up to 30 minutes after discontinuation; translingual spray, 30 to 60 minutes; transmucosal tablet, 5 hours; ointment, 3 to 6 hours; oral (sustained-release), 4 to 8 hours; and transdermal, 18 to 24 hours.

Indications, dosage, and action
Prophylaxis for anginal attacks
• *Adult dosage:* One sustained-release tablet or capsule (1.3 to 9 mg) q 8 to 12 hours or 1 to 3 mg transmucosally every 3 to 5 hours during waking hours. The starting dose for 2% ointment is ½″ ointment, increasing in ½″ increments until headache occurs and then decreasing to previous dose. Range of dosage with ointment is 2″ to 5″. Usual dose is 1″ to 2″.

Alternatively, a transdermal disk or pad delivering 0.1 to 0.6 mg/hour may be applied to a hairless site once daily. However, to prevent toler-

ance, topical forms shouldn't be worn overnight.
• *Action:* Reduces cardiac oxygen demand by decreasing left ventricular end-diastolic pressure (preload) and, to a lesser extent, systemic vascular resistance (afterload). Also increases blood flow through the collateral coronary vessels.

Treatment and prevention of acute angina
• *Adult dosage:* One sublingual 0.15- to 0.6-mg tablet (0.4 mg is most common) dissolved under tongue or in buccal pouch as soon as anginal attack begins or before stressful events that may cause angina. May repeat q 5 minutes to a maximum of three doses within a 15-minute period. Or spray one or two doses of Nitrolingual into mouth, preferably onto or under tongue. May repeat q 3 to 5 minutes to a maximum of three doses within a 15-minute period.

Hypertension, CHF, angina associated with surgery
• *Adult dosage:* Initial infusion rate is 5 mcg/minute. May be increased by 5 mcg/minute q 3 to 5 minutes until response is noted. If 20 mcg/minute doesn't produce desired response, dosage may be increased by as much as 20 mcg/minute q 3 to 5 minutes.
• *Antianginal and vasodilating action:* Relaxes vascular smooth muscle of venous bed and, to a lesser extent, arterioles. This effect decreases both venous filling pressure (preload) and arterial resistance (after-

load). Myocardial workload is reduced, and myocardial oxygen consumption decreases.

Contraindications and cautions

• Avoid use in head trauma or cerebral hemorrhage because of potential for increased ICP.
• Don't use in severe anemia because nitrate ions can readily oxidize hemoglobin to methemoglobin.
• Don't use I.V. nitroglycerin in patients with hypotension or uncorrected hypovolemia because it may cause severe hypotension and shock.
• Don't use I.V. nitroglycerin in constrictive pericarditis or pericardial tamponade because it may cause hypotension, reduce preload, and decrease cardiac output.
• Know that because nitroglycerin may exaggerate outflow obstructions, it's contraindicated in hypertrophic obstructive cardiomyopathy, except for diagnostic use.
• Use cautiously in patients with glaucoma.
• Use cautiously during the initial days after acute MI because the drug may decrease right ventricular filling pressure, leading to hemodynamic and clinical deterioration.
• Use with caution in mitral stenosis, which may excessively reduce preload.
• Know that tolerance to effects of the drug can develop, and cross-tolerance between the nitrates and nitrites has been demonstrated. Tolerance is usually associated with a high or sustained plasma drug concentration. Patients taking oral isosorbide dinitrate or topical nitroglycerin have not exhibited cross-tolerance to sublingual nitroglycerin.
• Know that development of tolerance can be prevented by using the lowest effective dose and maintaining an intermittent dosing schedule. A nitrate-free interval of at least 8 hours daily (for example, by removing the transdermal nitroglycerin patch in the early evening and reapplying it the next morning) also helps prevent tolerance.
• The drug should be discontinued if rash, dermatitis, blurred vision, or dry mouth occurs.
• Be aware that methemoglobinemia may occur in individuals receiving large doses of nitroglycerin.
• Because it's unknown whether this drug is excreted in breast milk, use caution in administering it to a breast-feeding woman.
• Pregnancy risk category C

Life-threatening adverse reactions

• Profound hypotension

Common adverse reactions

• Orthostatic hypotension, tachycardia, flushing, palpitations
• Headache (sometimes throbbing), dizziness

Infrequent adverse reactions

• Fainting
• Weakness, blurred vision
• Nausea, vomiting
• Cutaneous vasodilation, skin irritation (with topical form)
• Sublingual burning, dry mouth (with sublingual form)

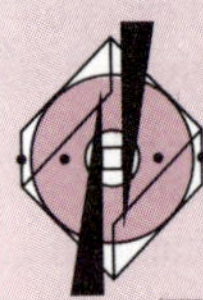

Administration guidelines

Plastics to avoid when infusing nitroglycerin

Nitroglycerin binds to polyvinyl chloride (PVC) plastic, which is commonly found in I.V. infusion bags and tubing. Soft, pliable plastics commonly contain PVC; glass and harder plastics, such as polypropylene and polyolefin, don't bind to the drug. To minimize drug loss and ensure proper dosage, follow these guidelines when administering nitroglycerin:

• Reconstitute the drug in a glass bottle or container using D_5W. Never use an I.V. bag.
• Avoid using I.V. filters because they're made of plastic.
• Use the administration sets provided by the drug manufacturer.
• Avoid using extension tubing unless it's made from non-PVC plastic.
• Use the same type of tubing when changing I.V. lines.

If you can't avoid using PVC plastic tubing, carefully titrate dosage to clinical response. Binding is not constant or self-limiting, but most of the binding occurs early in the infusion. Expect frequent dosage adjustments when a new administration set is used.

• Hypersensitivity reactions (rash, dermatitis)

Interactions

• *Alcohol:* Concomitant use may cause additive hypotensive effects.
• *Antihypertensives, phenothiazines:* Risk of severe hypotension.

• *Ergot alkaloids:* Concomitant use may precipitate angina. Oral nitroglycerin may increase the bioavailability of ergot alkaloids.
• *Heparin:* Concomitant I.V. administration with I.V. nitroglycerin may require increased heparin dosage. Monitor PTT and expect dosage to be adjusted accordingly. When discontinuing nitroglycerin, check PTT.

Interventions

Preparation and administration

• For I.V. infusion, use special nonabsorbent tubing. (See *Plastics to avoid when infusing nitroglycerin.*)
• Always use an infusion pump. The dosage should be titrated to the desired patient response.
• During infusion, closely monitor vital signs. Pay attention to blood pressure, especially if the drug is being given to a patient with MI.
• Don't mix nitroglycerin with other drugs.
• The sublingual and translingual forms should be used to relieve acute anginal attacks (signaled by anginal pain or its equivalent, or excessive dyspnea). Use these forms prior to exercise or any stress or activity that induces angina (such as sexual activity) or at bedtime if angina is nocturnal. Administer the ordered sublingual tablet at the first sign of an attack. If the patient complains of a tingling sensation with the tablet placed sublingually, tell him to try holding it in his buccal pouch. (See *Taking nitroglycerin at home).*

Safety tip. If serious adverse reactions develop in a patient using ointment or a transdermal system, remove the product at once or

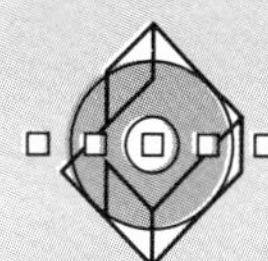

Patient-teaching checklist

Taking nitroglycerin at home

In addition to explaining the drug's action and dosage, teach the patient who will continue nitroglycerin therapy after discharge to follow these important guidelines.

Taking oral nitroglycerin
□ Even when you're feeling well, take your medication as prescribed.
□ Take oral tablets with a full (8-oz) glass of water on an empty stomach, either 30 minutes before or 1 to 2 hours after meals.

Taking sublingual tablets
□ Sit down, wet the sublingual tablet with your saliva, place it under your tongue, and let it dissolve. Don't chew, crush, or swallow sublingual tablets.
□ If angina or shortness of breath continues, you may repeat the dose every 5 minutes for a maximum of three doses. If you don't experience relief, notify your doctor immediately or have someone take you to the nearest emergency department.
□ Upon first opening a bottle of sublingual tablets, write the date on the side of the bottle. Replace this bottle 6 months from that date to ensure potency of tablets. The expiration date printed on the label is only good if the bottle hasn't been opened. Also, discard the bottle if the tablets become crushed. Don't transfer the tablets to another container.

Taking transmucosal tablets
□ While sitting down, place the buccal form of nitroglycerin between your upper lip and gum above your incisors or between your cheek and gum and let it dissolve. Either way, don't swallow or chew the tablet because this will make it ineffective.
□ If angina continues, repeat the dose every 5 minutes for a maximum of three doses. If you don't experience relief, notify your doctor immediately or have someone take you to the nearest emergency department.

Using translingual spray
□ While sitting down, remove the plastic cover from the nitroglycerin spray container. Don't shake the container; hold it upright.
□ With the container held close to your mouth, press the button to spray onto or under your tongue. Don't inhale the spray. Release the button and close your mouth.
□ After spraying the nitroglycerin, wait about 10 seconds before swallowing.
□ If angina or shortness of breath continues, you may take one spray every 5 minutes for a maximum of three doses. If your chest pain isn't relieved after three sprays in a 15-minute period, notify your doctor immediately or have someone drive you to the nearest emergency department.

(continued)

Taking nitroglycerin at home *(continued)*

Applying topical nitroglycerin
☐ Spread the prescribed amount of nitroglycerin ointment in a uniform thin layer on any hairless body area. Don't rub it in.
☐ Cover with plastic film to aid absorption and protect your clothing.
☐ If you're using the Tape-Surrounded AppliRuler (TSAR) system, measure the prescribed length in inches, squeezing the tube to retain a uniform thickness. Fold the paper ruler in half to spread the ointment over its surface, and then open and place it on your skin in a dry, hairless area. Keep the TSAR on your skin to protect your clothing and to ensure that the ointment remains in place. (If desired, you may apply it at your wrist and cover it with a terrycloth wristband.)
☐ Remove all excess nitroglycerin ointment from the previous site before applying the next dose.
☐ Don't get ointment on your fingers.

Applying transdermal patch
☐ Apply the patch to any clean, dry, hairless body area that's free of scars, cuts, or irritation, except the distal parts of your arms or legs.
☐ Apply a new patch if the first one loosens or falls off.
☐ Apply each dose to a different area of skin to prevent skin irritation.
☐ Be sure to remove the old patch before applying a new one.

Minimize adverse reactions
☐ Remember to change positions slowly, especially from lying flat to sitting upright. Dangle your legs over the bedside for a few minutes before standing to minimize dizziness. Lie down immediately if dizziness or faintness occurs.
☐ Avoid driving or operating machinery until you've adjusted to the drug's effects.
☐ To minimize dizziness, avoid alcoholic beverages, long periods of standing, and excessive exercise.
☐ Be aware that initially a headache may occur following each dose of nitroglycerin. Take a mild pain-reliever, such as acetaminophen or aspirin, as needed. If the headaches don't subside, check with your doctor.

Other instructions
☐ Don't eat, drink, smoke, or use chewing tobacco while a buccal or sublingual tablet is dissolving.
☐ Store nitroglycerin in a cool, dark place in a tightly closed container.
☐ Never store nitroglycerin in a closed car or glove compartment.
☐ Don't carry the nitroglycerin bottle close to your body because the heat may accelerate the drug's decomposition. Instead, carry the bottle in a jacket pocket or purse.
☐ Use caution when wearing a transdermal patch of nitroglycerin near a microwave oven. Leaking radiation may heat the patch's metallic backing and cause burns.
☐ To determine the number of doses left in the container, place it in a bowl filled with water. When it almost floats to the top of the water, you know it's time to obtain a new container.
☐ Check with your doctor or pharmacist before taking OTC medications.

wipe the ointment from his skin. Take care to avoid contact with the ointment.

Monitoring and supportive care
• When administering nitroglycerin to patients during the initial days following acute MI, monitor hemodynamic and clinical status carefully.
• Monitor blood pressure and the intensity and duration of the patient's response to the drug.
• If the drug causes headache (especially likely with initial doses), aspirin or acetaminophen may be indicated. Nitroglycerin dosage may need to be reduced temporarily.

Safety tip. Remember that although nitroglycerin may cause a local burning sensation, many brands no longer produce this sensation and it shouldn't be used as an indication of tablet potency.
• Remember that nitroglycerin may cause orthostatic hypotension.
• Be sure to remove a transdermal patch before defibrillation. Because of the patch's aluminum backing, electric current could cause the patch to explode.
• You can interchange the various brands of transdermal nitroglycerin to achieve the prescribed dose. Standardized labels specify the amount of nitroglycerin released over 24 hours.
• To prevent withdrawal symptoms, expect dosage to be reduced gradually after long-term use of oral or topical preparations.

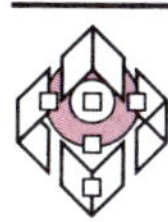 **MedTest**

1. If your patient develops tolerance to his nitroglycerin, manage it best by:
    a. increasing his dosage.
    b. substituting a different administration form of the drug.
    c. allowing an 8-hour nitrate-free interval daily.
    d. changing to a different nitrate preparation.

2. When taking the transmucosal form of nitroglycerin, the patient should:
    a. place the tablet under his upper lip or in the buccal pouch and allow it to dissolve.
    b. place the tablet between his lower lip and gum, and moisten it frequently by touching it with his tongue to aid dissolution.
    c. wet the tablet with saliva and place it under his tongue, allowing 3 to 5 minutes for dissolution before taking any food or fluids.
    d. place the tablet in his buccal pouch and wait 3 to 5 minutes before chewing and swallowing it.

3. If your patient is using nitroglycerin spray, teach him to:
    a. inhale the spray.
    b. release the spray onto or under his tongue.
    c. swallow immediately after spraying the dose into his mouth.
    d. sniff three to five times after spraying the dose into his nares.

Nitroprusside sodium

Also known by the brand names Nipride and Nitropress, nitroprusside is a vasodilator that's classified therapeutically as an antihypertensive agent. It's available as a powder for injection in 50-mg vials.

Pharmacokinetics
- *Absorption:* Because this drug is not absorbed, it's administered I.V., reducing blood pressure almost immediately.
- *Distribution:* Unknown.
- *Metabolism:* Metabolized rapidly in erythrocytes and tissues and converted to cyanide and then to thiocyanate in liver. Thiocyanate is therapeutically inactive but adds to drug toxicity.
- *Excretion:* Excreted primarily in urine as metabolites.

Indications, dosage, and action
Hypertensive emergencies
- *Adult and pediatric dosage:* I.V. infusion titrated to blood pressure; average dosage is 3 mcg/kg/minute, with a range of 0.5 to 10 mcg/kg/minute. Maximum rate is 10 mcg/kg/minute; infusions at the maximum rate shouldn't exceed 10 minutes.
- *Antihypertensive action:* Acts directly on vascular smooth muscle (equally on arteries and veins), causing peripheral vasodilation.

Contraindications and cautions
- Don't use in compensatory hypertension secondary to arteriovenous shunt or coarctation of the aorta because a decrease in blood pressure may be harmful to these patients.
- Use cautiously in renal insufficiency because thiocyanate, one of the metabolites of nitroprusside, is excreted by the kidneys and may accumulate.
- Use with caution in hepatic insufficiency because drug metabolism may be impaired.
- Use with caution in hypothyroidism because thiocyanate inhibits iodine uptake and binding.
- Use cautiously in patients with low vitamin B_{12} concentrations because the drug may interfere with vitamin B_{12} distribution and metabolism.
- Discontinue this drug if metabolic acidosis or drug tolerance occurs; either may indicate cyanide toxicity.
- Be aware that elderly patients may be more sensitive to the drug's antihypertensive effects.
- Because it's not known whether nitroprusside is distributed in breast milk, administer it with caution to breast-feeding women.
- Pregnancy risk category C

Life-threatening adverse reactions
- Severe hypotension
- Loss of consciousness, coma
- Cyanide toxicity

Common adverse reactions
- Headache, dizziness, diaphoresis (Whether they occur individually or in different combinations, these adverse reactions usually indicate an overdose.)

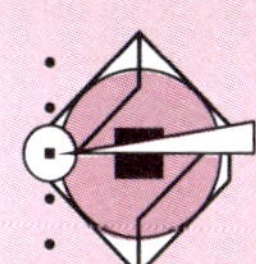

Interactions alert

Life-threatening hazards of multidrug therapy with nitroprusside

Interacting drug	Effects
Antihypertensive agents (such as hydralazine)	Cause severe additive hypotension and myocardial ischemia
Ganglionic-blocking agents (such as mecamylamine)	Increase risk of severe hypotension
General anesthetics (such as halothane)	Increase risk of severe hypotension
Negative inotropic agents (such as propranolol)	Increase risk of severe hypotension

Infrequent adverse reactions

• Distant heart sounds, palpitations, dyspnea, shallow breathing, hypotension (Whether they occur individually or in different combinations, these adverse reactions usually indicate an overdose.)
• Pulmonary shunting
• Ataxia, restlessness, muscle twitching, weak pulse, absent reflexes, widely dilated pupils
• Vomiting, nausea, abdominal pain
• Worsened renal insufficiency
• Metabolic acidosis
• Pink skin color

Interactions

For dangerous interactions, see *Life-threatening hazards of multidrug therapy with nitroprusside*.

Interventions

Preparation and administration

• Before giving this drug, obtain baseline vital signs and find out what parameters the doctor wants to achieve. (See *Giving I.V. nitroprusside*, page 242.)

Safety tip. Keep the patient supine when initiating nitroprusside therapy or titrating dosage to minimize orthostatic hypotension.
• Know that nitroprusside may lose its potency if given with other drugs. (See *Nitroprusside combinations to avoid*, page 243.)

Monitoring and supportive care

• Nitroprusside can cause cyanide toxicity, especially with excessive doses (totaling 10 mg/kg or more), with rapid infusion (rate exceeding 10 mcg/kg/minute), or with prolonged infusion. Therefore, check serum thiocyanate levels every 72 hours. Levels above 100 mcg/ml are associated with cyanide toxicity, which can produce profound metabolic acidosis, profound hypotension, dyspnea, ataxia, vomiting, seizures,

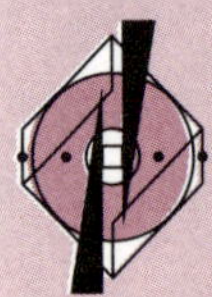

Administration guidelines

Giving I.V. nitroprusside

Follow these instructions when preparing and administering I.V. nitroprusside.

Prepare the setup
• Use only D₅W for reconstitution. Fresh solutions should have a faint brownish tint.
• Because of the solution's sensitivity to light, wrap the I.V. container in foil. However, you don't need to wrap the tubing or drip chamber.
• Discard the solution after 24 hours.

Administer the I.V. solution
• If possible, administer the drug piggyback through a peripheral I.V. line with no other medication, using an infusion pump.
• Don't adjust the rate of the main I.V. line while the drug is infusing because even small boluses can cause severe hypotension.
• Monitor the drug's effectiveness by checking the patient's blood pressure q 5 minutes at the start of the infusion and q 15 minutes thereafter.
• When nitroprusside is no longer required, taper the dose slowly. Never stop the drug abruptly.

and coma. If such signs occur, discontinue the infusion, notify the doctor and reevaluate therapy.
• Monitor acid-base balance and venous oxygen levels.
• Be aware that hypertensive patients are highly sensitive to nitroprusside, as are patients taking other antihypertensive drugs. Monitor blood pressure frequently; if hypotension occurs, monitor ECG for ischemic changes.
• This drug is sometimes used with a direct-acting cardiac stimulant such as dopamine in patients with refractory heart failure.
• Ask the patient to report any CNS symptoms (such as headache or dizziness) promptly.

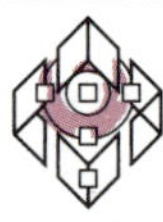

MedTest

1. When preparing nitroprusside, you should:

   a. dilute it in sterile 0.9% NaCl solution.

   b. protect the I.V. container from light with foil wrap.

   c. discard the prepared solution if it has a brownish color.

   d. use a special tubing resistant to light and to drug interaction.

2. While administering nitroprusside, you should monitor the patient's blood pressure:

   a. q 5 minutes at the start of the infusion and then q 15 minutes for the duration.

   b. q 5 minutes throughout the infusion period.

   c. q 1 to 2 minutes initially, then q 5 minutes for an hour, and then q 15 minutes.

   d. q 3 to 5 minutes × 4, then q 15 minutes × 4, and then hourly.

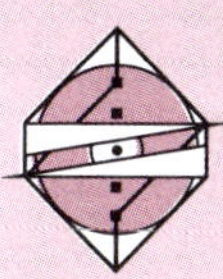

Incompatibility warning
Nitroprusside combinations to avoid

Nitroprusside ions can react with minute quantities of a wide variety of inorganic and organic substances, including benzyl alcohol. These mixtures form highly colored products — usually blue, green, or dark red — and require discarding the solution. Because of the potential for reduced or lost potency, don't mix nitroprusside with most other drugs. If you *must* mix nitroprusside with another drug, be sure to consult the pharmacist for specific compatibility information.

3. Concerned that your patient receiving nitroprusside may develop cyanide toxicity, you:

   a. check his serum thiocyanate levels q 12 hours.
   b. monitor his cardiac rate and rhythm.
   c. assess for dyspnea, ataxia, and vomiting.
   d. assess for shallow respirations, bradycardia, and pink color.

Norepinephrine bitartrate

Also known by the brand name Levophed, norepinephrine is a direct-acting adrenergic that's classified therapeutically as a vasopressor. It's available for I.V. infusion in 1-mg/ml vials.

Pharmacokinetics
• *Absorption:* Pressor effect occurs rapidly after I.V. infusion but stops within 1 to 2 minutes after infusion is stopped.
• *Distribution:* Localizes in sympathetic nerve tissues.
• *Metabolism:* Metabolized in the liver and other tissues to inactive compounds.
• *Excretion:* Excreted in urine primarily as sulfate and glucuronide conjugates. Small amounts excreted unchanged in urine.

Indications, dosage, and action
Restoring blood pressure in acute hypotensive states
• *Adult dosage:* 8 to 12 mcg/minute by I.V. infusion initially, titrated to maintain desired blood pressure; maintenance dosage is 2 to 4 mcg/minute.
• *Pediatric dosage:* 2 mcg/minute or 2 mcg/m^2/minute I.V. infusion initially, titrated to maintain desired blood pressure. For advanced cardiac life support, initial infusion rate is 0.1 mcg/kg/minute.
• *Vasopressor action:* Stimulates alpha-adrenergic receptors, constricting both capacitance and resistance blood vessels. This results in increased total peripheral resistance and increased systolic and diastolic blood pressure. The drug also has a direct stimulating effect on beta$_1$-adrenergic receptors of the heart, producing a positive inotropic response. Its main therapeutic effects are vasoconstriction and cardiac stimulation.

It may produce a reflex decrease in heart rate.

Contraindications and cautions
• Don't use in patients with peripheral or mesenteric vascular thrombosis (because drug may worsen ischemia or extend area of infarction), profound hypoxia or hypercapnia, or hypovolemia or in those undergoing general anesthesia with cyclopropane or other inhalation hydrocarbon anesthetics (because drug increases the risk of inducing cardiac arrhythmias).
• Administer cautiously to hypertensive or hyperthyroid patients because of the increased risk of adverse reactions.
• Give cautiously to patients with known hypersensitivity to sulfites; the commercially available formulation contains sodium metabisulfite.
• Discontinue the drug if hypersensitivity or thrombosis occurs.
• Change sites if infiltration occurs.
• Know that elderly patients are more sensitive to the drug's effects.
• Use with caution in children.
• Because it's unknown whether this drug is excreted in breast milk, use caution when administering to a breast-feeding woman.
• Pregnancy risk category D

Life-threatening adverse reactions
• Severe hypertension, ischemic injury from potent vasoconstrictor action and tissue hypoxia, VT, fibrillation
• Cerebral hemorrhage

Common adverse reactions
• Headache

Infrequent adverse reactions
• Precordial pain, severe hypertension, severe peripheral and visceral vasoconstriction, arrhythmias, bradycardia
• Respiratory difficulty
• Anxiety, weakness, dizziness, restlessness, anxiety, insomnia, tremor, seizures
• Nausea, vomiting
• Decreased urine output
• Photophobia
• Metabolic acidosis, hyperglycemia
• Sweating, severe local irritation and necrosis with extravasation
• Hyperthermia, pallor

Interactions
• *Alpha-adrenergic blocking agents:* May antagonize drug effects.
• *Anticholinergics such as atropine:* Concomitant use blocks the reflex bradycardia caused by norepinephrine and enhances its pressor effects.
• *Beta blockers:* Concomitant use may increase potential for hypertension.
• *Diuretics:* May decrease pressor response.
• *Ergot alkaloids, general anesthetics, guanethidine, MAO inhibitors, methyldopa, tricyclic antidepressants:* Risk of hypertensive crisis. Avoid concomitant use.

Interventions
Preparation and administration
• Protect stored vials of solution from light. Discard solution that's discolored or contains a precipitate.
• Avoid mixing with other drugs. Iron salts, alkaline solutions, and oxidizing agents cause rapid decomposition of norepinephrine. Check with a

pharmacist before mixing with other drugs or I.V. solutions.

• Prepare infusion solution by adding 4 mg of norepinephrine to 1 liter of D_5W. The resultant solution contains 4 mcg/ml. Or prepare according to hospital protocol. (See *Preparing and infusing I.V. norepinephrine*.)

• Monitor infusion rate.

• If prolonged I.V. therapy is necessary, change the injection site frequently.

Monitoring and supportive care

• Correct blood volume depletion before administering this drug. Norepinephrine is not a substitute for blood, plasma, fluid, or electrolyte replacement.

• Check the I.V. site frequently for signs of extravasation. Also check for blanching along the course of the infused vein, because it may progress to superficial sloughing. To treat, use a fine needle to infiltrate the site promptly with 10 to 15 ml of 0.9% NaCl solution containing 5 to 10 mg of phentolamine.

Safety tip. Some doctors add phentolamine (5 to 10 mg) to each liter of infusion solution to prevent sloughing, should extravasation occur.

• Monitor the patient constantly during administration of norepinephrine. Take baseline blood pressure and pulse rate before therapy, repeat q 2 minutes until stabilization, and then repeat q 5 minutes during drug administration.

• Monitor intake and output.

• Norepinephrine reduces renal blood flow, which may cause de-

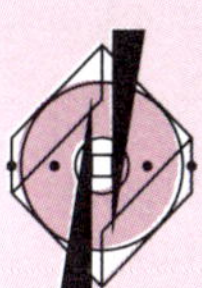

Administration guidelines
Preparing and infusing I.V. norepinephrine

Observe these guidelines if your patient requires I.V. norepinephrine therapy.

Diluting norepinephrine

• Before use, dilute norepinephrine in 5% dextrose solution.

• Don't dilute norepinephrine with NaCl alone. Studies have shown that dextrose helps prevent norepinephrine oxidation, so admixtures prepared in dextrose-containing solutions have better stability.

Infusing the solution

• Use a central line or a large vein, such as a vein in the antecubital fossa, to minimize the risk of extravasation.

• To regulate the infusion flow rate, administer the solution using an infusion pump or controller and a piggyback setup. This setup also will allow the main I.V. infusion to continue if norepinephrine is discontinued.

• Piggyback the infusion into a D_5W solution, 0.9% NaCl injection, or lactated Ringer's injection.

• Never leave the patient unattended during the infusion.

• Stop the infusion and notify the doctor immediately if extravasation occurs.

creased urine output initially. Report this sign to the doctor immediately.

• In addition to vital signs, monitor the patient's mental status, skin temperature of his extremities, and skin color (especially of his earlobes, lips, and nail beds).

• During infusion, frequently monitor ECG, cardiac output, CVP, and PAWP. Titrate the infusion rate according to these findings and the doctor's guidelines.

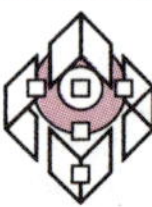 **Safety tip.** In patients with previously normal blood pressure, adjust the flow rate to maintain blood pressure at low-normal levels (usually 80 to 100 mm Hg systolic); in hypertensive patients, maintain systolic pressure at no less than 40 mm Hg below the preexisting pressure.

• Withdraw the drug gradually; recurrent hypotension may follow abrupt withdrawal.

Safety tip. Monitor vital signs even after the drug is stopped. Watch for a severe drop in blood pressure.

MedTest

---

1. The recommended dilution for norepinephrine is:

  a. 4 mg to 250 ml of D_5W to equal 16 mcg/ml.

  b. 4 mg to 500 ml of D_5W and 0.45% NaCl to equal 8 mcg/ml.

  c. 4 mg to 1,000 ml of D_5W to equal 4 mcg/ml.

  d. 4 mg to 1,000 ml of 0.9% NaCl solution to equal 4 mcg/ml.

2. To check for extravasation of norepinephrine, you would assess the site for:

  a. coldness and swelling.

  b. warmth and swelling.

  c. redness along the course of the infused vein.

  d. blanching along the course of the infused vein.

3. When administering norepinephrine, you should monitor blood pressure:

  a. q 2 to 3 minutes throughout the infusion.

  b. q 5 minutes throughout the infusion.

  c. q 2 minutes until stabilization and then q 5 minutes.

  d. q 5 minutes until stabilization and then q 15 minutes.

Pentoxifylline

Also known by the brand name Trental, pentoxifylline is a xanthine derivative that's classified therapeutically as a hemorrheologic agent. It's available in 400-mg extended-release tablets.

Pharmacokinetics

• *Absorption:* Absorbed almost completely from the GI tract but undergoes first-pass hepatic metabolism. Absorption is slowed by food. Peak concentrations occur in 2 to 4 hours.

• *Distribution:* Distribution is unknown; drug is bound to erythrocyte membranes.

• *Metabolism:* Metabolized extensively by erythrocytes and the liver to active metabolites.

• *Excretion:* Metabolites excreted mainly in urine; less than 4%, in feces. Half-life of unchanged drug is 30 to 45 minutes; half-life of metabolites is 1 to 1½ hours. Clinical effect requires up to 4 weeks of daily therapy.

Indications, dosage, and action
Intermittent claudication from chronic occlusive vascular disease
• *Adult dosage:* 400 mg P.O. t.i.d. with meals.
• *Hemorrheologic action:* Improves capillary blood flow by increasing erythrocyte flexibility and reducing blood viscosity.

Contraindications and cautions
• Don't give to patients with known hypersensitivity to this drug or other xanthine derivatives, such as caffeine, theophylline, or theobromine.
• Use cautiously in patients at high risk for hemorrhage, such as surgical patients or those with peptic ulcers.
• Discontinue if adverse reactions persist after dosage reduction.
• Be aware that elderly patients are at higher risk for adverse reactions.
• Because pentoxifylline enters breast milk, recommend an alternative feeding method for breast-feeding mothers.
• Pregnancy risk category C

Life-threatening adverse reactions
None noted

Common adverse reactions
None noted at standard doses

Infrequent adverse reactions
• Mild hypotension, arrhythmias, tachycardia, palpitations, flushing, edema, dyspnea, increased PT
• Headache, dizziness, tremor, agitation, nervousness, drowsiness, insomnia
• Dyspepsia, nausea, vomiting, belching, flatus, bloating

Interactions
• *Anticoagulants:* Increased anticoagulant effect.

Interventions
Preparation and administration
• Don't crush or break extended-release tablets; make certain the patient swallows them whole. (See *Taking pentoxifylline at home,* page 248.)

Safety tip. Administer the drug with meals to minimize GI distress.

Monitoring and supportive care
• Monitor PT, especially in patients taking anticoagulants such as warfarin.
• If GI or CNS adverse reactions occur, the dosage may be decreased to b.i.d. If adverse reactions persist, drug should be discontinued.
• Be aware that this drug is useful in patients who aren't good candidates for surgery.
• Advise patients to avoid smoking because nicotine causes vasoconstriction, which can worsen the condition.
• Explain the need for continuing therapy for at least 8 weeks; warn the patient not to discontinue the drug during this period without medical approval.

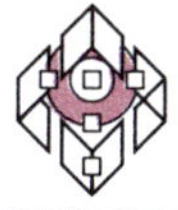 **MedTest**

---

1. Pentoxifylline increases capillary blood flow by:
    a. relaxing smooth muscle and vasodilating vessels.
    b. increasing erythrocyte flexibility.

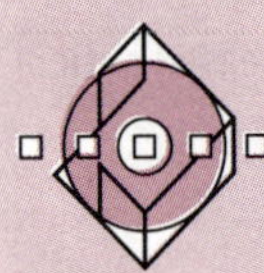

Taking pentoxifylline at home

In addition to explaining the drug's action and dosage, teach the patient who will continue pentoxifylline therapy after discharge to follow these important guidelines.

Take your medication correctly
☐ Take pentoxifylline with meals to minimize any stomach upset the drug may cause.
☐ Swallow the tablets whole. Don't break, crush, or chew them.
☐ Take pentoxifylline as prescribed even when you're feeling well. Be aware that the drug may take 2 to 4 weeks to produce optimal effects.
☐ Continue taking the drug even if unpleasant adverse reactions occur. But make sure you discuss these reactions with your doctor because your dosage may need to be adjusted.

Other instructions
☐ Lie down immediately if dizziness occurs.
☐ Avoid driving or operating machinery if this drug causes dizziness.
☐ Avoid smoking because nicotine causes blood vessels to narrow, which can worsen your condition.
☐ If you experience stomach upset, ask your doctor about the possibility of taking pentoxifylline with an antacid.
☐ Store pentoxifylline at room temperature and protect it from moisture, direct light, and air.

c. osmotically diluting blood volume.
d. increasing blood viscosity.

2. Pentoxifylline should be taken:
a. without regard to meals.
b. on an empty stomach to improve absorption.
c. with meals to reduce GI distress.
d. 1 hour after meals to slow absorption.

3. If GI or CNS adverse reactions occur, your first action should be to:
a. stop the drug immediately.
b. cut the dosage in half.

c. administer the drug with an antacid.
d. change the frequency to b.i.d.

Phenoxybenzamine hydrochloride

Also known by the brand names Dibenzyline and (in Australia) Dibenyline, phenoxybenzamine is an alpha-adrenergic blocking agent that's classified therapeutically as an antihypertensive for pheochromocytoma and as a cutaneous vasodilator. It's available in 10-mg capsules.

Pharmacokinetics
• *Absorption:* After oral administration, phenoxybenzamine is absorbed variably from the GI tract; its effects begin gradually over several hours.
• *Distribution:* Highly lipid-soluble and may accumulate in fat after large doses.
• *Metabolism:* By dealkylation, probably in the liver. It's unknown whether metabolites are active or inactive.
• *Excretion:* Excreted in urine and bile. Half-life is 24 hours, and effects last 3 to 4 days. Alpha-adrenergic blocking effects may persist for up to 7 days.

Indications, dosage, and action
Adjunctive treatment of pheochromocytoma
• *Adult dosage:* Initially, 10 mg P.O. b.i.d.; then increased every other day until desired response is achieved. Usual maintenance dosage is 20 to 40 mg b.i.d or t.i.d. daily.
• *Pediatric dosage:* Initially, 0.2 mg/kg or 6 mg/m^2 P.O. daily in a single dose. Maintenance dosage is 0.4 to 1.2 mg/kg or 12 to 36 mg/m^2 daily.
• *Antihypertensive action:* Noncompetitively blocks alpha-adrenergic receptors, causing long-acting sympathetic blockade.

Adjunctive treatment of Raynaud's syndrome, frostbite, and acrocyanosis
• *Adult dosage:* Initially, 10 mg P.O. b.i.d., then increased by 10 mg q 4 days to a maximum of 60 mg/day.
• *Cutaneous vasodilating action:* Blocks epinephrine- and norepinephrine-induced vasoconstriction.

Contraindications and cautions
• Use with caution in CHF, CAD, coronary or cerebrovascular insufficiency, or advanced renal disease because hypotension may exacerbate these conditions.
• Be cautious when giving to elderly patients, who are more apt to have marked cerebral or coronary atherosclerosis or renal insufficiency.
• Administer cautiously to children.
• Recommend an alternative to breast-feeding because it's not known whether phenoxybenzamine is distributed in breast milk.
• Pregnancy risk category C

Life-threatening adverse reactions
• Shock

Common adverse reactions
• Orthostatic hypotension, tachycardia
• Impotence, inhibition of ejaculation
• Nasal stuffiness, dry mouth, miosis

Infrequent adverse reactions
• Lethargy, drowsiness
• Vomiting, abdominal distress

Interactions
• *Alpha-adrenergics:* May block the effects of alpha-adrenergic agonists.
• *Antihypertensives:* Excessive hypotension. Use together cautiously.
• *Epinephrine:* Alpha-adrenergic blockade produced by phenoxybenzamine results in unopposed beta-adrenergic stimulation by epinephrine. The result is "epinephrine reversal": hypotension and tachycardia.

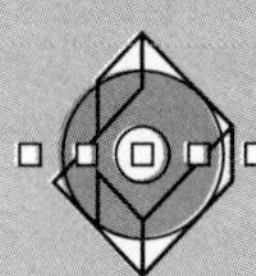

Patient-teaching checklist

Taking phenoxybenzamine at home

In addition to explaining the drug's action and dosage, teach the patient who will continue phenoxybenzamine therapy after discharge to follow these important guidelines.

Take your medication correctly
☐ To prevent stomach upset, take phenoxybenzamine with milk or food.
☐ Take the drug at the same time each day.
☐ Expect frequent dosage changes at the beginning of therapy. The prescribed dosage is small initially and is increased gradually until the desired effect is obtained.
☐ Take phenoxybenzamine as prescribed, even when you're feeling well. Be aware that the drug may take several weeks to produce optimal effects.

Watch for adverse reactions
☐ Be sure to discuss any adverse reactions with your doctor. Continue taking the drug even if unpleasant reactions occur.
☐ Know that nasal congestion, inhibition of ejaculation, and impotence usually decrease with continued therapy.
☐ Remember to change positions slowly, especially from lying flat to sitting upright. Dangle your legs over the bedside for a few minutes before standing. This will help to minimize dizziness.
☐ Lie down immediately if dizziness, light-headedness, or faintness occurs.
☐ Avoid drinking alcoholic beverages while taking this drug.

Other instructions
☐ Minimize prolonged standing, excessive exercise, and your exposure to hot weather because dizziness, light-headedness, or fainting is more likely to occur.
☐ Avoid driving or operating machinery until after you've adjusted to the drug's effects.
☐ If you experience stomach upset, discuss the possibility of dividing your dosage into several smaller doses taken with milk throughout the day.
☐ Relieve dry mouth with sugarless gum, hard candy, or ice chips.
☐ Check with your doctor or pharmacist before taking any OTC medications.
☐ Store phenoxybenzamine at room temperature and protect it from moisture, direct light, and air.

Interventions

Preparation and administration
• Administer the drug with milk or food or in divided doses to reduce GI irritation. (See *Taking phenoxybenzamine at home.*)

Monitoring and supportive care
• During dosage adjustment, monitor pulse rate and rhythm; check blood pressure in recumbent and standing

positions. When the patient is stabilized, continue to monitor his heart rate and blood pressure periodically.
• Monitor respiratory status carefully; symptoms of pneumonia and asthma may be aggravated.
• If faintness or dizziness occurs, place the patient in Trendelenburg's position and notify the doctor of vital signs and clinical status.
• Know that propranolol is commonly used with phenoxybenzamine to block tachycardia associated with pheochromocytoma.
• Small initial doses are usually increased gradually until the desired effect is obtained. Observe the patient after each dosage increase for at least 4 days.
• Know that the optimal effect may require several weeks; monitor the patient closely for adverse reactions.
• Nasal congestion and impaired male sexual function usually subside during continued therapy.

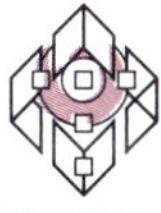 **MedTest**

---

1. Phenoxybenzamine is pharmacologically classified as:
    a. an alpha-adrenergic blocker.
    b. a beta-adrenergic blocker.
    c. a dopaminergic blocker.
    d. an ACE inhibitor.

2. Common adverse effects of phenoxybenzamine include:
    a. nausea and vomiting.
    b. flatulence and constipation.
    c. impotence and ejaculation inhibition.
    d. bradycardia and AV block.

3. If your patient experiences nasal stuffiness while taking phenoxybenzamine, you would:
    a. stop the drug immediately.
    b. tell the patient it will go away when his course of treatment is completed.
    c. have his dosage decreased.
    d. tell him it will probably subside as therapy continues.

Phentolamine mesylate

Also known by the brand names Regitine and (in Canada) Rogitine, phentolamine is an alpha-adrenergic blocker that's therapeutically classified as an antihypertensive agent for pheochromocytoma and as a cutaneous vasodilator. It's available for injection in concentrations of 5 mg/ml in 1-ml vials and (in Australia) in concentrations of 10 mg/ml in 1-ml vials.

Pharmacokinetics

• *Absorption:* Antihypertensive effect is immediate after I.V. administration.
• *Distribution:* Unknown.
• *Metabolism:* Unknown.
• *Excretion:* About 10% of a given dose is excreted unchanged in urine. Drug has a short duration of action; plasma half-life is 19 minutes.

Indications, dosage, and action
Aid for diagnosing pheochromocytoma
- *Adult dosage:* 5 mg I.V. or I.M.
- *Pediatric dosage:* 1 mg I.V., 3 mg I.M., or 0.1 mg/kg or 3 mg/m^2 I.V.
- *Action:* Competitively blocks effects of pheochromocytoma-produced catecholamines on alpha-adrenergic receptors.

Control or prevention of paroxysmal hypertension before or during pheochromocytomectomy
- *Adult dosage:* 5 mg I.M. or I.V. 1 to 2 hours preoperatively, repeated as necessary; 5 mg I.V. during surgery if indicated.
- *Pediatric dosage:* 1 mg, 0.1 mg/kg, or 3 mg/m^2 I.M. or I.V. 1 to 2 hours preoperatively, repeated as necessary; 1 mg, 0.1 mg/kg, or 3 mg/m^2 I.V. during surgery if indicated.
- *Antihypertensive action:* Blocks alpha-adrenergic receptors, causing arterial dilation and decreased peripheral resistance.

Prevention of dermal necrosis and sloughing or extravasation after I.V. norepinephrine
- *Adult and pediatric dosage:* Inject 5 to 10 mg in 10 ml of 0.9% NaCl solution into the affected area, or add 10 mg to each liter of I.V. fluids containing norepinephrine.
- *Action:* Blocks catecholamine-induced vasoconstriction.

Contraindications and cautions
- Don't use in patients with CAD or recent MI because the drug may exacerbate these conditions.
- Use cautiously in patients with gastritis or peptic ulcer.
- Drug should be discontinued if severe hypotension develops.
- Use with caution in patients receiving other antihypertensives.
- Administer cautiously to elderly patients.
- Administer cautiously to children under age 18.
- Be aware that it's not known if phentolamine is distributed in breast milk. Use cautiously in breast-feeding women.
- Pregnancy risk category C

Life-threatening adverse reactions
- Shock

Common adverse reactions
- Hypotension, arrhythmias, palpitations, tachycardia
- Dizziness, weakness, flushing
- Nausea, vomiting, diarrhea
- Nasal stuffiness

Infrequent adverse reactions
- Angina pectoris
- Lethargy
- Abdominal pain, hyperperistalsis
- Hypoglycemia

Interactions
- *Epinephrine*: Alpha-adrenergic blockade provided by phentolamine results in unopposed beta-adrenergic stimulation by epinephrine. The result is "epinephrine reversal" — hypotension and tachycardia.

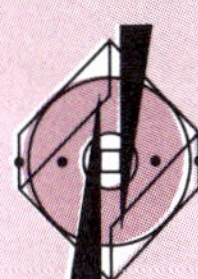

Administration guidelines

Using phentolamine to detect pheochromocytoma

If your patient is scheduled for a phentolamine test to aid in the diagnosis of pheochromocytoma, observe the following guidelines.

Preparing for the test
• When possible, withdraw sedatives, analgesics, and all other medications at least 24 hours (preferably 48 to 72 hours) before the test.
• Have the patient rest in a supine position until his blood pressure is stabilized.

Monitoring during the test
• When you're giving phentolamine I.V., inject the dose rapidly. A marked decrease in blood pressure will be seen immediately; the maximum effect will occur within 2 minutes.
• Record blood pressure immediately after I.V. injection, at 30-second intervals for the first 3 minutes, and at 1-minute intervals for the next 7 minutes.
• When you're giving phentolamine I.M., the maximum effect occurs within 20 minutes. Record blood pressure q 5 minutes for 30 to 45 minutes after injection.

Interpreting test results
• The test result is positive when the patient's systolic blood pressure drops at least 35 mm Hg and diastolic, at least 25 mm Hg.
• The test result is negative when the patient's blood pressure remains unchanged, increases, or decreases less than amounts given above.

Interventions

Preparation and administration
• If the patient is scheduled for the phentolamine test to detect pheochromocytoma, antihypertensive drugs should be withdrawn. The test is performed after blood pressure returns to pretreatment levels. At least 4 weeks before the test, rauwolfia alkaloids should be withdrawn. (See *Using phentolamine to detect pheochromocytoma.*)

Monitoring and supportive care
• Know that usual doses of phentolamine have little effect on the blood pressure of normal individuals or patients with essential hypertension.
• Tell the patient to report adverse reactions at once.
• Advise patients not to take sedatives or narcotics for at least 24 hours before a phentolamine test.
• Know that phentolamine has been used alone or with papaverine as an adjunctive treatment for males with impotence (neurogenic or vascular). Patients are taught to self-administer this drug by intercavernosal injection.

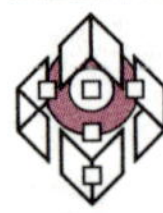 **MedTest**

1. Phentolamine is classified pharmacologically as:
   a. a dopaminergic blocking agent.
   b. a beta$_1$- and beta$_2$-blocking agent.
   c. a cardioselective beta$_1$-blocking agent.
   d. an alpha-adrenergic blocking agent.

2. The plasma half-life of phentolamine after I.V. injection is:
   a. 5 to 10 minutes.
   b. 19 minutes.
   c. 1 to 2 hours.
   d. 6 hours or more.

3. To prevent extravasation or sloughing from I.V. norepinephrine, phentolamine may be:
   a. administered I.M. before norepinephrine is started.
   b. infiltrated into the tissues surrounding the site when the I.V. catheter is inserted.
   c. added to the norepinephrine infusion (10 mg/liter).
   d. put through the I.V. catheter if extravasation is suspected.

Phenylephrine hydrochloride

Also known by the brand name Neo-Synephrine, phenylephrine is an adrenergic that's classified therapeutically as a vasoconstrictor. It's available for injection in 10-mg/ml vials.

Pharmacokinetics
- *Absorption:* Pressor effects occur almost immediately after I.V. injection and persist 15 to 20 minutes; after I.M. injection, onset occurs within 10 to 15 minutes and effects persist for 30 minutes to 2 hours; after S.C. injection, onset occurs within 10 to 15 minutes and effects persist for 50 to 60 minutes.
- *Distribution:* Unknown.
- *Metabolism:* Metabolized in liver and intestine by enzyme MAO to inactive metabolites, found in urine.
- *Excretion:* Unknown.

Indications, dosage, and action
Hypotensive emergencies during spinal anesthesia
- *Adult dosage:* 0.1 to 0.2 mg I.V. initially; subsequent doses should also be low (0.1 mg).
- *Pediatric dosage:* 44 to 88 mcg/kg I.M. or S.C.

Prevention of hypotension during anesthesia
- *Adult dosage:* 2 to 3 mg S.C. or I.M. given 3 or 4 minutes before anesthesia.

Mild to moderate hypotension
- *Adult dosage:* 1 to 5 mg S.C. or I.M. (initial dose should not exceed 5 mg). Additional doses may be given in 1 to 2 hours if needed. Or 0.1 to 0.5 mg by slow I.V. injection (initial dose should not exceed 0.5 mg). Additional doses may be given q 10 to 15 minutes.
- *Pediatric dosage:* 0.1 mg/kg or 3 mg/m^2 I.M. or S.C.

PSVT
• *Adult dosage:* Initially, 0.5 mg by rapid I.V.; subsequent doses may be increased in increments of 0.1 to 0.2 mg. Maximum dose shouldn't exceed 1 mg.

Adjunctive treatment of severe hypotension or shock
• *Adult dosage:* 0.1 to 0.18 mg/minute by I.V. infusion. After blood pressure stabilizes, maintain infusion at 0.04 to 0.06 mg/minute, adjusted to patient response.
• *Vasopressor action:* Stimulates alpha-adrenergic receptors to constrict resistance and capacitance blood vessels. This results in increased total peripheral resistance, increased systolic and diastolic blood pressure, and decreased blood flow to vital organs, skin, and skeletal muscle.

Phenylephrine may also act indirectly by releasing norepinephrine from its storage sites. Phenylephrine doesn't stimulate $beta_1$-receptors except in large doses. Tachyphylaxis (tolerance) may follow repeated injections.

Contraindications and cautions
• Don't use in severe CAD, CV disease (including MI), or peripheral or mesenteric vascular thrombosis because drug may increase ischemia or extend the area of infarction.
• Avoid use in severe hypertension or VT.
• Don't use with local anesthetics on fingers, toes, ears, nose, or genitalia.
• Use with extreme caution in hyperthyroidism, bradycardia, partial AV block, myocardial disease, diabetes mellitus, angle-closure glaucoma, severe arteriosclerosis, acute pancreatitis, or hepatitis (drug may worsen ischemia in liver or pancreas).
• Administer cautiously to patients with known hypersensitivity to sulfites because phenylephrine contains sulfite preservatives.
• Discontinue the drug if hypersensitivity or cardiac arrhythmias occur.
• Administer with extreme caution to elderly or debilitated patients. Effects may be exaggerated.
• Be aware that phenylephrine may cause contraction of the pregnant uterus and constriction of uterine blood vessels.
• Know that infants and children may be more susceptible than adults to the drug's effects.
• Because it's not known if phenylephrine is distributed in breast milk, use with caution in breast-feeding women.
• Pregnancy risk category C

Life-threatening adverse reactions
• Arrhythmias, severe hypertension

Common adverse reactions
• Restlessness, light-headedness, weakness, headache

Infrequent adverse reactions
• Precordial pain or discomfort, peripheral and visceral vasoconstriction, reflex bradycardia, tachycardia, decreased cardiac output, hypertension, palpitations, angina
• Respiratory distress
• Insomnia, excitability, anxiety, nervousness, dizziness, tremor, paresthe-

sia in extremities and coolness in skin (after injection)
- Vomiting
- Local tissue sloughing with extravasation, blanching of skin
- Tolerance with prolonged use

Interactions
- *Alpha-adrenergic blockers, antihypertensives, diuretics, guanadrel, guanethidine, nitrates, rauwolfia alkaloids:* Decreased pressor response or arrhythmias may result when phenylephrine is used with these agents.
- *Doxapram, ergot alkaloids, mazindol, mecamylamine, methyldopa, trimethaphan:* Increased pressor response. Observe the patient and monitor his blood pressure closely.
- *Nitrates:* Concomitant use may reduce antianginal effects.
- *Thyroid hormones:* Use of phenylephrine with thyroid hormones may increase the effects of either drug.

   For dangerous interactions, see *Life-threatening hazards of multidrug therapy with phenylephrine.*

Interventions
Preparation and administration
- Use a central venous catheter or a large vein, such as one located in the antecubital fossa, to minimize the risk of extravasation. The preferred dilution is to add 10 mg of the drug to 500 ml of D_5W or 0.9% NaCl solution. Begin the infusion at 100 to 180 mcg/minute. When blood pressure is stabilized at the desired level, reduce the flow rate to a maintenance level of 40 to 60 mcg/minute.

- Use an infusion pump to regulate the infusion flow rate.

◆ **Safety tip.** To treat local ischemia due to extravasation, infiltrate the site promptly and liberally with 10 to 15 ml of 0.9% NaCl solution containing 5 to 10 mg of phentolamine through a fine needle. Topical nitroglycerin has also been used.
- Prolonged exposure to air or strong light may cause oxidation and discoloration. Don't use the solution if it is brown or contains a precipitate.

Monitoring and supportive care
- During I.V. administration, monitor pulse rate, blood ressure, and CVP q 2 to 5 minutes.
- Control the flow rate and dosage to prevent excessive blood pressure increases. I.V. overdoses can induce ventricular arrhythmias.
- Avoid an excessive rise in blood pressure. Maintain blood pressure at slightly below the patient's normal level. In previously normotensive patients, maintain systolic blood pressure at 80 to 100 mm Hg; in previously hypertensive patients, maintain systolic blood pressure at 30 to 40 mm Hg below their usual levels; or follow prescribed guidelines for the specific patient.
- Correct hypovolemic states before administering the drug. Don't use phenylephrine in place of fluid, blood, plasma, or electrolyte replacement.
- Know that this drug is longer-acting than ephedrine and epinephrine. It causes little or no CNS stimulation.
- With prolonged I.V. infusions, avoid abrupt withdrawal. During infusion,

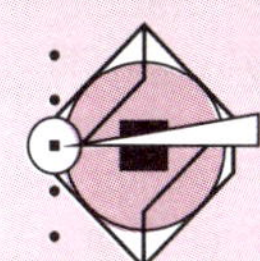

Interactions alert

Life-threatening hazards of multidrug therapy with phenylephrine

Interacting drug	Effects
Digitalis glycosides (such as digoxin)	Increase risk of life-threatening arrhythmias
Ergonovine maleate, parenteral (ergot alkaloid)	Increases risk of severe hypertension
General anesthetics (such as cycloprorane or halothane)	Increase risk of life-threatening arrhythmias
Levodopa (antiparkinsonian agent)	Increases risk of life-threatening arrhythmias
MAO inhibitors (such as isocarboxazid)	Increase risk of life-threatening arrhythmias and hypertensive crisis
Oxytocic agents (such as oxytocin)	Increase risk of severe, prolonged hypertension
Sympathomimetics (such as epinephrine)	Increase risk of life-threatening arrhythmias
Tricyclic antidepressants (such as amitryptyline)	Increase risk of life-threatening arrhythmias and increased pressor response

frequently monitor ECG, blood pressure, cardiac output, CVP, PAWP, pulse rate, urine output, and color and temperature of extremities. Titrate the infusion rate according to findings and the doctor's guidelines.

• Know that phenylephrine is chemically incompatible with oxidizing agents.

• Be aware that phenylephrine is also used to prolong spinal anesthesia and for vasoconstriction in regional anesthesia.

• Know that phenylephrine (ophthalmic) is used to provide mydriasis without cycloplegia, to treat adhesions of the iris, as initial therapy for malignant glaucoma, and to treat conjunctival congestion.

• Be aware that phenylephrine (nasal) is used to relieve nasal, sinus, and eustachian tube congestion.

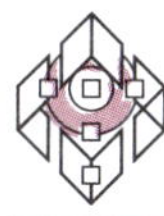

MedTest

1. When administering phenylephrine I.V., you should monitor the patient's blood pressure, pulse rate, and CVP:

   a. q 2 to 5 minutes.

b. q 2 minutes for 15 minutes and then q 5 minutes until infusion is discontinued.
c. q 5 minutes for 1 hour, then q 15 minutes throughout the infusion.
d. q 15 minutes × 4, then q 30 minutes × 4, then q 1 hour × 4, then q 4 hours.

2. In a previously normotensive patient receiving phenylephrine, you'd aim to maintain systolic blood pressure at:
    a. 80 to 100 mm Hg.
    b. 30 to 40 points below normal for this patient.
    c. the patient's normal level.
    d. 10 to 20 mm Hg above normal for this patient.

3. When discontinuing a phenylephrine infusion, you should:
    a. shut off the infusion; the drug weans itself.
    b. increase the flow rate as prescribed for 10 minutes and then discontinue.
    c. administer a prescribed I.M. bolus to sustain the patient after the infusion is discontinued.
    d. withdraw the drug gradually, monitoring blood pressure and patient response.

Phenytoin

Also known by the brand names Dilantin and Di-Phen, phenytoin is a hydantoin derivative. It's classified therapeutically as an anticonvulsant but at times is used to treat ventricular arrhythmias. The drug is available in 50-mg chewable tablets; as an oral suspension in concentrations of 30 mg/5 ml and 125 mg/5 ml; in 30- and 100-mg extended-release capsules; in 30- and 100-mg prompt-release capsules; and for injection in 50-mg/ml vials.

Pharmacokinetics

• *Absorption:* Absorbed slowly from the small intestine. Extended-release capsules yield peak serum concentrations at 4 to 12 hours; prompt-release products peak at 1½ to 3 hours. I.M. doses are absorbed erratically; 50% to 75% of I.M. dose is absorbed in 24 hours.
• *Distribution:* Widespread through the body. Drug is about 90% protein-bound (less so in malnourished and uremic patients).
• *Metabolism:* By the liver to inactive metabolites.
• *Excretion:* Inactive metabolites excreted in urine.

Indications, dosage, and action

Ventricular arrhythmias unresponsive to lidocaine or procainamide, or induced by digitalis glycosides
• *Adult dosage:* Loading dose is 1 g P.O. divided over first 24 hours, followed by 500 mg daily for 2 days, and then maintenance dosage of 200 to 400 mg P.O. daily; I.V. dose is 10 to 15 mg/kg over 1 hour, followed by maintenance dosage of 400 to 600 mg/day. Infusion rate shouldn't exceed 25 mg/minute.

Alternate method is to give 100 mg I.V. q 15 minutes until adverse effects develop, arrhythmias are controlled, or 1 g has been given.

Also may administer entire loading dose of 1 g I.V. slowly at 25 mg/minute. I.M. administration isn't recommended because of pain and erratic absorption.

• *Pediatric dosage:* 2 to 4 mg/kg P.O. or slow I.V. daily, or 250 mg/m^2 daily given as single dose or divided in two doses.

• *Antiarrhythmic action:* Normalizes sodium influx to Purkinje's fibers in patients with digitalis glycoside–induced arrhythmias.

Contraindications and cautions

• Avoid use in hypersensitivity to hydantoins or phenacemide.

• Don't use I.V. phenytoin in patients with sinus bradycardia, SA or AV block, or Stokes-Adams syndrome.

• Use cautiously in acute intermittent porphyria and hepatic or renal dysfunction. This is especially true for malnourished or uremic patients, who have higher serum drug levels (free or unbound drug) because of decreased protein binding.

• Use with caution in myocardial insufficiency or respiratory depression.

• Use with caution in elderly or debilitated patients, who may require lower doses.

• Use cautiously in patients taking other hydantoin derivatives.

• Discontinue the drug if signs of hypersensitivity, hepatotoxicity, or blood dyscrasias occur, or if lymphadenopathy occurs.

• Know that a special pediatric-strength suspension is available (30 mg/5 ml). Take extreme care to use correct strength. Don't confuse with adult strength (125 mg/5 ml).

• Because phenytoin is excreted in breast milk, recommend an alternative feeding method during therapy.
• Pregnancy risk category D

Life-threatening adverse reactions

• CV collapse
• Toxic hepatitis
• Thrombocytopenia, leukopenia, agranulocytosis, pancytopenia
• Stevens-Johnson syndrome, toxic epidermal necrolysis

Common adverse reactions

• Ataxia, slurred speech, confusion
• Nausea, vomiting, gingival hyperplasia (especially in children)
• Nystagmus, diplopia
• Hirsutism

Infrequent adverse reactions

• Hypotension
• Dizziness, insomnia, nervousness, twitching, headache
• Jaundice
• Blurred vision
• Hyperglycemia
• Scarlatiniform or morbilliform rash; bullous or purpuric dermatitis; lupus erythematosus; photosensitivity; purple glove syndrome; local pain, necrosis, and inflammation at injection site; hypertrichosis; exfoliative dermatitis
• Periarteritis nodosa, lymphadenopathy, osteomalacia

Interactions

• *Allopurinol, amiodarone, antihistamines, chloramphenicol, chlorpheniramine, cimetidine, cycloserine,*

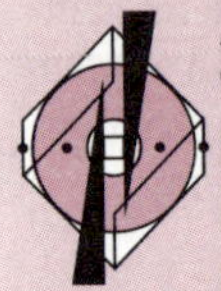

Administration guidelines

Preparing and infusing I.V. phenytoin

Phenytoin sodium is a highly insoluble drug. It's prepared in a special vehicle containing propylene glycol and alcohol, and the pH is adjusted to about 12. The manufacturer states that phenytoin shouldn't be added to any other drugs or I.V. solutions.

Unfortunately, this means that the drug should only be given by I.V. push, which is inconvenient and associated with CV adverse reactions if it's injected too fast. To avoid these problems, investigators have studied the solubility of phenytoin in I.V. solutions. They have concluded that phenytoin infusions can be safely prepared if the following guidelines are followed:

• Always use an in-line filter.

• Prepare solutions immediately before use.

• Infuse the drug within 1 hour.

• Use 0.9% NaCl injection or lactated Ringer's injection as a diluent and to flush existing line.

• Keep the phenytoin concentration at 100 mg/25 or 50 ml, and never prepare a solution with a concentration of less than 100 mg/dl

Because of the potential for phenytoin precipitation, always consult a pharmacist before mixing phenytoin with any other drugs or I.V. solutions.

diazepam, disulfiram, ethanol (acute), ibuprofen, imipramine, influenza vaccine, isoniazid, miconazole, oral anticoagulants, phenyl- *butazone, salicylates, sulfamethoxazole, trimethoprim, valproate:* Monitor for increased phenytoin activity and toxicity.

• *Antacids, antineoplastics, barbiturates, calcium, calcium gluconate, carbamazepine, charcoal, dexamethasone, diazoxide, ethanol (chronic), folic acid, loxapine, nitrofurantoin, pyridoxine, theophylline:* Monitor for decreased phenytoin activity.

• *Corticosteroids, cyclosporine, dicumarol, digitoxin, disopyramide, dopamine, doxycycline, estrogens, furosemide, haloperidol, levodopa, meperidine, methadone, metyrapone, oral contraceptives, quinidine, sulfonylureas:* Phenytoin may decrease the effects of these drugs by stimulating hepatic metabolism.

• *Oral tube feedings with Isocal or Osmolite:* May interfere with absorption of oral phenytoin. Schedule feedings as far as possible from drug administration.

Interventions

Preparation and administration

• Use only clear solution for injection. A slight yellow color is acceptable. Never use cloudy solution. (See *Preparing and infusing I.V. phenytoin.*)

 Safety tip. Check the patency of the I.V. catheter before administering. Extravasation can cause severe local tissue damage.

• Know that only extended-release capsules are approved for once-daily administration; all other forms are given in divided doses q 8 to 12 hours.

• Administer oral forms with food or milk to minimize GI distress.

• Oral or nasogastric feedings may interfere with absorption of oral suspension. Separate doses from feedings as much as possible.

• During continuous tube feeding, flush the tube thoroughly with water before and after a dose. When administering the drug via the feeding tube, use the injectable form of the drug instead of the oral suspension to enhance absorption.

Monitoring and supportive care
• When giving I.V., monitor ECG, blood pressure, and respiratory status.

• Monitor serum phenytoin levels. Therapeutic levels range from 10 to 20 mcg/ml, but signs of toxicity can occur at levels as low as 5 to 10 mcg/ml. Lateral nystagmus may occur at levels above 20 mcg/ml; ataxia usually occurs at levels above 30 mcg/ml; significantly decreased mental capacity occurs at 40 mcg/ml.

• Monitor CBC and serum calcium levels q 6 months, and periodically monitor hepatic function. The doctor may prescribe folic acid and vitamin B_{12} supplements if megaloblastic anemia is evident.

• If a rash appears, notify the doctor, who may discontinue the drug. If the rash is scarlet or resembles measles, you may resume the drug after the rash clears. If the rash reappears, discontinue therapy. If the rash is exfoliative, purpuric, or bullous, don't resume the drug.

• Phenytoin may color urine pink, red, or reddish brown.

• Tell the patient to use the same brand of phenytoin consistently.

Changing brands may change the therapeutic effect.

• Tell the patient to take phenytoin with food or milk to minimize GI distress.

• Warn the patient not to discontinue the drug, except with medical supervision. Also advise him to avoid hazardous activities that require alertness until the drug's CNS effects have been determined and to avoid drinking alcoholic beverages, which can decrease the drug's effectiveness and increase its adverse effects.

• Encourage good oral hygiene to minimize gingival hyperplasia and gum sensitivity.

• Know that phenytoin may raise blood glucose levels by inhibiting pancreatic insulin release, lower serum levels of protein-bound iodine and free thyroxine without producing signs of hypothyroidism, cause a slight decline in urine 17-hydroxysteroid and 17-ketosteroid levels, increase urine 6-β hydroxycortisol excretion and serum levels of ALP or γ-glutamyltransferase, and decrease values for the 1-mg dexamethasone suppression or metyrapone test.

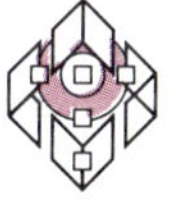 **MedTest**

1. Your patient is receiving a peripheral I.V. infusion of D_5W. In order to administer I.V. phenytoin, you should:
   a. start another line.
   b. arrange for insertion of a central line.
   c. first clear the line with 0.9% NaCl solution.

d. mix the phenytoin in a separate 50-ml minibag of D_5W and infuse it over 20 to 30 minutes.

2. Warn the patient that this drug may:
    a. cause headaches until he adjusts to it.
    b. make his mouth dry.
    c. result in constipation.
    d. turn his urine, pink, red, or reddish brown.

3. Phenytoin's CV use is to treat:
    a. ventricular arrhythmias unresponsive to lidocaine or procainamide.
    b. arrhythmias induced by beta blockers.
    c. supraventricular arrhythmias.
    d. heart block and Stokes-Adams syndrome.

Pravastatin sodium

Also known by the brand name Pravachol, pravastatin is a 3-hydroxy-3-methylglutaryl-coenzyme A (HMG-CoA)-reductase inhibitor that's classified therapeutically as an antilipemic agent. It's available in 10- and 20-mg tablets.

Pharmacokinetics

• *Absorption:* Rapidly absorbed, with peak plasma levels in 1 to 1½ hours. Average oral absorption is 34%, with absolute bioavailability of 17% because of first-pass metabolism. Although food reduces bioavailability, drug effects are the same if drug is taken with meals or 1 hour p.c.

• *Distribution:* Plasma levels are proportional to dose but don't necessarily correlate perfectly with lipid-lowering effects. About 50% is bound to plasma proteins.
• *Metabolism:* Metabolized by the liver; at least six metabolites have been identified. Some are active.
• *Excretion:* Drug and metabolites are excreted by the liver and kidneys.

Indications, dosage, and action
Reduction of LDL and total cholesterol in primary hypercholesterolemia (types IIa and IIb)
• *Adult dosage:* Initially, 5 to 10 mg daily h.s. Adjust dosage q 4 weeks based on patient tolerance and response; maximum daily dosage is 40 mg. Most elderly patients respond to a daily dosage of 20 mg or less.
• *Action:* Inhibits the enzyme HMG-CoA reductase. This hepatic enzyme is an early (and rate-limiting) step in the synthetic pathway of cholesterol.

Contraindications and cautions
• Don't use in patients with active liver disease or conditions associated with unexplained persistent elevations of serum transaminase levels.
• Know that liver function tests should be performed frequently at the start of therapy and periodically thereafter.
• Use with caution in patients with a history of liver disease or of heavy alcohol ingestion.
• Advise women not to breast-feed while taking pravastatin because it's excreted in breast milk.
• Don't administer to pregnant women or women of childbearing age unless there is no risk of pregnancy.

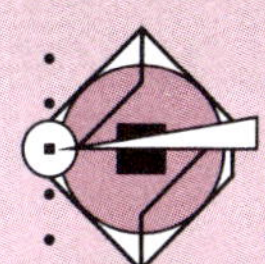

Interactions alert

Life-threatening hazards of multidrug therapy with pravastatin

Interacting drug	Effects
Erythromycin (antibiotic)	Increases risk of rhabdomyolysis
Fibric acid derivatives (such as clofibrate)	Increase risk of rhabdomyolysis
Immunosuppressive agents (such as cyclosporine)	Increase risk of rhabdomyolysis
Niacin in high doses	Increases risk of rhabdomyolysis

- Pregnancy risk category X

Life-threatening adverse reactions
- Hepatitis
- Rhabdomyolysis

Common adverse reactions
None noted with standard dosages

Infrequent adverse reactions
- Chest pain
- Cough
- Headache, fatigue, dizziness
- Nausea, vomiting, diarrhea, heartburn, liver dysfunction, elevated serum transaminase levels
- Rhinitis
- Rash
- Common cold, influenza, localized muscle pain, myalgia

Interactions
- *Cholestyramine, colestipol:* Concomitant administration decreases absorption of pravastatin. Administer pravastatin 1 hour before or 4 hours after these drugs.
- *Chronic alcohol abuse, hepatotoxic drugs:* Increased risk of hepatotoxicity. Avoid concomitant use.
- *Gemfibrozil:* Decreases protein-binding and urinary clearance of pravastatin. Avoid concomitant use.

For dangerous interactions, see *Life-threatening hazards of multidrug therapy with pravastatin.*

Interventions
Preparation and administration
- Administer the recommended dose in the evening, preferably at bedtime. The drug may be given without regard to meals. (See *Taking pravastatin at home,* page 264.)

Monitoring and supportive care
- Expect liver function tests to be performed frequently at the start of therapy and periodically thereafter.

Safety tip. Clinical evidence of liver dysfunction may occur in up to 1.3% of patients. If this hap-

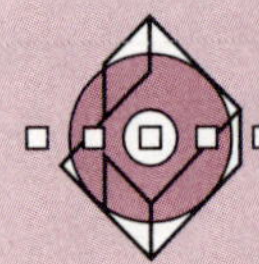

Patient-teaching checklist

Taking pravastatin at home

In addition to explaining the drug's action and dosage, teach the patient who will continue pravastatin therapy after discharge to follow these important guidelines.

Take your medication correctly
☐ Take pravastatin in the evening, preferably at bedtime.
☐ Take pravastatin as prescribed even when you're feeling well.
☐ Continue taking the drug even if unpleasant adverse reactions occur. When you stop taking it, your blood lipid levels may increase again. Make sure you discuss any adverse reactions, especially muscle aches and pains, with your doctor.

Modify your lifestyle
☐ Restrict alcohol intake because of the drug's possible effect on the liver.
☐ Take steps to correct any cardiac risk factors that you may have, such as obesity (lose weight), smoking (engage in a smoking cessation program), and sedentary lifestyle (start an exercise program). These risk factors, if not corrected, may make the drug less effective.
☐ Adhere to a low-fat, low-cholesterol diet because pravastatin is most effective when used in conjunction with dietary restrictions.

Other instructions
☐ Adhere to scheduled testing for serum cholesterol, HDL and LDL (lipid) levels, and triglyceride levels to monitor the effectiveness of the drug regimen.

pens, the doctor will discontinue the drug. Monitor this patient closely. A liver biopsy may be performed if enzyme levels remain elevated.

• Watch for signs of myositis. Some cases of myopathy and markedly elevated CK levels (which may lead to rhabdomyolysis and renal failure secondary to myoglobinuria) have been reported.

• The drug should be temporarily discontinued in any patient with an acute condition that suggests a developing myopathy or in patients having risk factors that may predispose them to rhabdomyolysis (including severe acute infection; severe endocrine, metabolic, or electrolyte disorders; hypotension; major surgery; or uncontrolled seizures).

• Pravastatin therapy should be initiated only after dietary and other non-pharmacologic therapies have proved ineffective.

• Tell patients to continue a low-cholesterol diet during therapy.

• Make dosage adjustments q 4 weeks. If cholesterol levels fall below the target range, reduce the dosage.

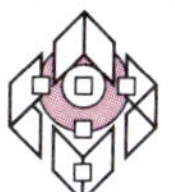 **MedTest**

1. Pravastatin is therapeutically classified as:
   a. a vasodilator.
   b. an antiarrhythmic.
   c. an antilipemic.
   d. a thrombolytic.

2. The patient should take pravastatin:
   a. first thing in the morning.
   b. with the midday meal.
   c. with the largest meal.
   d. in the evening, preferably h.s.

3. Advise the patient receiving pravastatin to restrict his intake of:
   a. caffeine-containing beverages and foods.
   b. salt and high-sodium foods.
   c. dairy products.
   d. alcoholic beverages.

Prazosin hydrochloride

Also known by the brand name Minipress, prazosin is an alpha-adrenergic blocker that's classified therapeutically as an antihypertensive agent. It's available in 1-, 2-, and 5-mg capsules. (See *Prazosin alternatives: Doxazosin and terazosin,* page 266.)

Pharmacokinetics

• *Absorption:* Variable from the GI tract. Antihypertensive effect begins in about 2 hours, peaking within 4 hours.

• *Distribution:* Distributed throughout body and highly protein-bound (approximately 97%).

• *Metabolism:* Metabolized extensively in the liver to active metabolites.

• *Excretion:* Over 90% of given dose excreted in feces via bile; remainder excreted in urine. Plasma half-life is 2 to 4 hours.

Indications, dosage, and action
Mild to moderate hypertension; reducing afterload in chronic CHF

• *Adult dosage:* Initial dose is 1 mg P.O. h.s. to prevent first-dose syncope. Then increase dosage to 1 mg P.O. b.i.d. or t.i.d. Gradually titrate dosage according to patient's response. Maximum daily dosage is 20 mg. All dosage increases are also initiated first as a bedtime dose. Usual maintenance dosage is 6 to 15 mg daily in divided doses. A few patients have required dosages larger than this (up to 40 mg daily). If other antihypertensive or diuretic agents are added to prazosin therapy, reduce dosage of prazosin to 1 or 2 mg t.i.d., and then gradually increase as necessary.

• *Antihypertensive action:* Selectively and competitively inhibits alpha-adrenergic receptors, reducing peripheral vascular resistance and blood pressure. Antihypertensive effect lasts less than 24 hours. Peak effects are seen after 4 to 6 weeks of continuous therapy.

Contraindications and cautions

• Use cautiously in patients taking other antihypertensive drugs.

Prazosin alternatives: Doxazosin and terazosin

Like prazosin, doxazosin mesylate and terazosin hydrochloride are selective competitive inhibitors of alpha$_1$-adrenergic postsynaptic receptors. They relax the smooth muscle in both arteries and veins and reduce peripheral vascular resistance and blood pressure.

Compared to these two drugs, prazosin has a short plasma half-life of 2 to 4 hours and must be taken two or three times a day for optimal effect. Doxazosin, on the other hand, has a half-life of about 11 hours; terazosin, a half-life of about 12 hours. They can be taken once a day and may increase compliance in some patients.

In some hypertensive patients, alpha$_1$-adrenergic blockers may be the preferred first-line drugs. Unlike beta-adrenergic blockers, these drugs can be safely used in patients with bronchospastic disease, heart block, or impaired renal function. And unlike thiazides, these drugs don't cause electrolyte imbalances or elevate triglyceride or cholesterol levels. Terazosin has recently been approved to enhance urine flow in men with benign prostatic hyperplasia; hypertensive males with this disorder may obtain added benefit from terazosin therapy.

Doxazosin mesylate

Known by the brand name Cardura, doxazosin is available in 1-, 2-, 4-, and 8-mg tablets. The usual initial adult dosage is 1 mg P.O daily. The effect on standing and supine blood pressure is determined 2 to 6 hours and then 24 hours after dosing. If necessary, the dosage is then increased to 2 mg daily. To minimize adverse reactions, titrate dosage slowly (usually, increase dosage only q 2 weeks). Daily dosage may be increased to 4 mg and then 8 mg if necessary. Maximum daily dosage is 16 mg, but dosage exceeding 4 mg is associated with a greater incidence of adverse reactions.

Terazosin hydrochloride

Known by the brand name Hytrin, terazosin is available in 1-, 2-, 5-, and 10-mg tablets. The usual adult dosage initially is 1 mg P.O. h.s. Adjust dosage and schedule according to patient response. The recommended range is 1 to 5 mg daily or divided b.i.d. If therapy is discontinued for several days or longer, reinstitute the initial dosage regimen of 1 mg h.s. Slowly increase dosage until desired blood pressure is attained. Doses over 20 mg don't appear to affect blood pressure further.

Possible disadvantages

One potential disadvantage of alpha$_1$-adrenergic blockers is that patients commonly experience orthostatic hypotension and syncope at the start of therapy. This "first-dose" phenomenon can be reduced by starting therapy with a low dosage. To prevent possible injury, teach your patients to take their first dose h.s., and remind them to rise slowly when getting out of bed.

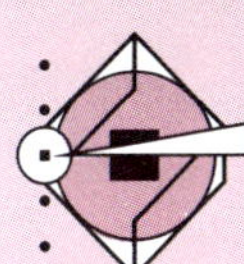

Life-threatening hazards of multidrug therapy with prazosin

Interacting drug	Effects
Antihypertensive agents (such as amlodipine and hydralazine)	May cause severe hypotension
Beta blockers (such as propranolol)	May cause severe hypotension

- Use with caution in chronic renal failure.
- Know that elderly patients may require lower doses.
- Because small amounts of prazosin are excreted in breast milk, recommend an alternative feeding method to breast-feeding mothers.
- Pregnancy risk category C

Life-threatening adverse reactions

- Syncope, which increases the risk of accidental falls and head injury

Common adverse reactions

- Palpitations
- Dizziness, headache, drowsiness, lack of energy, weakness

Infrequent adverse reactions

- Orthostatic hypotension, edema
- First-dose syncope, depression
- Nausea, vomiting, diarrhea, abdominal cramps, constipation
- Priapism, impotence, urinary frequency
- Blurred vision, dry mouth

Interactions

- *Highly protein-bound drugs:* Because prazosin is highly bound to plasma proteins, it may interact with other highly protein-bound drugs.

  For dangerous interactions, see *Life-threatening hazards of multidrug therapy with prazosin.*

Interventions

Preparation and administration

- Administer initial dose and any dose increases h.s. (See *Taking prazosin at home,* page 268.)

Monitoring and supportive care

- Monitor the patient's blood pressure and pulse rate frequently.
- First-dose phenomenon (dizziness, light-headedness, and syncope) may occur within 30 minutes to 1 hour after the initial dose. It may be severe, resulting in loss of consciousness, if the initial dose is greater than 2 mg. The effect is transient and may be diminished by giving the drug h.s.; it is more common during febrile illness and more severe if the patient is hyponatremic.

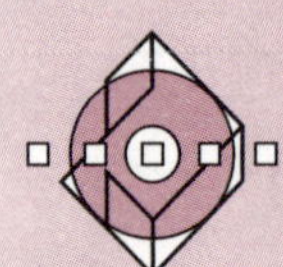

Patient-teaching checklist

Taking prazosin at home

In addition to explaining the drug's action and dosage, teach the patient who will continue prazosin therapy after discharge to follow these important guidelines.

Take your medication correctly
☐ Prazosin may be taken with or without food.
☐ Take the first dose and any dosage increases at bedtime because the drug may make you dizzy. Dizziness will be less noticeable if you are sleeping.
☐ Take prazosin as prescribed even when you're feeling well.
☐ Take your blood pressure or have it checked at a nearby blood pressure station frequently (at least once a week), if so advised. Report any significant changes to your doctor.

Watch for adverse reactions
☐ Continue taking this drug even if adverse reactions occur because abrupt discontinuation may cause your blood pressure to become abnormally elevated. However, make sure you discuss any adverse reactions with your doctor.

☐ Remember to change positions slowly, especially from lying flat to sitting upright. Dangle your legs over the bedside for a few minutes before standing. This will minimize the lightheadedness or dizziness that can result from taking this drug.
☐ Lie down immediately if dizziness or faintness occurs.
☐ To reduce the risk of prazosin-induced dizziness, light-headedness, or fainting, restrict your intake of alcoholic beverages and avoid prolonged standing, excessive exercise, and exposure to hot weather.

Other instructions
☐ Avoid driving or operating machinery until after you've adjusted to the drug's effects.
☐ To relieve dry mouth, use sugarless chewing gum, hard candy, or ice chips.
☐ Check with your doctor or pharmacist before taking OTC medications.

Safety tip. Always increase the dosage gradually, beginning with the bedtime dose, and have the patient sit or lie down if he experiences dizziness.
• Know that prazosin's effect is most pronounced on diastolic blood pressure.

• Prazosin also has been used with diuretics and digitalis glycosides to treat severe CHF, to manage the signs and symptoms of pheochromocytoma preoperatively, and to treat ergotamine-induced peripheral ischemia.

• Prazosin alters the results of screening tests for pheochromocytoma and causes increases in levels of the urinary metabolite of norepinephrine and vanillylmandelic acid; it may cause a positive antinuclear antibody titer and liver function test abnormalities. A transient fall in leukocyte count and increased serum uric acid and BUN levels may also occur.

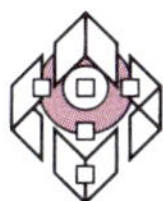 **MedTest**

1. Prazosin is excreted primarily in:
   a. urine.
   b. feces.
   c. bile.
   d. respiratory moisture and sweat.

2. A common adverse effect of prazosin is:
   a. dizziness.
   b. nausea.
   c. edema.
   d. depression.

3. Prazosin should be administered:
   a. with food.
   b. without regard to food.
   c. on arising.
   d. h.s.

Probucol

Also known by the brand names Lorelco and (in Australia) Lurselle, probucol is a bis-phenol derivative that's classified therapeutically as a cholesterol-lowering agent. It's available in 250- and 500-mg tablets.

Pharmacokinetics
• *Absorption:* GI absorption limited (2% to 8%) and variable. When taken with food, probucol produces higher blood levels and is less variable. Blood levels increase during first 3 to 4 months and then remain constant; clinical response usually occurs in 1 to 3 months.
• *Distribution:* Lipid-soluble and accumulates slowly in adipose tissue.
• *Metabolism:* Unknown.
• *Excretion:* Eliminated via bile in feces; half-life ranges from 24 hours to over 500 hours because drug slowly leaches out of adipose tissue. Probucol is still detected in blood 6 months after last dose.

Indications, dosage, and action
Primary hypercholesterolemia
• *Adult dosage:* 500 mg P.O. b.i.d. with morning and evening meals. Don't exceed 1 g/day. Not recommended for children.
• *Action:* Lowers cholesterol levels by inhibiting cholesterol transport from the intestine. It may also inhibit early stages of cholesterol synthesis but has little effect on triglycerides. Drug seems to be more effective in patients with mild cholesterol elevations than in those with severe hypercholesterolemia. It's a second-line agent for total lipid, LDL, and total cholesterol reduction. It also reduces HDL levels, in particular HDL_2, by 20% to 30%. Probucol is the drug of choice for the rare homozygote with familial hypercholesterolemia because homozygotes lack LDL-receptor activity.

Contraindications and cautions
- Avoid use of probucol in patients with recent or progressive myocardial damage or cardiac arrhythmias because of the risk of serious cardiac toxicity. ECG monitoring before and during probucol therapy is advised.
- Don't use in patients with preexisting prolonged QT intervals.
- Discontinue the drug if cardiac arrhythmias or prolonged QT intervals occur.
- Because it's not known if probucol is excreted in breast milk, recommend against its use during breast-feeding.
- Advise patients wishing to conceive to stop the drug at least 6 months before attempting conception and to use birth control throughout the waiting period because the drug is detectable in the blood for 6 months after the last dose.
- Pregnancy risk category B

Life-threatening adverse reactions
- Cardiac arrhythmias
- Angioedema

Common adverse reactions
- Diarrhea, flatulence, abdominal pain, nausea, vomiting
- Hyperhidrosis

Infrequent adverse reactions
- Prolonged QT interval on ECG, arrhythmias
- Headache, dizziness, insomnia, tinnitus, paresthesia, peripheral neuritis
- Indigestion, GI bleeding
- Impotence, nocturia
- Conjunctivitis, tearing, blurred vision, diminished sense of taste and smell
- Eosinophilia, thrombocytopenia, decreased hemoglobin and hematocrit levels
- Fetid sweat, rash, pruritus, ecchymoses, petechiae

Interactions
- *Antiarrhythmics likely to prolong the QT interval (such as quinidine), diuretics:* Avoid concomitant use.
- *Beta blockers, calcium channel blockers, class Ia antiarrhythmics, digitalis glycosides, phenothiazines, tricyclic antidepressants:* Increased risk of arrhythmias.
- *Clofibrate:* Concomitant use may decrease HDL cholesterol levels.

Interventions
Preparation and administration
- Administer probucol with food to enhance absorption. (See *Taking probucol at home.*)

Monitoring and supportive care
- Monitor ECG before and during drug therapy.
- Monitor serum total cholesterol, LDL, HDL, and triglyceride levels periodically throughout therapy.
- **Safety tip.** Don't use probucol in patients with low or falling HDL levels.
- Don't exceed a dosage of 1 g daily.
- Probucol alters serum levels of bilirubin, glucose, CK, AST, ALT, uric acid, ALP, and BUN, as well as eosinophil, hematocrit, and hemoglobin counts.

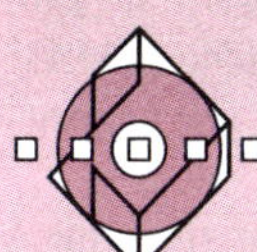

Patient-teaching checklist

Taking probucol at home

In addition to explaining the drug's action and dosage, teach the patient who will continue probucol therapy after discharge to follow these important guidelines.

Take your medication correctly
- [ ] Take probucol with food to enhance absorption.
- [ ] Take probucol as prescribed even when you're feeling well.
- [ ] Continue taking the drug even if unpleasant adverse reactions occur. When you stop taking it, your blood lipid levels may increase again. Be sure to discuss any adverse reactions, especially an irregular pulse, with your doctor.

Watch for other adverse reactions
- [ ] Lie down immediately if you experience dizziness.
- [ ] Avoid driving or operating machinery until after you've adjusted to the drug's effects.
- [ ] If the drug causes insomnia, avoid late-evening doses.

Other instructions
- [ ] Take steps to correct any cardiac risk factors that you may have, such as obesity (lose weight), smoking (engage in a smoking cessation program), and sedentary lifestyle (incorporate an exercise program into your schedule). These risk factors, if uncorrected, may make the drug less effective.
- [ ] Adhere to a low-fat, low-cholesterol diet because probucol is most effective when used in conjunction with dietary restrictions.
- [ ] Comply with scheduled tests to monitor serum total cholesterol, LDL, HDL, and triglyceride levels.

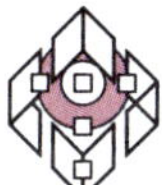

MedTest

1. When should you administer probucol, and why?
   a. Before meals to enhance absorption
   b. With meals to prevent gastric distress
   c. With meals to enhance drug absorption
   d. After meals to prevent gastric distress

2. A common adverse effect of probucol is:
   a. dizziness.
   b. hyperhidrosis.
   c. blurred vision.
   d. pruritus.

3. What special concern does probucol pose for women who wish to conceive?
   a. Probucol will cross the placenta and deposit in fetal fat.
   b. Six months should elapse between discontinuation of probucol

and attempts to become pregnant because of persistent drug blood levels.

c. The patient must use contraceptives for 1 year after discontinuation of probucol therapy.

d. Women of child-bearing age cannot be given probucol because it will never fully leave their body and thus poses a threat to the fetus.

Procainamide hydrochloride

Also known by the brand names Procan SR, Pronestyl, and Pronestyl-SR, procainamide is a procaine derivative that's classified therapeutically as a ventricular antiarrhythmic and a supraventricular antiarrhythmic agent. It's available in 250-, 375-, and 500-mg tablets; 250-, 500-, 750-mg, and 1-g sustained-release tablets; 250-, 375-, and 500-mg capsules; and for injection in 1-g vials containing 100 mg/ml (10 ml) and 500 mg/ml (2 ml) concentrations.

Pharmacokinetics

• *Absorption:* Rate and extent of GI absorption vary. With tablets and capsules, peak plasma levels occur in about 1 hour. Extended-release tablets provide a sustained rate of release and absorption throughout the small intestine. With I.M. injection, onset of action occurs in 10 to 30 minutes, with peak levels in about 1 hour.

• *Distribution:* About 15% binds to plasma proteins.

• *Metabolism.* Acetylated in liver to form N-acetylprocainamide (NAPA), which also exerts antiarrhythmic activity.

• *Excretion.* Excreted in the urine. Procainamide's half-life is about $2\frac{1}{2}$ to $4\frac{3}{4}$ hours. NAPA's half-life is about 6 hours. Usual therapeutic range for serum procainamide concentrations is 4 to 8 mcg/ml. The therapeutic range for serum procainamide and NAPA levels combined is 10 to 30 mcg/ml.

Indications, dosage, and action
PVCs, VT, atrial fibrillation or flutter unresponsive to quinidine; PAT

• *Adult dosage:* 100 mg q 5 minutes by slow I.V. push, no faster than 50 mg/minute, until arrhythmias disappear, adverse reactions develop, or 1 g has been given. When arrhythmias disappear, give continuous infusion of 1 to 4 mg/minute. Usual effective loading dose is 500 to 600 mg. If arrhythmias recur, repeat bolus dose as above and increase infusion rate. For oral therapy, initiate dosage at 50 mg/kg/day in divided doses q 3 hours until therapeutic levels are reached. Once patient is stable, sustained-release form may be given q 6 hours.

Loading dose for atrial fibrillation or PAT: 1 to 1.25 g P.O. If arrhythmias persist after 1 hour, give additional 750 mg. If no change occurs, give 500 mg to 1 g q 2 hours until arrhythmias disappear or adverse reactions occur.

Loading dose for VT: 1 g P.O. Maintenance dosage is 50 mg/kg/day given at 3-hour intervals; average is 250 to

500 mg q 4 hours but may require 1 to 1.5 g q 4 to 6 hours.

Sustained-release tablets may be used for maintenance dosing when treating VT, atrial fibrillation, and PAT. Dosage is 500 mg to 1 g q 6 hours.

• *Antiarrhythmic action:* A class Ia antiarrhythmic agent, procainamide depresses phase O of the action potential. It also possesses anticholinergic activity. It controls atrial tachyarrhythmias by relaxing the velocity, prolonging the effective refractory period, and increasing the action potential duration in the atria, ventricles, and His-Purkinje system. Suppression of automaticity in the His-Purkinje system and ectopic pacemakers accounts for the drug's effectiveness in treating ventricular premature beats. Procainamide prolongs the PR and QT intervals (this effect may be used as an index of drug effectiveness and toxicity). The QT interval is not prolonged to the extent achieved with quinidine.

Procainamide exerts a peripheral vasodilatory effect; with I.V. administration, it may cause hypotension.

Contraindications and cautions

• Don't use in patients with complete AV block with an AV junctional or idioventricular rhythm, unless the patient has an artificial pacemaker.

• Avoid use in patients with prolonged QT interval or QRS duration because of the risk of inducing serious arrhythmias.

• Don't use in patients with digitalis toxicity because the drug may further depress conduction.

• Don't use in patients with torsades de pointes because the drug may exacerbate this arrhythmia.

• Avoid use in myasthenia gravis because the drug may exacerbate muscle weakness.

• Don't use in patients with hypersensitivity to procainamide or related compounds (such as procaine).

• Use cautiously in incomplete AV block or bundle-branch heart block because the drug may further depress conduction.

• Use cautiously in CHF because the drug may worsen this condition.

• Use with caution in patients with renal or hepatic dysfunction because the drug or its active metabolite may accumulate, causing toxicity.

• Discontinue procainamide if granulocytopenia or lupuslike syndrome occurs, unless the drug's benefits outweigh the risks.

• Be aware that elderly patients may require reduced dosage. Because of highly variable metabolism, monitor serum drug levels.

• Know that the manufacturer hasn't established dosage guidelines for children. For treating arrhythmias, the suggested dosage is 40 to 60 mg/kg of standard tablets or capsules P.O. daily, given in four to six divided doses; or 3 to 6 mg/kg I.V. over 5 minutes, followed by a drip of 0.02 to 0.08 mg/kg/minute.

• Recommend an alternative feeding method for breast-feeding women because procainamide and NAPA are distributed in breast milk.

• Pregnancy risk category C

Life-threatening adverse reactions

- Ventricular fibrillation, severe hypotension
- Seizures
- Neutropenia, agranulocytosis

Common adverse reactions

- Bradycardia
- Nausea, vomiting, anorexia, diarrhea
- Positive antinuclear antibody (ANA) titer (60%)
- Fever

Infrequent adverse reactions

- Second-degree AV block
- Hallucinations, confusion, depression, seizures
- Bitter taste (with oral form)
- Thrombocytopenia, neutropenia, agranulocytosis, hemolytic anemia
- Maculopapular rash
- Myalgia, lupus-like syndrome (especially after prolonged administration)

Interactions

- *Anticholinergics:* Additive anticholinergic effects.
- *Anticholinesterase agents:* Anticholinesterase dosage may need to be increased.
- *Cholinergic agents (such as neostigmine and pyridostigmine):* Concomitant use may negate the effects of cholinergic agents, requiring increased dosage.
- *Neuromuscular blocking agents:* Increased skeletal muscle relaxant effects. Monitor patient closely.

For dangerous interactions, see *Life-threatening hazards of multidrug therapy with procainamide.*

Interventions

Preparation and administration

- Note that the vials for I.V. injection contain 1 g of the drug: 100 mg/ml (10 ml) or 500 mg/ml (2 ml).

Safety tip. Use an infusion pump to monitor the infusion precisely.

- Know that procainamide solution for injection may become discolored. If so, check with the pharmacist.
- Be aware of physical incompatibility between procainamide and some other drugs or solutions. (See *Procainamide combinations to avoid,* page 276.)

Monitoring and supportive care

- Know that the I.V. drug form is more likely to cause adverse cardiac reactions, which may lead to severe hypotension.
- Monitor blood pressure and ECG continuously during I.V. administration. Watch for prolonged QT interval and QRS duration, heart block, or increased arrhythmias. If these occur, withhold the drug, obtain a rhythm strip, and notify the doctor immediately.

Safety tip. Withhold the drug if the QRS duration increases 50% above baseline, or 25% above baseline in patients with complete bundle-branch heart block.

- Remember that if procainamide is administered too rapidly I.V., hypotension can occur.

Safety tip. Keep the patient supine for I.V. administration to prevent orthostatic hypotension.

- Monitor serum electrolyte levels, especially potassium. Hypokalemia predisposes patients to arrhythmias.

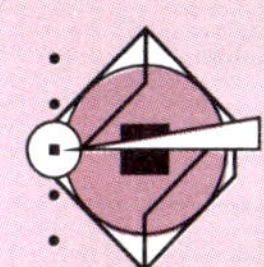

Interactions alert

Life-threatening hazards of multidrug therapy with procainamide

Interacting drug	Effects
Antiarrhythmic agents (such as amiodarone)	May cause additive or antagonistic cardiac effects, with possible additive toxic effects
Antihypertensive agents (such as diltiazem)	May cause additive antihypertensive effects
Histamine-receptor antagonists (such as cimetidine and ranitidine)	Increase risk of procainamide toxicity

• Baseline and periodic determinations of ANA titers, lupus erythematosus (LE) cell preparations, and CBCs may be indicated, especially during the first 3 months of therapy, because procainamide has been associated with lupus-like syndrome.

• Know that a positive ANA titer is common in about 60% of patients who don't have symptoms of lupus-like syndrome. This response is related to prolonged use, not to dosage.

Safety tip. Watch closely for adverse reactions and notify the doctor if they occur. Instruct the patient to report fever, rash, muscle pain, diarrhea, bleeding, bruises, or pleuritic chest pain. (See *Taking antiarrhythmics at home,* page 74.)

• Dosage should be decreased in hepatic or renal dysfunction. The half-life of procainamide is increased as much as threefold in these patients.

• After prolonged atrial fibrillation, restoration of normal rhythm may result in thromboembolism because of thrombi dislodging from the atrial wall. Anticoagulation is usually advised before restoration of normal sinus rhythm.

• In treating atrial fibrillation or flutter, the ventricular rate may accelerate because of the drug's anticholinergic effects. To prevent this effect, a digitalis glycoside is given before procainamide therapy begins.

• Monitor therapeutic serum levels of procainamide, which range from 3 to 10 mcg/ml (most patients are controlled at 4 to 8 mcg/ml). Toxicity may occur at levels greater than 16 mcg/ml).

• Also monitor NAPA levels; some clinicians think that combined procainamide and NAPA levels should be 10 to 30 mcg/ml.

• In prolonged use of the oral form, perform ECGs occasionally to determine continued need for the drug.

• Be aware and warn patient that after taking the sustained-release form of the drug, the wax matrix capsule is not absorbed and may appear in fe-

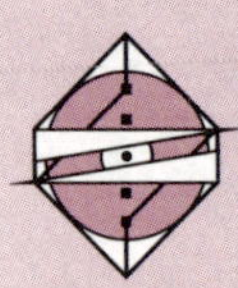

Incompatibility warning

Procainamide combinations to avoid

Procainamide should be mixed in 0.45% or 0.9% NaCl injection because the drug decomposes rapidly in D_5W. Other evidence suggests that procainamide forms a complex with dextrose that may decrease its pharmacologic activity.

Procainamide has been reported to be physically incompatible with some drugs, such as bretylium, esmolol, and milrinone. The incompatibility depends on several factors, such as drug concentrations, specific diluents used, resulting pH, and temperature. Be sure to consult the pharmacist before mixing procainamide with any other drug or drug solution to avoid possible loss of potency.

ces; despite this, the drug has been absorbed.

• Procainamide will invalidate bentiromide test results; discontinue at least 3 days before a bentiromide test. Procainamide may alter edrophonium test results and may cause positive ANA titers, positive direct antiglobulin (Coombs') tests, and ECG changes. The physiologic effects of the drug may result in decreased leukocyte and platelet counts and increased levels of bilirubin, LD, ALP, ALT, and AST.

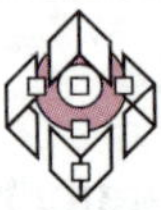

MedTest

1. For life-threatening arrhythmias, the initial dose of procainamide should be administered:
   a. by rapid I.V. bolus.
   b. by slow I.V. push, no faster than 50 mg/minute.
   c. by infusion, using a pump or controller.
   d. I.M., massaging the site well.

2. When giving the sustained-release tablet form, be aware and warn patient that:
   a. profound hypotension frequently occurs while the dosage is being adjusted, so he should change positions and move about cautiously.
   b. a wax-matrix capsule may appear in his stools. However, the drug has been absorbed.
   c. ECG abnormalities and arrhythmias commonly occur during the initial period, requiring cardiac monitoring throughout this adjustment.
   d. embolization of mural thrombi may occur with this drug, so anticoagulant therapy will be started.

3. An extremely common effect of procainamide is:
   a. a positive ANA titer.
   b. depression.
   c. a bitter taste.
   d. agranulocytosis.

Propafenone hydrochloride

Also known by the brand name Rhythmol, propafenone is a sodium channel antagonist that's classified therapeutically as an antiarrhythmic (class Ic). It's available in 150- and 300-mg tablets.

Pharmacokinetics
• *Absorption:* Well absorbed from GI tract; absorption not affected by food. Because of significant first-pass effect, bioavailability is limited; however, it increases with dosage. Absolute bioavailability is 3.4% with 150-mg tablet and 10.6% with 300-mg tablet.
• *Distribution:* Peak levels occur about 3½ hours after administration.
• *Metabolism:* Metabolized by the liver. Two active metabolites have been identified. Some patients (10% of all patients and all patients receiving quinidine) metabolize the drug more slowly.
• *Excretion:* Excreted by kidneys. Elimination half-life is 2 to 10 hours in patients with normal metabolism (about 90% of patients); it can be 10 to 32 hours in patients with slow metabolism.

Indications, dosage, and action
Suppression of life-threatening arrhythmias
• *Regular adult dosage:* Initially, 150 mg P.O. q 8 hours. Dosage may be increased to 225 mg q 8 hours after 3 or 4 days. If necessary, increase dosage to 300 mg q 8 hours. Maximum daily dosage is 900 mg.

• *Dosage in hepatic failure:* The manufacturer recommends that patients with hepatic impairment receive 20% to 30% of the usual dosage.
• *Antiarrhythmic action:* Reduces the inward sodium current in myocardial cells and Purkinje fibers; also has weak beta-adrenergic blocking effects. It slows the upstroke velocity of the action potential (phase 0 depolarization); slows conduction of the AV node, His-Purkinje system, and intraventricular conduction system; and prolongs the refractory period in the AV node.

Contraindications and cautions
• Avoid use in uncontrolled CHF, bradycardia, significant hypotension, or cardiogenic shock.
• Don't use in SA, AV, or intraventricular conduction disorders (such as SSS or AV block) unless the patient has an artificial pacemaker.
• Avoid use in patients who have symptoms of electrolyte disturbances.
• Use cautiously in bronchospasm or bronchospastic disease because of the drug's beta-blocking properties.
• Use all class Ic antiarrhythmics cautiously because many have demonstrated proarrhythmic effects. Limit use to patients with life-threatening arrhythmias.
• Propafenone may alter both the pacing and sensing thresholds of artificial pacemakers. Pacemakers should be monitored and reprogrammed as necessary.
• Use cautiously in patients with a history of CHF. Because sympathetic stimulation may be important to continued function of the failing heart, the beta-blocking effects of pro-

pafenone may be detrimental to
these patients.
• Because propafenone is extensively
metabolized in the liver and excreted by the kidneys, use with caution
in hepatic or renal disease.
• Perform CBCs in patients with unexplained fever or decreased WBC
count to rule out possible agranulocytosis or granulocytopenia, especially
during the first 3 months of therapy.
• In elderly patients and patients
with substantial heart disease, increase the dosage more gradually
during the initial phase of treatment.
• Because it's not known whether
the drug is excreted in breast milk,
recommend alternative infant feeding methods during therapy.
• Pregnancy risk category C

Life-threatening adverse reactions
• CHF, proarrhythmic events (such
as VT and PVCs)

Common adverse reactions
• Dyspnea
• Dizziness, fatigue
• Constipation, nausea, vomiting
• Unusual taste

Infrequent adverse reactions
• Angina, atrial fibrillation, bradycardia, bundle-branch heart block, CHF,
chest pain, edema, first-degree AV
block, hypotension, prolonged QRS
duration, intraventricular conduction delay, palpitations
• Anxiety, ataxia, drowsiness, headache, insomnia, syncope, tremor,
weakness

• Anorexia, abdominal pain or
cramps, diarrhea, dyspepsia, flatu-
lence, dry mouth
• Blurred vision
• Diaphoresis, rash
• Joint pain

Interactions
• *Cimetidine:* Decreased metabolism
of propafenone, increasing its plasma levels. Monitor patient closely.
• *Quinidine:* Slows the metabolism
of propafenone, increasing its half-
life. Avoid concomitant use.

For dangerous interactions, see
*Life-threatening hazards of multi-
drug therapy with propafenone.*

Interventions
Preparation and administration
• Administer the drug with food to
minimize adverse GI reactions. (See
Taking antiarrhythmics at home,
page 74.)

Monitoring and supportive care
• Continuously monitor ECG during
initiation of therapy and dosage adjustments. If PR interval or QRS duration increases by more than 25%, the
dosage may need to be reduced.
• Be aware that propafenone pharmacokinetics are complex. Studies
have shown that a 3-fold increase in
daily dosage (from 300 to 900 mg/
day) may produce a 10-fold increase
in plasma levels.
• Expect the dosage to be increased
stepwise at 3- to 4-day intervals
because this time period is required
to achieve a steady state.
• Know that some patients metabolize propafenone rapidly, and early
studies indicate that the drug may

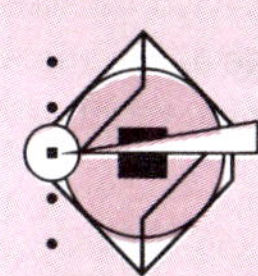

Interactions alert

Life-threatening hazards of multidrug therapy with propafenone

Interacting drug	Effects
Beta blockers (such as propranolol)	Increase risk of CHF
Digitalis glycosides (such as digoxin)	Increase risk of digitalis toxicity
Local anesthetics (such as lidocaine)	Increase risk of CNS toxicity
Oral anticoagulants (such as warfarin)	Increase risk of hemorrhage

have a plasma half-life of 5 to 6 hours in patients with fast metabolism and 17 hours or more in patients with slow metabolism.

- Dosage should be individualized for each patient.
- During concomitant use with digoxin, frequently monitor ECG and serum digoxin levels because propafenone increases serum digoxin levels by 35% to 85%.
- Be aware that the drug may slow conduction and increase the PR interval and QRS duration but that ECG changes alone can't be used to predict plasma concentration or drug efficacy.
- Assess the patient for and instruct him to report any signs of infection, such as sore throat, chills, or fever.

Safety tip. CBC should be performed on a patient demonstrating unexplained signs and symptoms of infection.

- Know that increased liver enzyme levels have been reported in fewer than 0.2% of patients.

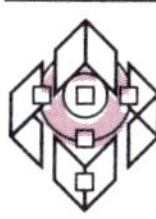

MedTest

1. Propafenone is pharmacologically classified as:
   a. a calcium channel blocker.
   b. a potassium channel blocker.
   c. a sodium channel antagonist.
   d. an ACE inhibitor.

2. Common adverse effects of propafenone include:
   a. nausea and vomiting.
   b. AV and bundle-branch heart blocks.
   c. headache and dizziness.
   d. atrial fibrillation or palpitations.

3. Propafenone should be administered:
   a. p.c. to enhance absorption.
   b. with food to minimize adverse GI reactions.
   c. a.c. to eliminate adverse reactions.
   d. h.s. to minimize postural hypotension.

Propranolol

Also known by the brand names Inderal, Inderal LA, and Ipran, and (in Canada) Apo-Propranolol, Detensol, Novopranol, and PMS-Propranolol, propranolol is a beta-adrenergic blocker. It's classified therapeutically as an antihypertensive, antianginal, and antiarrhythmic as well as an adjunctive therapeutic agent for MI. It's available in 10-, 20-, 40-, 60-, 80-, and 90-mg tablets; in 60-, 80-, 120-, and 160-mg sustained-release capsules; in an oral solution containing 4, 8, or 80 mg/ml; and for injection in 1-mg/ml vials.

Pharmacokinetics
• *Absorption:* Almost completely absorbed from the GI tract, but first-pass metabolism limits bioavailability to about 10%. Absorption enhanced when given with food. Peak plasma concentrations occur 60 to 90 minutes after administration of regular-release tablets.
• *Distribution:* More than 90% protein-bound.
• *Metabolism:* Metabolized to active metabolites.
• *Excretion:* 96% to 99% of given dose is excreted in urine as metabolites; remainder, in feces as unchanged drug and metabolites. Biological half-life is about 4 hours.

Indications, dosage, and action
Hypertension
• *Adult dosage:* Initially, 80 mg P.O. daily in two to four divided doses or one 80-mg sustained-release capsule daily. Increase at 3- to 7-day intervals to maximum daily dosage of 640 mg. Usual maintenance dosage is 160 to 480 mg daily.
• *Antihypertensive action:* Blocks beta-adrenergic receptors, reducing cardiac output and sympathetic outflow from the CNS. It also suppresses renin release.

Angina pectoris
• *Adult dosage:* 10 to 20 mg t.i.d. or q.i.d., or one 80-mg sustained-release capsule daily. Dosage may be increased at 7- to 10-day intervals. The average optimum dosage is 160 to 240 mg daily.
• *Antianginal action:* Blocks beta-adrenergic receptors and decreases cardiac output, myocardial workload, and myocardial oxygen consumption.

Supraventricular, ventricular, and atrial arrhythmias; catecholamine-induced tachyarrhythmias
• *Adult dosage:* 1 to 3 mg I.V. diluted in 50 ml of D_5W or 0.9% NaCl solution infused slowly, not to exceed 1 mg/minute. After 3 mg have been infused, another dose may be given in 2 minutes; subsequent doses, no sooner than q 4 hours. Usual maintenance dosage is 10 to 80 mg P.O. t.i.d. or q.i.d.
• *Antiarrhythmic action:* Slows heart rate and prevents exercise-induced increases in heart rate. It decreases myocardial contractility, cardiac output, and SA and AV node conduction velocity. It also has a membrane-stabilizing effect.

Reduction of infarct size and mortality after MI

• *Adult dosage:* 180 to 240 mg P.O. daily in divided doses. Usually administered in three to four doses daily, beginning 5 to 21 days after infarct.

• *MI prophylactic action:* Reduction of infarct size is believed to result from reduced myocardial oxygen consumption and redistribution of collateral blood flow to areas of ischemia. The exact mechanism by which propranolol lowers mortality after MI is unknown.

Contraindications and cautions

• Don't use in overt cardiac failure, sinus bradycardia, second- or third-degree AV block (unless a functional artificial pacemaker is in place), bronchial asthma, cardiogenic shock, or Raynaud's syndrome because the drug may worsen these conditions.

• Use cautiously in left ventricular dysfunction because beta-adrenergic blockade may precipitate CHF.

• Use cautiously in pulmonary disease.

• Use cautiously in diabetes mellitus, hypoglycemia, or hyperthyroidism because propranolol may mask tachycardia (but not dizziness and sweating) due to hypoglycemia.

• Use cautiously in impaired hepatic function.

• Know that propranolol may mask common signs of shock.

• Discontinue propranolol if signs of heart failure or bronchospasm occur.

• Be aware that elderly patients may require lower maintenance doses of propranolol because they are more prone to develop adverse reactions.

• Propranolol is distributed in breast milk; recommend an alternative infant feeding method during therapy.

• Pregnancy risk category C

Life-threatening adverse reactions

• CHF
• Bronchospasm

Common adverse reactions

• Bradycardia, hypotension
• Increased airway resistance
• Fatigue, lethargy

Infrequent adverse reactions

• CHF, intensification of AV block, peripheral vascular insufficiency
• Light-headedness, mental depression, vivid dreams, hallucinations
• Nausea, vomiting, epigastric distress, abdominal cramping, diarrhea, constipation
• Impotence
• Agranulocytosis, nonthrombocytopenic purpura, thrombocytopenic purpura
• Alopecia, rash
• Fever, arthralgia

Interactions

• *Aminophylline:* Propranolol may attenuate the bronchodilating effects of aminophylline. Use together cautiously.

• *Antihypertensive agents:* Propranolol potentiates antihypertensive effects of other antihypertensive agents, especially catecholamine-depleting agents such as reserpine.

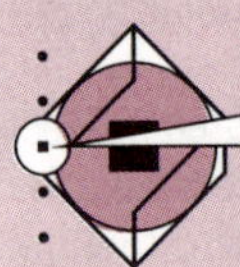

Interactions alert

Life-threatening hazards of multidrug therapy with propranolol

Interacting drug	Effects
Antiarrhythmic agents (such as lidocaine or quinidine)	Cause additive cardiac toxicity
Digitalis glycosides (such as digoxin)	Potentiate bradycardia and myocardial depressant effects of propranolol
Epinephrine (sympathomimetic agent)	May cause severe vasoconstriction
Phenothiazines (such as chlorpromazine)	May cause additive hypotension

• *Atropine, tricyclic antidepressants, and other drugs with anticholinergic effects:* May antagonize propranolol-induced bradycardia.
• *Cimetidine:* Inhibits propranolol's metabolism. Monitor for greater beta-blocking effect.
• *Glucagon, isoproterenol:* Antagonize propranolol's effect.
• *Insulin, oral antidiabetic drugs:* Can alter requirements for these drugs in previously stabilized diabetics. Monitor for hypoglycemia.
• *Isoproterenol, MAO inhibitors:* Propranolol may antagonize beta-adrenergic stimulating effects of sympathomimetic agents such as isoproterenol.
• *NSAIDs:* May antagonize propranolol's antihypertensive effects.
• *Tubocurarine:* High doses of propranolol may potentiate neuromuscular blocking effect of tubocurarine and related compounds.

(For dangerous interactions, see *Life-threatening hazards of multidrug therapy with propranolol.*)

Interventions
Preparation and administration
• Always check the patient's apical pulse before giving this drug. If you detect extremes in pulse rates, withhold the drug and call the doctor. (See *Taking beta-adrenergic blockers at home,* page 63.)
• This drug should be given with meals to enhance absorption.
• To administer the concentrated oral form, carefully measure the dose and mix it with an appropriate liquid. (See *Giving the concentrated oral form of propranolol,* page 283.)

Monitoring and supportive care

• Check blood pressure, ECG, and heart rate and rhythm frequently, especially during I.V. administration.

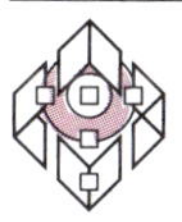 **Safety tip.** If the patient develops severe hypotension, notify the doctor. He may prescribe a vasopressor.

Safety tip. In diabetic patients, assess for diaphoresis or CNS signs of hypoglycemia, such as mental status changes, restlessness, anxiety, or dizziness.

• Propranolol is used to prevent frequent, severe, uncontrollable, or disabling migraine or vascular headaches.

• Propranolol should never be given as an adjunct in the treatment of pheochromocytoma unless the patient is pretreated with alpha-adrenergic blocking agents.

• Know that propranolol may elevate serum transaminase, ALP, and LD levels, and may elevate BUN levels in patients with severe heart disease.

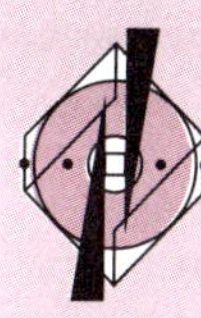

Administration guidelines

Giving the concentrated oral form of propranolol

When giving propranolol in its concentrated oral form, follow these guidelines:

• Measure your dose with the specially marked dropper that comes with the bottle.

• Mix the drug with some water, juice, or carbonated beverage.

• After the patient drinks all the liquid containing the medication, rinse the glass with a little more liquid and have him drink that as well.

• Know that you may mix doses with a small amount of applesauce or pudding.

• Mix only the amount of propranolol that you need for the dose; don't keep any that's left over after the patient has taken the drug.

MedTest

1. Which group of patients requires a lower dosage of propranolol?

  a. Pregnant women
  b. Those with renal impairment
  c. Elderly patients
  d. Those with hepatic impairment

2. When should you administer propranolol and why?

  a. Before meals to enhance absorption
  b. With meals to prevent nausea
  c. With meals to enhance absorption
  d. After meals to prevent GI distress

3. Your diabetic patient is taking propranolol, which can mask beta-adrenergic signs of hypoglycemia. Which hypoglycemic indicator may not be present as a clue for the patient?

  a. Mental status changes
  b. Dizziness
  c. Restlessness
  d. Rapid heart rate

Quinidine

A cinchona alkaloid that's classified therapeutically as an antiarrhythmic agent, quinidine is available in different salts. Quinidine bisulfate is known by the brand names Biquin Durules (in Canada) and Kinidin Durules (in Australia); quinidine gluconate, by the brand names Duraquin, Quinaglute Dura-Tabs, and Quinalan, and (in Canada) Quinate. Quinidine polygalacturonate is known by the brand name Cardioquin; quinidine sulfate, by the brand names CinQuin, Quinidex Extentabs, Quinora, and (in Canada) Apo-Quinidine and Novoquinidin.

Quinidine bisulfate is available in 250-mg tablets; gluconate, in 324- and 330-mg sustained-release tablets, and for injection in vials containing 80 mg/ml; polygalacturonate, in 275-mg tablets; and sulfate, in 100-, 200-, and 300-mg tablets, 300-mg sustained-release tablets (in Canada), 200- and 300-mg capsules (in Canada), and for injection in vials of 200 mg/ml (in Canada).

Pharmacokinetics
• *Absorption:* Well absorbed from GI tract, but serum drug levels vary greatly among individuals. Onset of sulfate is 1 to 3 hours. For sustained-release forms, onset may be slower. Peak plasma levels occur in 3 to 4 hours for quinidine gluconate and in 6 hours for quinidine polygalacturonate.
• *Distribution:* Concentrates in heart, liver, kidneys, and skeletal muscles. Distribution volume decreases in patients with CHF, who may require dosage reduction. About 80% of drug is bound to plasma proteins; unbound (active) fraction may increase in patients with hypoalbuminemia.
• *Metabolism:* 60% to 80% metabolized in the liver to two metabolites that may have some pharmacologic activity.
• *Excretion:* 10% to 30% excreted in urine within 24 hours as unchanged drug. Elimination half-life averages 6½ hours. Duration of effect ranges from 6 to 8 hours.

Indications, dosage, and action
Atrial flutter or fibrillation
• *Adult dosage:* 200 mg of quinidine sulfate (or equivalent) P.O. q 2 to 3 hours for five to eight doses with subsequent daily increases until sinus rhythm is restored or toxic effects develop. Conventional maintenance dosage is 300 to 400 mg q 6 hours. Maximum dosage is 3 g daily.

PACs, PVCs, paroxysmal AV junctional rhythm, atrial tachycardia, VT, and cardioversion maintenance
• *Adult dosage:* After the patient receives a test dose of 200 mg P.O., monitor vital signs before therapy with 200 to 400 mg of quinidine sulfate (or equivalent) P.O. q 4 to 6 hours. Or 600 mg of quinidine gluconate I.M. initially, then up to 400 mg q 2 hours p.r.n. Or (rarely used) 800 mg of quinidine gluconate I.V. diluted in 40 ml of D_5W, infused at 16 mg (1 ml)/minute.

For maintenance therapy, sustained-release forms may be used. The patient will receive 600 mg of quinidine sulfate in sustained-release form (in Canada) or 324 to

648 mg of quinidine gluconate in sustained-release form q 8 to 12 hours.
• *Pediatric dosage:* After receiving a test dose of 2 mg/kg, the patient will be given 3 to 6 mg/kg P.O. q 2 to 3 hours for five doses daily.
• *Antiarrhythmic action:* A class Ia antiarrhythmic, quinidine depresses phase O of the action potential. It decreases myocardial excitability and conduction velocity and may depress myocardial contractility. It reduces conduction velocity in the atria, ventricles, and His-Purkinje system. It helps control atrial tachyarrhythmias by prolonging the effective refractory period and increasing the action potential duration in the atria, ventricles, and His-Purkinje system, thereby causing tissue to remain refractory even after returning to resting membrane potential. Quinidine's anticholinergic effects shorten the effective refractory period of the AV node. Digitalis glycosides should be administered for atrial tachyarrhythmias before quinidine therapy, to prevent VT.

Quinidine suppresses automaticity in the His-Purkinje system and ectopic pacemakers and helps treat PVCs. Because the drug prolongs the QRS duration and QT interval, ECGs may be used to evaluate drug effectiveness and toxicity.

Contraindications and cautions

• Don't use in complete AV block with an AV junctional or idioventricular rhythm because of the potential for asystole.
• Avoid use in patients with arrhythmias caused by digitalis toxicity, AV conduction disorders, or intraventricular conduction defects because quinidine increases the QT interval and QRS duration. Such conduction delays and proarrhythmic effects are potentially serious, possibly leading to complete AV block, VT, ventricular fibrillation, or asystole.
• Don't use in myasthenia gravis because the drug's anticholinergic effects may exacerbate muscle weakness.
• Use with caution in patients with incomplete AV block because complete AV block may occur.
• Use cautiously in CHF or hypotension because the drug may worsen these conditions.
• Use cautiously in elderly patients and in those with renal or hepatic dysfunction because toxic drug accumulation may result.
• Use with caution in patients with asthma, weakness, or febrile infection because these conditions may mask hypersensitivity reactions to the drug.
• Expect drug discontinuation if the following problems develop — blood dyscrasias; hepatic or renal dysfunction; syncope; cardiotoxicity, including conduction defects (50% widening of the QRS complex, 25% widening in the presence of an intraventricular conduction defect, or QT interval prolonged beyond 500 milliseconds); ventricular flutter or VT; frequent PVCs; or complete AV block.
• Because the drug is excreted in breast milk, avoid use in breast-feeding women.
• Pregnancy risk category C

Life-threatening adverse reactions
- PVCs, torsades de pointes, ventricular fibrillation, severe hypotension, aggravated CHF
- Respiratory arrest
- Hemolytic anemia, thrombocytopenia, agranulocytosis
- Angioedema

Common adverse reactions
- SA and AV block, VT, ECG changes (particularly widening QRS complex, notched P waves, widened QT interval, and ST-segment depression)
- Vertigo, headache, light-headedness
- Diarrhea, nausea, vomiting
- Tinnitus (with excessive dosage)
- Fever or cinchonism (overdose)

Infrequent adverse reactions
- Acute asthma attack
- Confusion, restlessness, cold sweat, pallor, fainting, dementia
- Anorexia, abdominal pain, hepatotoxicity, including granulomatous hepatitis
- Excessive salivation, blurred vision
- Rash, petechial hemorrhage of buccal mucosa, pruritus
- Lupus-like syndrome

Interactions
- *Alkalinizing agents, amiodarone, cimetidine:* Increase serum quinidine levels. Monitor for increased effect.
- *Anticholinergic drugs:* Concomitant use may add to anticholinergic effects.
- *Anticholinesterases and cholinergic drugs:* Quinidine may interfere with the effects of these drugs.
- *Antihypertensive agents:* Concomitant use may worsen hypotension (mainly when administered I.V.).
- *Barbiturates, phenytoin, rifampin:* Increase the rate of quinidine metabolism, leading to decreased quinidine levels. Monitor for reduced quinidine effect.
- *Nifedipine:* May lower quinidine blood levels. Monitor quinidine levels carefully.

For dangerous interactions, see *Life-threatening hazards of multidrug therapy with quinidine.*

Interventions
Preparation and administration
- Check the patient's apical pulse rate, blood pressure, and ECG tracing before therapy. If you detect extremes in pulse rate, withhold the drug and notify the doctor at once. (See *Taking antiarrhythmics at home,* page 74.)

Safety tip. Never use discolored (brownish) quinidine solution.
- Administer the drug with food or milk to reduce GI symptoms.
- For maintenance therapy, give only by oral or, rarely, I.M. route.
- Dosage requirements vary. Some patients may require the drug q 4 hours; others, q 6 hours.

Safety tip. Titrate dosage by observing clinical response, the ECG, and blood levels. Reduce the dose if the QRS complex widens or the QT interval is prolonged.

Monitoring and supportive care
- Monitor the ECG, especially when large doses of the drug are being administered.

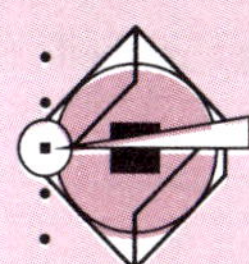

Interactions alert

Life-threatening hazards of multidrug therapy with quinidine

Interacting drug	Effects
Antiarrhythmic agents (such as flecainide and procainamide)	May cause additive or antagonistic cardiac effects and additive toxic effects that may lead to life-threatening arrhythmias such as torsades de pointes
Digitalis glycosides (such as digoxin)	Increase risk of digitalis toxicity
Neuromuscular blocking agents (such as pancuronium bromide)	May potentiate effects of neuromuscular blocking agents and increase risk of respiratory arrest
Phenothiazines (such as chlorpromazine)	May cause additive cardiac depressant effects
Reserpine (rauwolfia alkaloid)	May cause additive cardiac depressant effects
Verapamil (calcium channel blocker)	May result in significant hypotension in patients with idiopathic hypertrophic cardiomyopathy
Warfarin (oral anticoagulant)	Increases risk of hemorrhage

• Because conversion of chronic atrial fibrillation may be associated with embolism, an anticoagulant should be administered before quinidine therapy begins.

• When changing administration routes, the dosage should be altered to compensate for variations in quinidine base content.

• Monitor liver function tests during the first 4 to 8 weeks of therapy.

• Assess for and instruct patient to report rash, fever, unusual bleeding, bruising, ringing in the ears, or visual disturbances.

• GI adverse reactions, especially diarrhea, may be signs of toxicity or may occur in the absence of toxicity. Check serum quinidine levels; suspect toxicity when they exceed 8 mcg/ml. Minimize GI symptoms by administering quinidine with food.

• Keep in mind that quinidine may cause hemolysis in patients with G6PD deficiency.

• Quinidine is hemodialyzable. The dosage may need to be adjusted in patients undergoing dialysis.

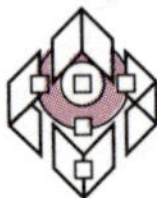

MedTest

1. Quinidine is used to treat:
   a. bradyarrhythmias.
   b. AV block of varying degrees.
   c. atrial and ventricular tachyarrhythmias.
   d. CHF.

2. Oral quinidine preparations
should generally be administered:
   a. a.c. to enhance absorption.
   b. with meals to reduce GI symptoms.
   c. p.c. to reduce gastric distress.
   d. h.s. to limit postural hypotension.

3. Check serum quinidine levels for
possible toxicity if your patient develops:
   a. hypotension.
   b. acute asthma attacks.
   c. ECG changes.
   d. diarrhea.

Reserpine

Known by the brand names Novore-
serpine (in Canada), Sandril, Ser-
palan, Serpanray, Serpasil, Serpate,
and Zepine, reserpine is a rauwolfia
alkaloid and peripherally acting anti-
adrenergic agent that's classified
therapeutically as an antihypertensive and antipsychotic agent. It's
available in 0.1-, 0.25-, and 1-mg tablets.

Pharmacokinetics
• *Absorption:* Oral form absorbed
rapidly.
• *Distribution:* High concentrations
found in adipose tissue.
• *Metabolism:* Extensively metabolized to inactive compounds.
• *Excretion:* Slowly excreted along
with unchanged drug in urine and feces. Onset takes 2 to 3 weeks; antihypertensive effects may persist for several days to weeks after discontinuation of long-term therapy. Mean half-
life is 33 hours.

Indications, dosage, and action
**Mild to moderate essential hyper-
tension**
• *Adult dosage:* Initial and maintenance dosages are both 0.25 mg/day.
Some clinicians recommend an initial dosage of 0.1 mg/day. Maximum
dosage is 0.25 mg/day.
• *Antihypertensive action:* Blocks
catecholamine uptake into adrenergic nerve terminals. Neurotransmit-
ters are gradually depleted, resulting
in peripheral adrenergic blockade.
Reserpine may also deplete some neu-
rotransmitters in the CNS and alter
sympathetic outflow to the periphery.

Contraindications and cautions
• Don't use in patients receiving elec-
troconvulsive therapy for depression
because cerebral depletion of seroto-
nin and catecholamines may worsen
depression and predispose them to
seizures and extrapyramidal reactions.
• Don't use in mental depression, ulcerative colitis, or peptic ulcer disease because reserpine may exacerbate these conditions.

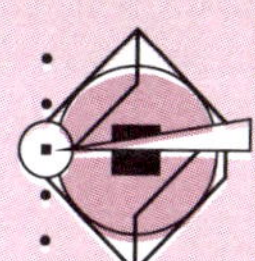

Interactions alert

Life-threatening hazards of multidrug therapy with reserpine

Interacting drug	Effects
CNS depressants (such as diazepam)	Increase risk of severe CNS depression
Digitalis glycosides (such as digoxin)	Increase risk of life-threatening arrhythmias
Quinidine (antiarrhythmic agent)	Increases risk of life-threatening arrhythmias

- The drug should be discontinued if signs of drug-induced mental depression develop.
- Use cautiously in patients with epilepsy or impaired renal function because the drug may worsen these conditions.
- Be aware that lower dosages may be necessary in elderly patients because of decreased drug clearance.
- Because drug is distributed in breast milk, avoid use in breast-feeding women.
- Pregnancy risk category C

Life-threatening adverse reactions

None reported

Common adverse reactions

- Orthostatic hypotension, bradycardia
- Depression, drowsiness, nervousness, paradoxical anxiety, nightmares
- Nausea, vomiting
- Dry mouth, nasal stuffiness
- Breast engorgement, gynecomastia

Infrequent adverse reactions

- Arrhythmias
- Dyspnea
- Syncope, mental confusion, extrapyramidal symptoms, sedation
- Hyperacidity, diarrhea, GI bleeding
- Dysuria, impotence
- Glaucoma, miosis, uveitis, optic atrophy, conjunctival congestion
- Pruritus, skin flushing, rash
- Hypothermia, leg pain, weight gain

Interactions

- *Alcohol:* May potentiate CNS depressant effects of alcohol.
- *Antihypertensive agents, diuretics:* Increased risk of hypotension.
- *Levodopa:* May diminish effects of levodopa.
- *MAO inhibitors:* May cause excitability and hypertension. Use together cautiously.

For dangerous interactions, see *Life-threatening hazards of multidrug therapy with reserpine.*

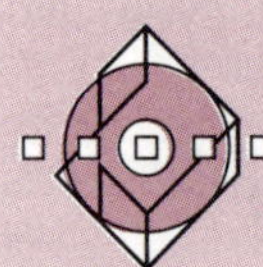

Patient-teaching checklist

Taking reserpine at home

In addition to explaining the drug's action and dosage, teach the patient who will continue reserpine therapy after discharge to follow these important guidelines.

Take your medication correctly
☐ Take reserpine with meals.
☐ Check your blood pressure or have it checked at a nearby blood pressure station frequently (at least once a week) if so instructed by your doctor. Report any significant changes.
☐ Take reserpine as prescribed even when you're feeling well.
☐ Continue taking the drug even if unpleasant adverse reactions occur. But make sure you discuss these adverse reactions, especially mental depression or nightmares, with your doctor.

Minimize adverse reactions
☐ Remember to change positions slowly (especially from lying flat to sitting upright) and to dangle your legs over the bedside for a few minutes before standing to minimize light-headedness due to the drug.
☐ Lie down immediately if dizziness or faintness occurs.
☐ Avoid driving or operating machinery if dizziness occurs.

☐ Be aware that this drug can cause breast engorgement, breast enlargement in males, and impotence. If you notice these reactions, discuss them with your doctor.

Other instructions
☐ Notify your doctor promptly if you are planning to get pregnant or if you become pregnant unexpectedly because of this drug's potential harm to the fetus. The drug will need to be discontinued and another antihypertensive agent substituted.
☐ Weigh yourself daily and notify your doctor if you gain more than 3 lb (1.5 kg).
☐ Relieve a dry mouth with sugarless chewing gum, hard candy, or ice chips.
☐ Notify your doctor if you need relief for nasal stuffiness.
☐ Check with your doctor or pharmacist before taking OTC medications.
☐ Store reserpine at room temperature and protect it from moisture, light, and air.

Interventions
Preparation and administration
• Administer reserpine with meals. (See *Taking reserpine at home.*)

Monitoring and supportive care
• Monitor the patient's blood pressure and pulse rate frequently.
• Drowsiness and dizziness are common in early therapy; assist the patient with ambulation.

- Watch the patient closely for signs of mental depression, and ask him if he's experiencing nightmares; report these findings to the doctor.
- Be aware that the effects of this drug may last for 10 days after it's discontinued.
- Tell the patient to notify the doctor immediately if she becomes pregnant or plans to become pregnant.
- Know that reserpine therapy alters the detection of urinary corticosteroids by colorimetric assay and may interfere with excretion of urinary catecholamines and vanillylmandelic acid.

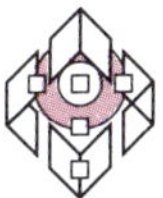 **MedTest**

1. Reserpine is an antihypertensive agent that's classified pharmacologically as:
   a. an ACE inhibitor.
   b. an anti-adrenergic agent.
   c. a beta blocker.
   d. a calcium channel blocker.

2. Common adverse effects of reserpine include:
   a. pruritus and skin flushing.
   b. diarrhea and rectal bleeding.
   c. mental confusion and sedation.
   d. dry mouth and nasal stuffiness.

3. Which adverse reactions are common in early reserpine therapy?
   a. Anorexia and dyspepsia
   b. Drowsiness and dizziness
   c. ECG changes and arrhythmias
   d. Dysuria and impotence

Simvastatin

Also known by the brand name Zocor, simvastatin is classified therapeutically as an antilipemic, cholesterol-lowering agent. It's available in 5-, 10-, 20-, and 40-mg tablets.

Pharmacokinetics
- *Absorption:* Readily absorbed, but extensive hepatic extraction limits plasma availability of active inhibitors to 5% of dose or less. Individual absorption varies considerably.
- *Distribution:* Parent drug and active metabolites over 95% bound to plasma proteins.
- *Metabolism:* Hydrolysis occurs in plasma; at least three major active metabolites have been identified.
- *Excretion:* Primarily in bile.

Indications, dosage, and action
Reduction of LDL and total cholesterol levels in primary hypercholesterolemia (types IIa and IIb)
- *Adult dosage:* Initially, 5 to 10 mg P.O. daily in the evening. Dosage should be adjusted q 4 weeks based on patient tolerance and response; maximum daily dosage is 40 mg.
- *Dosage in renal failure:* Patients with mild to moderate renal insufficiency should take the usual daily dosage. Patients with severe renal impairment should start therapy with 5 mg P.O. daily and should be closely monitored.
- *Antilipemic action:* Inhibits HMG-CoA reductase. This hepatic enzyme is an early (and rate-limiting) step in the synthetic pathway of cholesterol.

Contraindications and cautions
• Don't use in active liver disease or other conditions associated with persistent elevations of serum transaminase levels.
• Be aware that clinical evidence shows that liver dysfunction may occur in up to 1% of patients.
• Know that most elderly patients respond to a daily dosage of 20 mg or less.
• Because it's not known if simvastatin is excreted in breast milk, recommend an alternative feeding method during therapy.
• Don't give to women of childbearing age unless there's no risk of pregnancy.
• Pregnancy risk category X

Life-threatening adverse reactions
• Hepatotoxicity

Common adverse reactions
None reported at suggested dosages

Infrequent adverse reactions
• Upper respiratory infection
• Constipation, dyspepsia, flatulence, nausea, marked elevations of serum transaminase levels

Interactions
• *Chronic alcohol abuse, hepatotoxic drugs*: Increased risk of hepatotoxicity. Avoid concomitant use.
• *Digoxin:* Simvastatin may slightly elevate digoxin levels. Closely monitor serum digoxin levels.
• *Warfarin:* Anticoagulant effect may be slightly enhanced. Monitor patient's PT at start of therapy and during dosage adjustments.

For dangerous interactions, see *Life-threatening hazards of multidrug therapy with simvastatin.*

Interventions
Preparation and administration
• Administer this drug in the evening, usually with the evening meal, but you may give it without regard to meals. (See *Taking simvastatin at home,* page 294.)

Monitoring and supportive care
• Dosage adjustments should be made about q 4 weeks. If the cholesterol levels fall below the target range, the dosage should be reduced.
• Monitor liver function tests frequently at the start of therapy and periodically thereafter.
• Watch for signs of myositis. Myopathy, marked elevations of CK levels possibly leading to rhabdomyolysis, and renal failure secondary to myoglobinuria have been reported rarely.

Safety tip. Simvastatin should be temporarily discontinued in any patient with an acute condition that suggests a developing myopathy or anyone with risk factors that may predispose him to renal failure secondary to rhabdomyolysis. These factors include severe acute infection; severe endocrine, metabolic, or electrolyte disorders; hypotension; recent major surgery; or uncontrolled seizures.

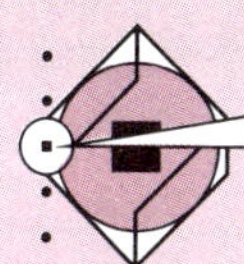

Interactions alert

Life-threatening hazards of multidrug therapy with simvastatin

Interacting drug	Effects
Erythromycin (antibiotic)	Increases risk of rhabdomyolysis
Fibric acid derivatives (such as clofibrate)	Increase risk of rhabdomyolysis
Immunosuppressant agents (such as cyclosporine)	Increase risk of rhabdomyolysis
Niacin (nicotinic acid, a B vitamin, in doses >1 g/day)	Increases risk of rhabdomyolysis

• Simvastatin should be initiated only after diet and other nonpharmacologic therapies have proved ineffective. Patients should continue a cholesterol-lowering diet during therapy.

• Know that as an expected pharmacologic effect, simvastatin will reduce total plasma cholesterol, VLDL, and LDL levels and may variably increase HDL levels. The ratios of total cholesterol to HDL, total cholesterol to LDL, and LDL to HDL will be reduced. Modest decreases in triglyceride levels may also occur.

• Monitor for toxic effects of the drug such as marked, persistent elevations of serum transaminase levels. During clinical trials, about 5% of patients had asymptomatic, marked elevations in the noncardiac fraction of CK levels.

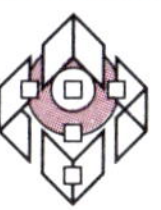

MedTest

1. Administer simvastatin:
   a. first thing in the morning.
   b. a.c.
   c. with meals.
   d. in the evening.

2. Laboratory findings in simvastatin toxicity include:
   a. reductions in total cholesterol, VLDL, and LDL levels.
   b. elevated BUN and serum creatinine levels.
   c. marked, persistent elevations in serum transaminase levels.
   d. liver biopsy findings.

3. Patients taking simvastatin should be cautioned to avoid:
   a. exposure to sunlight.
   b. alcohol intake.

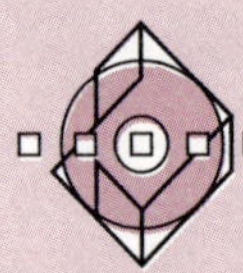

Taking simvastatin at home

In addition to explaining the drug's action and dosage, teach the patient who will continue simvastatin therapy after discharge to follow these important guidelines.

Take your medication correctly
☐ Take simvastatin in the evening.
☐ You can take simvastatin with or without food.
☐ Take simvastatin as prescribed even when you're feeling well.
☐ Continue taking the drug even if unpleasant adverse reactions occur because when you stop taking it, your blood cholesterol levels may increase again. But make sure you discuss any adverse reactions, especially signs of infection (fever, sore throat, malaise), muscle aches and pains, and seizures, with your doctor.

Modify your lifestyle
☐ Take steps to correct any cardiac risk factors that you may have, such as obesity (lose weight), smoking (engage in a stop-smoking program), and sedentary lifestyle (incorporate an exercise program into your routine). These risk factors may make the drug less effective.

☐ Adhere to a low-fat, low-cholesterol diet because simvastatin is most effective when used in conjunction with dietary restrictions.
☐ Restrict your use of alcohol because both alcohol and simvastatin can have adverse effects on liver function.

Other instructions
☐ Adhere to your doctor's schedule for testing serum cholesterol and triglyceride levels, which allows him to monitor the effectiveness of simvastatin therapy.
☐ If you wish to become pregnant or do become pregnant unexpectedly, notify your doctor promptly. The drug will have to be discontinued because it may harm the fetus.
☐ Check with your doctor or pharmacist before taking OTC medications.
☐ Store simvastatin at room temperature and protect it from moisture, direct light, and heat.

---

c. organ meats.
d. shellfish.

Sotalol

Also known by the brand names Betapace and (in Canada) Sotacor, sotalol is a beta blocker that's classified therapeutically as an antiarrhythmic with class II (beta-adrenergic blocking) and class III (prolongation of cardiac action potential duration) properties. In Canada, it's used for hypertension and angina. It's available in 80-, 160-, and 240-mg scored tablets.

Pharmacokinetics
• *Absorption:* After oral administration, bioavailability is 90% to 100%. Peak plasma concentrations are reached in 2½ to 4 hours and steady state plasma concentrations are attained within 2 to 3 days (after five to six doses when administered b.i.d.).
• *Distribution:* Crosses placenta, but crosses blood-brain barrier poorly.
• *Metabolism:* Doesn't bind to plasma protein and isn't metabolized.
• *Excretion:* In urine.

Indications, dosage, and action
Documented, life-threatening ventricular arrhythmias
• *Adult dosage:* Initially, 80 mg P.O. b.i.d. Dosage should be increased q 2 to 3 days as needed and tolerated; most patients respond to a daily dosage of 160 to 320 mg. A few patients with refractory arrhythmias have received as much as 640 mg daily.
• *Dosage in renal failure:* If creatinine clearance is 30 to 60 ml/minute/1.73 m^2, the dose will be given q 24 hours; 10 to 30 ml/minute/1.73 m^2, q 36 to 48 hours; less than 10 ml/minute/1.73 m^2, dosage individualized.
• *Antiarrhythmic action:* Class II (beta-blockade) effects are manifested by slowed heart rate, decreased AV node conduction, and increased AV node refractoriness. Class III electrophysiologic effects include prolongation of the atrial and ventricular (and AV accessory pathways, where present) action potential duration and effective refractory period.

Hypertension
Sotalol is used as an antihypertensive in Canada.
• *Adult dosage:* 80 mg P.O. b.i.d.; dosage increased at weekly intervals in increments of 80 mg b.i.d. as needed and tolerated. Most patients respond to a daily dosage of 160 to 320 mg; patients taking 320 mg or less daily may take drug as a single daily dose in the morning.
• *Action:* Competes with beta-adrenergic agonists (catecholamines) for available beta-receptor sites located on membranes of blood vessel smooth muscle. This results in vasodilation, reducing afterload and lowering blood pressure.

Angina
Sotalol is used as an antianginal agent in Canada.
• *Adult dosage:* 80 mg P.O. b.i.d.; dosage increased at weekly intervals in increments of 80 mg b.i.d. as needed and tolerated. Most patients respond to doses of 160 mg b.i.d.; maximum daily dosage is 480 mg.
• *Action:* By decreasing the heart rate and contractility, sotalol reduces myocardial oxygen consumption and thus relieves angina.

Contraindications and cautions
• Don't use in severe sinus node dysfunction, sinus bradycardia, or second- or third-degree AV block (unless a functioning pacemaker is present).
• Don't use in congenital or acquired QT syndrome, cardiogenic shock, CHF, bronchial asthma, or allergic

rhinitis because sotalol may worsen these conditions.
• Don't use in hypokalemia or hypomagnesemia because these conditions can worsen prolonged QT interval.
• Use cautiously and with dosage adjustments in patients with renal impairment.
• Use cautiously in patients with diabetes mellitus. Beta blockers may mask signs and symptoms of hypoglycemia.
• Because sotalol is excreted in breast milk, recommend an alternate feeding method during therapy.
• Pregnancy risk category B

Life-threatening adverse reactions
• Arrhythmias, CHF, AV block
• Bronchospasm
• CVA

Common adverse reactions
• Bradycardia (16%), chest pain (16%), palpitations, edema, ECG abnormalities, hypotension, arrhythmogenic effect
• Dyspnea (21%), pulmonary problems, upper respiratory tract problems
• Asthenia, headache, dizziness (20%), light-headedness, weakness, fatigue (20%), sleep problems, visual problems, syncope
• Nausea and vomiting, diarrhea, dyspepsia
• Rash
• Pain in extremities

Infrequent adverse reactions
• Presyncope, peripheral vascular insufficiency

• Asthma
• Depression, paresthesia, anxiety, altered level of consciousness, mood changes, appetite disorder
• Abdominal pain, colon problems, flatulence
• Urogenital problems, sexual dysfunction
• Fever, weight change, back pain

Interactions
• *Clonidine:* Beta blockers may enhance the rebound effect seen after withdrawal of clonidine. Sotalol should be discontinued several days before withdrawing clonidine.

For dangerous interactions, see *Life-threatening hazards of multidrug therapy with sotalol.*

Interventions
Preparation and administration
• Administer in the same manner consistently: either with or without food. Food can interfere with absorption but as long as sotalol is taken in the same way, this won't be a problem. (See *Taking antiarrhythmics at home,* page 74.)

Monitoring and supportive care
• Monitor ECG for QT-interval prolongation at initiation of therapy and during dosage adjustments (with patient hospitalized). Proarrhythmic events may occur at the start of therapy and during dosage adjustments. Equipment and personnel should be readily available for cardiac rhythm monitoring and interpretation of ECG waveforms.
• Adjust dosage slowly, allowing 2 to 3 days between dosage increments to adequately monitor QT intervals and

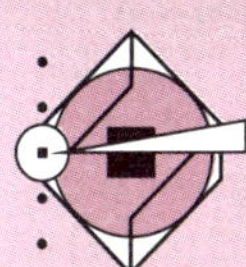

Interactions alert

Life-threatening hazards of multidrug therapy with sotalol

Interacting drug	Effects
Antiarrhythmic agents (such as flecainide)	Add to cardiac effects
Antihypertensive agents (such as reserpine)	Increase risk of hypotension
Calcium channel blockers (such as verapamil)	Increase risk of myocardial depression or AV conduction disturbances
General anesthetics (such as halothane)	Increase risk of myocardial depression

to allow plasma levels of the drug to reach a steady state.

• Although patients receiving I.V. lidocaine have started sotalol therapy without ill effects, other antiarrhythmic drugs should be withdrawn before sotalol therapy. Usually, sotalol therapy should be delayed until two or three half-lives of the withdrawn drug have elapsed. After withdrawal of amiodarone, sotalol shouldn't be administered until the QT interval normalizes.

• Monitor serum electrolyte levels regularly, especially if the patient is receiving diuretics. Electrolyte imbalances may enhance QT prolongation and increase the risk of serious arrhythmias.

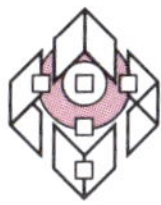

MedTest

1. A common adverse effect of sotalol is:
   a. asthma.
   b. bronchospasm.
   c. fever.
   d. dyspnea.

2. Administer sotalol:
   a. in the early morning.
   b. consistently, either with or without food.
   c. with food or milk.
   d. in the evening, preferably h.s.

3. Upon initiation of sotalol therapy and during dosage adjustment, you would closely monitor:
   a. blood pressure.

b. serum electrolyte levels.
c. ECG waveforms (QT interval).
d. PAWP and cardiac output.

Spironolactone

Also known by the brand names Aldactone, Novospiroton and Sincomen (in Canada), and Spirotone (in Australia), spironolactone is a potassium-sparing diuretic that's classified therapeutically for management of edema, as an antihypertensive for diagnosis of primary hyperaldosteronism, and for treatment of diuretic-induced hypokalemia. It's available in 25-, 50-, and 100-mg tablets.

Pharmacokinetics

• *Absorption:* About 90% absorbed after oral administration. Onset of action is gradual; maximum effect occurs on third day of therapy.
• *Distribution:* Spironolactone and its major metabolite, canrenone, are more than 90% plasma protein–bound.
• *Metabolism:* Rapidly and extensively metabolized to canrenone, its major active metabolite.
• *Excretion:* Canrenone and other metabolites excreted primarily in urine and in small amounts in feces via the biliary tract. Half-life of canrenone is 13 to 24 hours.

Indications, dosage, and action
Edema
• *Adult dosage:* 25 to 200 mg P.O. daily in divided doses.
• *Pediatric dosage:* 3.3 mg/kg or 60 mg/m^2 P.O. daily in divided doses initially.

• *Diuretic and potassium-sparing action:* Competitively inhibits aldosterone effects on the distal renal tubules, increasing sodium and water excretion and decreasing potassium excretion.

Hypertension
• *Adult dosage:* 50 to 100 mg P.O. daily in divided doses.
• *Antihypertensive action:* Spironolactone is a weak antihypertensive whose effect is caused by volume depletion; it may also block the effect of aldosterone on arteriolar smooth muscle.

Contraindications and cautions
• Don't use in patients with serum potassium levels above 5.5 mEq/liter.
• Don't use in patients receiving ACE inhibitors, other potassium-sparing diuretics, or potassium supplements because of the potential for hyperkalemia.
• Don't use in anuria, acute or chronic renal insufficiency, or diabetic nephropathy because of the risk of hyperkalemia.
• Use cautiously in severe hepatic insufficiency because electrolyte imbalance may precipitate hepatic encephalopathy.
• Use cautiously in diabetes because of the increased risk of hyperkalemia.
• Be aware that elderly patients are more susceptible to diuretic effects and may require lower dosages to prevent excessive diuresis.
• Because spironolactone's safety during breast-feeding hasn't been established, recommend an alternative feeding method during therapy.
• Pregnancy risk category C

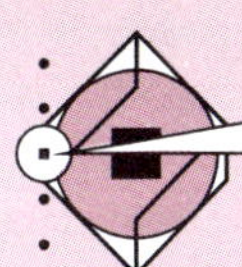

Interactions alert

Life-threatening hazards of multidrug therapy with spironolactone

Interacting drug	Effects
ACE inhibitors (such as captopril and enalapril)	Increase risk of hyperkalemia
Potassium-containing medications (such as parenteral penicillin G)	Increase risk of hyperkalemia
Potassium-sparing diuretics (such as amiloride)	Increase risk of hyperkalemia
Potassium supplements (such as potassium chloride)	Increase risk of hyperkalemia
Salt substitutes (such as Co-salt and Chlor-3 condiments)	Increase risk of hyperkalemia

Life-threatening adverse reactions
- Hyperkalemia

Common adverse reactions
None reported at standard dosages

Infrequent adverse reactions
- Headache
- Anorexia, nausea, diarrhea
- Hyperkalemia, dehydration, hyponatremia, transient rise in BUN level, acidosis
- Urticaria
- Gynecomastia in males, breast soreness and menstrual disturbances in females

Interactions
- *Antihypertensive agents:* May potentiate hypotension; this may be used to therapeutic advantage.
- *Digoxin:* May alter digoxin clearance and increase risk of toxicity. Monitor sodium digoxin levels.
- *NSAIDs, such as indomethacin or ibuprofen:* May impair renal function and thus affect potassium excretion.

For dangerous interactions, see *Life-threatening hazards of multidrug therapy with spironolactone.*

Interventions
Preparation and administration
- Give this drug on a consistent schedule, either with or without meals. (See *Taking spironolactone at home,* page 300.)

Monitoring and supportive care
- Monitor serum electrolyte levels, intake and output, weight, and blood pressure.
- Protect this drug from light.

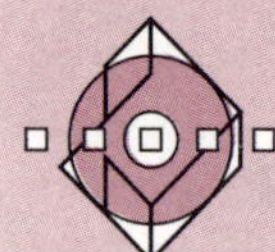

Taking spironolactone at home

In addition to explaining the drug's action and dosage, teach the patient who will continue spironolactone therapy after discharge to follow these important guidelines.

Take your medication correctly
☐ Take spironolactone on a consistent schedule, either with or without meals. Although food does aid absorption, taking the drug without food will be effective as long as you take it consistently without food.
☐ Also take the drug early in the day to prevent interruption of sleep caused by frequent urination at night.
☐ Take spironolactone as prescribed even when you're feeling well. Be aware that the drug may take up to 3 days to produce optimal effects.

Know when to call your doctor
☐ Continue taking the drug even if unpleasant adverse reactions occur because abrupt discontinuation can cause you to retain fluid or can raise your blood pressure. But make sure you discuss any adverse reactions with your doctor.
☐ Remember to report confusion, lethargy, muscle weakness, cramps, numbness or tingling feelings, diarrhea, and an irregular heartbeat to your doctor immediately; these may be signs of an abnormally high potassium level, which can occur with use of spironolactone.

☐ Check with your doctor if you become sick and have severe or continuing nausea, vomiting, or diarrhea. These problems may cause you to lose additional water, which could be harmful, or to lose excessive potassium, which could lessen the medicine's helpful effects.
☐ Monitor your fluid volume by weighing yourself daily and, if so instructed, by measuring and recording your intake and output because spironolactone can cause dehydration. Report a weight gain or loss exceeding 5 lb (2.3 kg) per week.

Other instructions
☐ Don't use potassium supplements, unless otherwise instructed; they can raise your potassium level above normal.
☐ Lie down immediately if dizziness or faintness occurs.
☐ If you're a man, be aware that this drug may cause breast swelling. This effect may or may not disappear when the drug is discontinued.
☐ Check with your doctor or pharmacist before taking OTC medications.
☐ Store spironolactone at room temperature and protect it from moisture, direct light, and heat.

- Be aware that adverse reactions are related to dosage levels and duration of therapy.
- Know that spironolactone therapy alters fluorometric determinations of plasma and urinary 17-hydroxycorticosteroid levels and may cause false elevations of serum digoxin levels on radioimmunoassay.

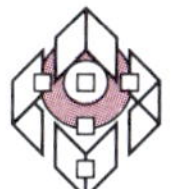

MedTest

---

1. Spironolactone is a diuretic that's further classified as:
   - **a.** acting on the loop of Henle.
   - **b.** a thiazide.
   - **c.** potassium sparing.
   - **d.** a carbonic anhydrase inhibitor.

2. Which adverse effect of spironolactone may not disappear after the drug is withdrawn?
   - **a.** Menstrual irregularities
   - **b.** Gynecomastia
   - **c.** Impotence
   - **d.** Anorexia

3. The maximum antihypertensive response to spironolactone can be expected to occur:
   - **a.** within 1 to 2 hours.
   - **b.** within 13 to 24 hours.
   - **c.** within 3 to 4 days.
   - **d.** within 2 weeks.

Streptokinase

Also known by the brand names Kabikinase and Streptase, streptokinase is classified therapeutically as a thrombolytic enzyme. It's available for injection in vials containing 100,000 IU (in Canada), 250,000 IU, 600,000 IU (in Canada), 750,000 IU, and 1,500,000 IU for reconstitution.

Pharmacokinetics
- *Absorption:* Plasminogen activation begins promptly after infusion or instillation of streptokinase; complete activation of fibrinolytic system occurs in 3 to 4 hours.
- *Distribution:* Doesn't cross placenta but antibodies to drug do.
- *Metabolism:* Insignificant.
- *Excretion:* Removed from circulation by antibodies and reticuloendothelial system. Half-life is biphasic. Terminal elimination half-life is 83 minutes. Fibrinolytic effect may persist for 12 to 24 hours after infusion is discontinued.

Indications, dosage, and action
Lysis of coronary artery thrombi after acute MI
- *Adult dosage:* 1,500,000 IU by I.V. infusion over 60 minutes. Alternatively, drug may be given by intracoronary injection. An intracoronary loading dose of 20,000 IU will be given via coronary catheter, followed by a maintenance dosage of 2,000 to 5,000 IU/minute for 60 minutes as an infusion.

Arteriovenous cannula occlusion
- *Adult dosage:* 250,000 IU in 2 ml of I.V. solution by infusion pump into each occluded limb of the cannula over 25 to 35 minutes. Clamp off cannula for 2 hours; then aspirate contents of cannula, flush with saline solution, and reconnect.

Venous thrombosis, pulmonary embolism, and arterial thrombosis and embolism
• *Adult dosage:* Loading dose of 250,000 IU by I.V. infusion over 30 minutes. Sustaining dosage: 100,000 IU/hour by I.V. infusion for 72 hours for deep vein thrombosis and 100,000 IU/hour over 24 to 72 hours by continuous I.V. infusion for pulmonary embolism.
• *Thrombolytic action:* Streptokinase promotes thrombolysis by activating plasminogen in two steps: 1) plasminogen and streptokinase form a complex, exposing plasminogen-activating sites and 2) cleavage of peptide bond converts plasminogen to plasmin, which hydrolyzes fibrin. The resulting lytic state inhibits further coagulation.

In treatment of acute MI, streptokinase prevents thrombus formation in microcirculation surrounding the necrotic area.

Contraindications and cautions
• Don't use streptokinase in patients with ulcerative wounds, active internal bleeding, recent trauma with possible internal injuries, visceral or intracranial neoplasm, ulcerative colitis, diverticulitis, severe hypertension, acute or chronic hepatic or renal insufficiency, uncontrolled hypocoagulation, chronic pulmonary disease with cavitation, subacute bacterial endocarditis or rheumatic valvular disease, diabetic hemorrhagic retinopathy, or recent cerebral embolism, thrombosis, or hemorrhage because excessive bleeding may occur.

• Administer streptokinase with extreme caution during pregnancy, for 10 days postpartum, and for 10 days after any intracranial, intraspinal, or intra-arterial diagnostic procedure or any surgery.
• Use caution when treating patients with arterial emboli originating in the left side of the heart because of the risk of cerebral infarction.
• The drug should be discontinued if an allergic reaction or severe bleeding occurs.
• Know that patients ages 75 and older have an increased risk of cerebral hemorrhage.
• Be aware that streptokinase may be ineffective in patients who have recently been treated with streptokinase or who have had a recent streptococcal infection.
• Pregnancy risk category C

Life-threatening adverse reactions
• Reperfusion arrhythmias
• Bleeding
• Anaphylaxis

Common adverse reactions
• Fever (up to 21%)

Infrequent adverse reactions
• Transient blood pressure changes
• Minor breathing difficulty, bronchospasms
• Nausea
• Hematuria
• Periorbital edema, gum bleeding
• Spontaneous bleeding, prolonged systemic hypocoagulability, bleeding or oozing from percutaneous trauma site
• Urticaria, ecchymosis

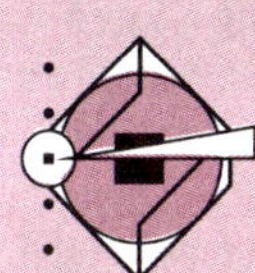

Life-threatening hazards of multidrug therapy with streptokinase

Interacting drug	Effects
Anticoagulants (such as heparin and warfarin)	Increase risk of bleeding
Antiplatelet drugs (such as aspirin)	Increase risk of bleeding

• Local phlebitis at injection site, musculoskeletal pain, drug hypersensitivity, angioedema

Interactions
• *Aminocaproic acid:* Inhibits streptokinase-induced activation of plasminogen.
• *Anticoagulants:* Increased risk of hemorrhage. However, heparin often is used concurrently. Monitor closely.
• *Aspirin, dipyridamole, drugs affecting platelet activity, NSAIDs*: Increased risk of bleeding. However, combined therapy with low-dose aspirin (81 to 325 mg) has improved short- and long-term results.

For dangerous interactions, see *Life-threatening hazards of multidrug therapy with streptokinase.*

Interventions
Preparation and administration
• Reconstitute a vial of the drug with 5 ml of 0.9% NaCl solution, and further dilute the solution to a total of 50 ml; roll gently to mix. Don't shake. Use immediately. Refrigerate the remainder and discard after 24 hours.
• Store powder at room temperature.

• Before using streptokinase to clear an occluded arteriovenous cannula, try flushing with heparinized NaCl solution. (See *Reconstituting streptokinase,* page 304.)

Monitoring and supportive care
• Before initiating therapy, check APTT, PT, thrombin time, fibrinogen level, hematocrit level, and platelet count.
• Monitor patient for excessive bleeding q 15 minutes for the first hour, q 30 minutes for the next 7 hours, and then once every shift. For minor bleeding (as at an I.V. site), apply pressure; for major bleeding (GI, retroperitoneal), stop therapy and notify the doctor. Pretreatment with heparin or drugs affecting platelet count results in a high risk of bleeding but may improve long-term results. Monitor closely.
• Have typed and crossmatched packed RBCs and whole blood ready to treat possible hemorrhage.

Safety tip. Keep aminocaproic acid available to treat bleeding.

• If minor bleeding can be controlled by local pressure, don't decrease the dose because that makes more plas-

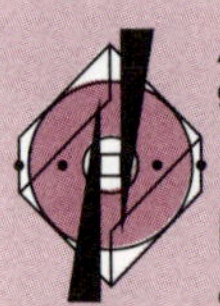

Administration guidelines

Reconstituting streptokinase

To reconstitute streptokinase, follow these four steps:
• Slowly add 5 ml of 0.9% NaCl solution or D₅W, directing the stream toward the side of the vial rather than into the powder.
• Gently roll and tilt the vial for reconstitution to liquid form. *Don't* shake the vial because this drug requires careful preparation to prevent undue foaming and increased flocculation.
• Slowly dilute the contents of the vial with an additional 45 ml of solution to a total of 50 ml. If necessary, redilute up to 500 ml in 50-ml increments.
• If you aren't administering the drug soon after reconstitution, store it at 35.6° to 39.2° F (2° to 4° C) and use within 24 hours.

minogen available for conversion to plasmin.

Safety tip. Maintain the involved extremity in straight alignment to prevent bleeding from the infusion site.

Safety tip. Monitor pulses and color of and sensation in extremities every hour.

• Keep venipuncture sites to a minimum and use pressure dressings on puncture sites for at least 30 minutes.
• Know that I.M. injections and other invasive procedures are contraindicated during streptokinase therapy.

Safety tip. Bruising is more likely during therapy; avoid unnecessary handling of the patient and pad the side rails of the bed.
• Keep a laboratory flow sheet on the patient's chart to monitor APTT, PT, and hemoglobin and hematocrit levels.

Safety tip. Watch for signs of hypersensitivity. Notify the doctor immediately. If a severe reaction occurs, stop the infusion immediately.
• Know that therapy need not be discontinued for minor allergic reactions that can be treated with antihistamines or corticosteroids.
• About one-third of patients experience a slight fever, and some have chills. You may give acetaminophen (but not aspirin or other salicylates) if the patient's temperature reaches 104° F (40° C). Patients may be pretreated with corticosteroids and may receive repeat doses during therapy to minimize pyrogenic or allergic reactions.
• Heparin by continuous infusion is usually started within an hour after stopping streptokinase. Use an infusion pump to administer heparin.
• Know that thrombolytic therapy in patients with acute MI may decrease infarct size, improve ventricular function, and decrease incidence of CHF. Streptokinase must be administered within 6 hours of the onset of symptoms for optimal effect.
• Know that antibodies to streptokinase can persist for 6 months or longer after the initial dose; if additional thrombolytic therapy is needed, alteplase or urokinase should be considered.
• Know that streptokinase increases thrombin time, APTT, and PT and

sometimes moderately decreases hematocrit levels.

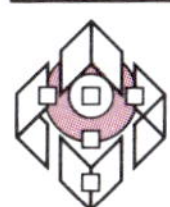 **MedTest**

1. Before initiating streptokinase therapy, you should determine:
    a. APTT, PT, and thrombin time.
    b. Lee-White coagulation and bleeding times.
    c. cardiac isoenzyme levels.
    d. ECG changes and cardiac rhythm.

2. If your patient receiving streptokinase develops a fever above 104° F (40° C), you should:
    a. stop therapy immediately.
    b. treat with aspirin.
    c. treat with ibuprofen.
    d. treat with acetaminophen.

3. If major bleeding occurs while the patient is receiving streptokinase, you should:
    a. discontinue therapy and notify the doctor.
    b. treat immediately with aminocaproic acid.
    c. administer packed RBCs.
    d. administer whole blood.

Timolol maleate

Also known by the brand names Blocadren and Apo-Timol (in Canada), timolol is a beta blocker that's classified therapeutically as an antihypertensive agent, an adjunct in treating MI, and an antiglaucoma agent. It's available in 5-, 10-, and 20-mg tablets.

Pharmacokinetics
• *Absorption:* About 90% of an oral dose is absorbed from GI tract; peak plasma concentration occurs in 1 to 2 hours.
• *Distribution:* Depending on assay method used, 10% to 60% protein-bound.
• *Metabolism:* About 80% metabolized in liver to inactive metabolites.
• *Excretion:* Timolol and its metabolites excreted primarily in urine; half-life is approximately 4 hours.

Indications, dosage, and action
Hypertension
• *Adult dosage:* Initially, 10 mg P.O. b.i.d. Usual daily maintenance dosage is 20 to 40 mg. Maximum daily dosage is 60 mg.
• *Antihypertensive action:* The exact mechanism of timolol's antihypertensive effect is unknown. Timolol may reduce blood pressure by blocking adrenergic receptors (thus decreasing cardiac output), by decreasing sympathetic outflow from the CNS, and by suppressing renin release.

Reduction of mortality and reinfarction after MI
• *Adult dosage:* 10 mg P.O. b.i.d. initiated within 4 weeks of MI.

Angina
• *Adult dosage:* 15 to 45 mg P.O. daily given t.i.d.
• *Antianginal and MI prophylactic action:* Decreases heart rate, peripheral vascular resistance, and myocardial work, thereby decreasing myocardial oxygen consumption. Mechanism by which it decreases mortality after MI is unknown.

Contraindications and cautions

- Don't use in severe bronchial asthma, allergic bronchospasm, severe COPD, severe bradycardia, overt cardiac failure, second- or third-degree AV block, or cardiogenic shock. The drug may worsen these conditions.
- Use cautiously in impaired hepatic or renal function because of the potential for drug accumulation.
- Use with caution in depressed left ventricular function because beta blockade may precipitate CHF.
- Use cautiously in diabetes mellitus because the drug may mask some signs of hypoglycemia.
- Discontinue if signs of heart failure or bronchospasm develop.
- Use cautiously in elderly patients, who may experience exacerbated adverse reactions. Also, the drug's half-life may be prolonged in elderly patients.
- Because timolol is distributed into breast milk, avoid using it in breast-feeding women.
- Pregnancy risk category C

Life-threatening adverse reactions

- CHF
- Bronchospasm

Common adverse reactions

- Bradycardia, cold extremities
- Increased airway resistance
- Dizziness, fatigue
- Nausea

Infrequent adverse reactions

- Hypotension, peripheral vascular insufficiency
- Pulmonary edema, wheezing, dyspnea
- Lethargy, vivid dreams
- Vomiting, diarrhea
- Impotence
- Rash, pruritus
- Fever

Interactions

- *Beta-adrenergic stimulants, methylxanthines such as theophylline*: Timolol may antagonize effects of xanthines or beta-adrenergic stimulants.
- *Digitalis glycosides:* Both drugs may prolong PR interval, cause excessive bradycardia, and increase potential for cardiac arrhythmias. Use together cautiously.
- *Indomethacin, NSAIDs:* Decreased antihypertensive effect. Monitor blood pressure.
- *Insulin, oral antidiabetic drugs:* Can alter requirements for these drugs in previously stabilized diabetic patients. Monitor for hypoglycemia.

  For dangerous interactions, see *Life-threatening hazards of multidrug therapy with timolol.*

Interventions

Preparation and administration

- Always check the patient's apical pulse rate before giving this drug. If you detect extremes in pulse rates, withhold the medication and notify the doctor. (See *Taking beta-adrenergic blockers at home,* page 63.)

Monitoring and supportive care

- Monitor blood pressure frequently.
- Dosage should be increased only after a 7-day interval on the previous dosage.
- This drug masks common signs of hypoglycemia such as tachycardia.

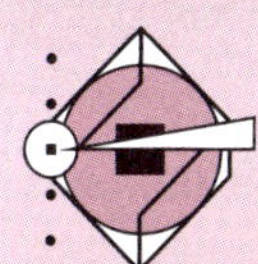

Life-threatening hazards of multidrug therapy with timolol

Interacting drug	Effects
Antihypertensive agents (such as reserpine)	Increase risk of hypotension
Calcium channel blockers (such as verapamil)	Increase risk of prolonged PR interval and decrease cardiac output
General anesthetics (such as halothane)	May cause excessive hypotension

Monitor for diaphoresis and CNS signs, such as mental status changes, restlessness, irritability, and dizziness.
• You may need to adjust the dosage for a patient with renal or hepatic impairment.
• Don't discontinue the drug abruptly. Reduce the dosage gradually over 1 to 2 weeks.
• Know that timolol also is used in an optical solution to treat glaucoma.
• Be aware that timolol may slightly increase BUN, serum potassium, uric acid, and blood glucose levels and may slightly decrease hemoglobin and hematocrit levels.

MedTest

1. Which of the following groups of patients may require adjustment of timolol dosage?
  a. Those with bronchial asthma
  b. Those with diabetes mellitus
  c. Those with cardiomyopathy
  d. Those with hepatic or renal impairment

2. Since timolol masks beta-adrenergic signs of hypoglycemia in the diabetic patient, you should monitor for CNS signs, such as:
  a. depression.
  b. euphoria.
  c. somnolence.
  d. restlessness.

3. Your patient's timolol is to be discontinued. This should be accomplished over a period of:
  a. 1 to 2 days.
  b. 3 to 5 days.
  c. 1 to 2 weeks.
  d. 1 to 2 months.

Tocainide hydrochloride

Also known by the brand name Tonocard, tocainide is a local anesthetic (amide type) that's classified therapeutically as a ventricular anti-arrhythmic agent. It's available in 400- and 600-mg tablets.

Pharmacokinetics

• *Absorption:* Rapidly and completely absorbed from GI tract; unlike lidocaine, it undergoes negligible first-pass effect in the liver. Peak serum levels occur in 30 minutes to 2 hours after oral administration. Bioavailability is nearly 100%.
• *Distribution:* Less lipophilic than lidocaine. Only 10% to 20% bound to plasma protein.
• *Metabolism:* In the liver to inactive metabolites.
• *Excretion:* In urine as unchanged drug and inactive metabolites (30% to 50%). Elimination half-life is 11 to 23 hours.

Indications, dosage, and action

Suppression of symptomatic ventricular arrhythmias, including frequent PVCs
• *Adult dosage:* Initially, 400 mg P.O. q 8 hours. Usual dosage is between 1,200 and 1,800 mg/day divided t.i.d.
• *Antiarrhythmic action:* Structurally similar to lidocaine, with similar electrophysiologic and hemodynamic effects. A class Ib antiarrhythmic, it suppresses automaticity and shortens the effective refractory period and action potential duration of His-Purkinje fibers and suppresses spontaneous ventricular depolarization. Tocainide doesn't significantly affect AV conduction or alter hemodynamics. It exerts its effects on the conduction system, causing inhibition of reentry mechanisms and cessation of ventricular arrhythmias;

these effects may be more pronounced in ischemic tissue.

Contraindications and cautions

• Don't use in patients with second- or third-degree AV block who don't have a pacemaker because the drug may further decrease conduction.
• Don't use in patients with hypersensitivity to amide-type anesthetic agents, including lidocaine.
• Use with caution in CHF.
• Use cautiously in atrial flutter or ventricular fibrillation because the drug may accelerate the ventricular rate.
• Use with caution in preexisting bone marrow failure or cytopenia because the drug may cause adverse hematologic effects.
• Use cautiously in severe renal or hepatic dysfunction because drug may accumulate and cause toxicity.
• Expect the drug to be discontinued if adverse hematologic, pulmonary, or cardiac reactions occur.
• Use with caution in elderly patients and monitor them closely.
• It's unknown whether tocainide is excreted in breast milk. As a precaution, recommend an alternative feeding method to breast-feeding women.
• Pregnancy risk category C

Life-threatening adverse reactions

• CHF, new or worsened arrhythmias
• Respiratory arrest, pulmonary edema or fibrosis, interstitial pneumonia
• Aplastic anemia, agranulocytosis

Common adverse reactions

• Dizziness
• Nausea (15%), vomiting
• Diaphoresis

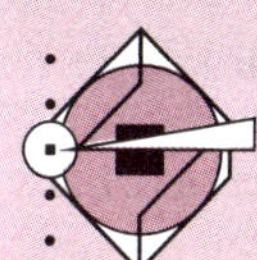

Interactions alert

Life-threatening hazards of multidrug therapy with tocainide

Interacting drug	Effects
Antiarrhythmic agents (such as quinidine)	Increase risk of life-threatening arrhythmias
Beta blockers (such as metoprolol)	May cause bradycardia and decreased myocardial contractility
Lidocaine (antiarrhythmic agent)	May cause CNS toxicity

Infrequent adverse reactions
- Hypotension, conduction disturbances, arrhythmias, bradycardia, palpitations, chest pain
- Cough, wheezing, dyspnea, pulmonary fibrosis
- Asthenia, light-headedness, tremors, restlessness, paresthesia, confusion, headache, altered mood, akinesia, anxiety
- Epigastric pain, constipation, diarrhea, anorexia
- Blurred vision
- Rash

Interactions
For dangerous interactions, see *Life-threatening hazards of multidrug therapy with tocainide.*

Interventions
Preparation and administration
- Minimize GI reactions by administering this drug with food. (See *Taking antiarrhythmics at home,* page 74.)

Monitoring and supportive care
- Use cautiously in patients with hepatic or renal impairment. Dosage adjustment may be necessary.
- Monitor blood levels; therapeutic levels range from 4 to 10 mcg/ml.
- Monitor blood counts periodically.
- Observe the patient for tremors, an early sign of toxicity.
- Be aware that tocainide may be used to ease transition from I.V. lidocaine to oral antiarrhythmic therapy. **Safety tip.** Monitor the patient and his ECG carefully during this transition period.
- Instruct the patient to report any unusual bleeding or bruising; signs of infection, such as fever, sore throat, stomatitis, or chills; or pulmonary symptoms, such as cough, wheezing, or exertional dyspnea.
- Know that elderly patients are more likely to experience dizziness and should have assistance while walking.

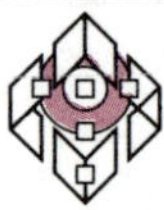 **MedTest**

1. Tocainide is an amide antiarrhythmic and may be used:
   a. instead of I.V. lidocaine.
   b. to ease transition from I.V. lidocaine to oral antiarrhythmic therapy.
   c. to treat supraventricular tachyarrhythmias.
   d. to manage AV blocks of all degrees.

2. Which of the following is an early sign of tocainide toxicity?
   a. Rash
   b. Anxiety
   c. Tremors
   d. Blurred vision

3. A patient who is given tocainide at the same time that he's receiving a lidocaine infusion may experience:
   a. CHF.
   b. urinary retention.
   c. CNS toxicity.
   d. respiratory arrest.

Torsemide

Also known by the brand name Demadex, torsemide is a loop diuretic similar to furosemide that's therapeutically classified as an antihypertensive agent and as a diuretic used for the treatment of edema associated with CHF, cirrhosis, or renal failure. It's available in 5-, 10-, 20-, and 100-mg tablets and for injection in 10-mg/ml vials containing 2 and 5 ml.

Pharmacokinetics
• *Absorption:* Rapidly absorbed following oral administration, with peak plasma levels reached in 1 to 2 hours.
• *Distribution:* Highly lipophilic; 97% to 99% is bound to plasma proteins. Peak blood level occurs 1 hour after oral administration; active-metabolite peak blood levels occur in 1 to 2 hours. Maximum diuresis occurs 15 to 40 minutes after I.V. administration and 1 to 4 hours after oral administration.
• *Metabolism:* By the liver. Three metabolites have been identified, two of which are active. Neither of these exerts a half-life longer than torsemide itself. In patients with hepatic dysfunction, torsemide levels peak later and half-life is increased.
• *Excretion:* About 27% of drug is excreted unchanged in urine, as are most of its active and inactive metabolites. Half-life is 3 to 4 hours, and duration of action, 6 hours.

Indications, dosage, and action
Mild to moderate essential hypertension
• *Adult dosage:* 2.5 to 5 mg P.O. daily in a single a.m. dose. (Increasing dose to 10 or 15 mg doesn't result in additional antihypertensive effect.) Maximal effect may not occur for 12 to 16 weeks.

Edema associated with CHF, cor pulmonale, or cirrhosis
• *Adult dosage:* 10 to 20 mg daily in a single a.m. dose I.V. or P.O., with incremental increases of 10 mg as

needed. In patients with cirrhosis, a daily dose as low as 5 mg is an effective recommended starting dose.

Edema associated with renal failure
• *Adult dosage:* 100, 200, or 400 mg daily in divided doses P.O., or 100 to 200 mg I.V.
• *Action:* Loop diuretics inhibit sodium and chloride reabsorption in the proximal (thick) part of the ascending loop of Henle, promoting the excretion of sodium, water, chloride, and potassium. Torsemide produces renal and peripheral vasodilation and may temporarily increase glomerular filtration rate and decrease peripheral vascular resistance.

Contraindications and cautions
• Don't use in anuria, hepatic coma, or electrolyte depletion.
• Use cautiously in patients with increasing BUN and serum creatinine levels or oliguria, despite the drug's use as a diuretic in patients with renal impairment.
• Use cautiously in patients allergic to sulfonamides, including furosemide, because cross-sensitivity may occur.
• Use with caution in patients with hepatic cirrhosis and ascites because electrolyte alterations may precipitate hepatic encephalopathy.
• Use cautiously in patients receiving digitalis glycosides because diuretic-induced hypokalemia may predispose them to digitalis toxicity.
• Be aware that rapid I.V. administration and high dosage may increase the risk of ototoxicity (although this hasn't been observed in clinical studies to date).
• Use cautiously in hepatic or renal disease.
• Know that elderly and debilitated patients require close observation because they're more susceptible to drug-induced diuresis. Reduced dosages may be indicated.
• Don't give to breast-feeding women.
• Pregnancy risk category B

Life-threatening adverse reactions
• Profound electrolyte and volume depletion, dehydration

Common adverse reactions
• Dehydration and severe electrolyte abnormalities

Infrequent adverse reactions
• Orthostatic hypotension
• Dizziness, headache, fatigue
• Electrolyte imbalances, including hyponatremia, hypochloremia, and hypokalemia
• Tinnitus
• Rash
• Muscle cramps, back pain

Interactions
• *Antihypertensive agents:* Increased risk of hypotension. Use together cautiously.
• *Digoxin:* Torsemide-induced hypokalemia may predispose patients to digitalis toxicity.
• *Indomethacin, NSAIDs, probenecid:* Inhibited diuretic response. Use cautiously.
• *Nephrotoxic* or *ototoxic drugs:* Concomitant administration with

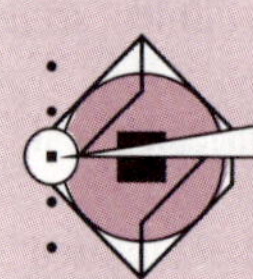

Interactions alert

Life-threatening hazards of multidrug therapy with torsemide

Interacting drug	Effects
Amphotericin B (antibiotic)	May cause severe potassium loss
Corticosteroids (such as prednisone)	May cause severe potassium loss
Lithium (antidepressant)	May cause severe potassium loss and increased lithium levels

such drugs may result in enhanced toxicity.

For dangerous interactions, see *Life-threatening hazards of multidrug therapy with torsemide.*

Interventions

Preparation and administration

• Give I.V. torsemide slowly, over 1 or 2 minutes. For intermittent infusion, give diluted drug through an intermittent infusion device or piggyback it into an I.V. line containing a free-flowing compatible solution. Infuse at the prescribed rate. Continuous infusion isn't needed.

• Give the oral form in the morning to prevent nocturia. If a second dose is necessary, give it in the early afternoon or by 6 p.m. at the latest to prevent nocturia. (See *Taking loop diuretics at home,* page 98.)

Monitoring and supportive care

• Monitor serum electrolyte, BUN, CO_2, and serum creatinine levels frequently, and monitor the patient for symptoms of dehydration or hypoten-

sion. Report such symptoms to the doctor because the drug may need to be discontinued if dehydration or hypotension occurs or if BUN and serum creatinine levels rise.

• Monitor for manifestations of overdose, including profound electrolyte and volume depletion.

• Torsemide potentiates the antihypertensive effect of most other antihypertensive agents and other diuretics; both actions are used to therapeutic advantage.

• Torsemide is longer acting and may affect potassium levels to a lesser degree than other loop diuretics. Still, monitor serum potassium levels and watch for signs of hypokalemia (for example, muscle weakness and cramps).

Safety tip. Patients also receiving digoxin have an increased risk of digitalis toxicity from the potassium-depleting effect of this diuretic. Monitor these patients carefully.

Safety tip. Consult with the doctor and dietitian to provide a high-potassium diet if indicated.

Foods rich in potassium include citrus fruits, tomatoes, bananas, dates, and apricots.
• Periodically monitor calcium, magnesium, uric acid, and triglyceride levels for elevations.
• Monitor for ototoxicity.

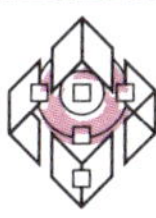 **MedTest**

1. Torsemide is pharmacologically classified as a:
  a. thiazide diuretic.
  b. potassium-sparing diuretic.
  c. mercurial diuretic.
  d. loop diuretic.

2. Torsemide's advantage over other drugs in its class may be that it:
  a. is less potassium wasting.
  b. requires lower dosages.
  c. is much longer acting.
  d. reaches maximal activity in a shorter time.

3. Which adverse reaction (though undocumented) should you watch for when giving torsemide at high doses or by rapid I.V. infusion?
  a. Orthostatic hypotension
  b. Ototoxicity
  c. Dizziness
  d. Hypokalemia

Triamterene

Also known by the brand name Dyrenium and (in Australia) Dytac, triamterene is a potassium-sparing diuretic that's classified therapeutically as a diuretic agent. It's available in 50- and 100-mg capsules.

Pharmacokinetics
• *Absorption:* Rapidly absorbed after oral administration, but extent of absorption varies. Diuresis usually begins in 2 to 4 hours.
• *Distribution:* About 67% protein-bound.
• *Metabolism:* By the liver.
• *Excretion:* Triamterene and its metabolites are excreted in urine; half-life of triamterene is 100 to 150 minutes.

Indications, dosage, and action
Diuresis
• *Adult dosage:* Initially, 100 mg P.O. b.i.d. p.c. Total daily dosage should not exceed 300 mg.
• *Diuretic action:* Acts directly on the distal renal tubules to inhibit sodium reabsorption and potassium excretion, reducing the potassium loss associated with other diuretics.

Triamterene is commonly used with other more effective diuretics to treat edema associated with excessive aldosterone secretion, hepatic cirrhosis, nephrotic syndrome, or CHF.

Contraindications and cautions
• Don't use in patients with serum potassium levels above 5.5 mEq/liter.
• Don't use in patients receiving ACE inhibitors, other potassium-sparing diuretics, or potassium supplements because of the potential for hyperkalemia.
• Don't use in anuria, acute or chronic renal insufficiency, or diabetic ne-

phropathy because the drug may worsen these conditions.
- Use cautiously in severe hepatic insufficiency because electrolyte imbalance may precipitate hepatic encephalopathy.
- Use with caution in diabetes mellitus because of the increased risk of hyperkalemia.
- Use with caution in debilitated or elderly patients and children; they may be more susceptible to hyperkalemia.
- Know that this drug may be excreted in breast milk; recommend alternative infant-feeding methods.
- Pregnancy risk category B

Life-threatening adverse reactions
- Hyperkalemia

Common adverse reactions
None reported at standard dosages

Infrequent adverse reactions
- Hypotension
- Dizziness
- Nausea, vomiting
- Sore throat, dry mouth
- Megaloblastic anemia related to low folic acid levels
- Dehydration, hyponatremia, transient rise in BUN levels, acidosis
- Photosensitivity, rash
- Muscle cramps

Interactions
- *ACE inhibitors, other potassium-sparing diuretics, potassium supplements:* Increased risk of hyperkalemia. Avoid concomitant use.
- *Indomethacin, NSAIDs:* May alter renal function, affecting potassium excretion. Avoid concomitant use.
- *Lithium:* May decrease lithium clearance.
- *Quinidine:* May interfere with some laboratory tests that measure quinidine levels. Inform laboratory that patient is taking triamterene.

Interventions
Preparation and administration
- Give this medication p.c. to prevent nausea. (See *Taking triamterene at home.*)

Monitoring and supportive care
- Monitor blood pressure and BUN and serum electrolytes levels.
- Know that triamterene is a potassium-sparing diuretic that's useful as an adjunct to other diuretic therapy. It's less potent than thiazide or loop diuretics.
- Know that triamterene is usually used with potassium-wasting diuretics. Its full effect is delayed 2 to 3 days when it's used alone.
- Assess for blood dyscrasias.
- Know that triamterene therapy may interfere with enzyme assays that use fluorometry, such as serum quinidine determinations.

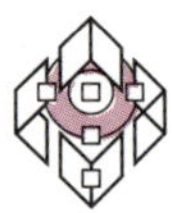 **MedTest**

---

1. Triamterene should be administered:
    a. a.c. to enhance absorption.
    b. with meals to enhance absorption.

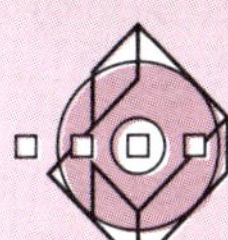

Patient-teaching checklist

Taking triamterene at home

In addition to explaining the drug's action and dosage, teach the patient who will continue triamterene therapy after discharge to follow these important guidelines.

Take your medication correctly

☐ Take triamterene after meals to prevent nausea.

☐ Take the drug early in the day to prevent disruption of sleep caused by frequent urination at night.

☐ Take triamterene as prescribed even when you're feeling well. Be aware that the drug may take up to 3 days to produce optimal effects.

Watch for adverse reactions

☐ Continue taking the drug even if unpleasant adverse reactions occur because abrupt discontinuation can cause you to retain fluid again. But make sure you discuss any adverse reactions with your doctor.

☐ Remember to report confusion, lethargy, muscle weakness, cramps, numbness and tingling, diarrhea, and an irregular heartbeat to your doctor immediately because these may be signs of an abnormally high potassium level, which can occur with use of triamterene.

☐ Monitor your fluid volume by weighing yourself daily and (if so instructed) measuring and recording your intake and output because triamterene can cause dehydration.

☐ Don't use potassium supplements because they can cause your potassium level to rise above normal levels.

☐ Lie down immediately if dizziness or faintness occurs.

☐ Avoid driving or operating machinery until you've adjusted to the drug's effects.

Other instructions

☐ Protect your skin from sunlight as much as possible because potassium-sparing diuretics such as triamterene may cause a rash, itching, redness or other discoloration of the skin, or even severe sunburn from brief exposure to sunlight. When sun exposure cannot be avoided, wear protective clothing, including a hat, and apply a sun block to your skin and lips that has a sun protection factor (SPF) of at least 15.

☐ Also check with your doctor or pharmacist before taking OTC medications.

☐ Store triamterene at room temperature and protect it from moisture, direct light, and heat.

---

c. p.c. to prevent nausea.
d. without regard to meals.

2. When initiating triamterene therapy, while adjusting dosage, and periodically throughout therapy, you should monitor:

   a. blood pressure and BUN and serum electrolyte levels.

b. cardiac rate and rhythm and ECG waveforms.
c. serum creatinine and creatinine clearance levels.
d. folic acid levels.

3. If the patient's folic acid level falls, he is at risk for:
  a. thrombocytopenia.
  b. agranulocytosis.
  c. hemolytic anemia.
  d. megaloblastic anemia.

Verapamil hydrochloride

Also known by the brand names Calan, Calan SR, Isoptin, Isoptin SR, Verelan, and (in Australia) Cordilox Oral and Veradil, verapamil is a calcium channel blocker that's classified therapeutically as an antianginal, antihypertensive, and antiarrhythmic agent. It's available in 40-, 80-, and 120-mg tablets; in 120-, 180-, and 240-mg extended-release tablets; in 120-, 180-, and 240-mg extended-release capsules; and for injection in 2.5-mg/ml vials.

Pharmacokinetics

• *Absorption:* Rapidly and completely absorbed from GI tract after oral administration; however, only 20% to 35% of drug reaches systemic circulation because of first-pass effect. When administered orally, peak effects occur within 1 to 2 hours with conventional tablets and within 4 to 8 hours with extended-release preparations. When administered I.V., effects occur within minutes after injection and usually persist 30 to 60 minutes (although they may last up to 6 hours).

• *Distribution:* Steady state distribution volume in healthy adults ranges from about 4.5 to 7 liters/kg but may increase to 12 liters/kg in patients with hepatic cirrhosis. About 90% of circulating drug is bound to plasma proteins.

• *Metabolism:* In the liver to active and inactive metabolites.

• *Excretion:* In urine as unchanged drug and active metabolites. Elimination half-life is normally 6 to 12 hours but increases to as much as 16 hours in patients with hepatic cirrhosis. In infants, elimination half-life may be 5 to 7 hours.

Indications, dosage, and action
Prinzmetal's, unstable, chronic, or stable angina

• *Adult dosage:* Initially, 80 mg P.O. t.i.d. or q.i.d. Dosage may be increased at weekly intervals. Some patients may require up to 480 mg daily.

• *Antianginal action:* Causes vasodilation, which reduces afterload and decreases myocardial oxygen consumption. In patients with Prinzmetal's variant angina, verapamil inhibits coronary artery spasm, resulting in increased myocardial oxygen delivery.

Acute supraventricular tachyarrhythmias

• *Adult dosage:* 0.075 to 0.15 mg/kg (5 to 10 mg) by I.V. push over 2 minutes with ECG and blood pressure monitoring. If no response occurs, a second dose of 10 mg (0.15 mg/kg)

may be given 15 to 30 minutes after the initial dose.
• *Pediatric dosage:* Ages 1 to 15, 0.3 to 1 mg/kg (2 to 5 mg) as I.V. bolus over 2 minutes. Dose shouldn't exceed 5 mg. Dose may be repeated in 30 minutes if no response occurs, but it shouldn't exceed 10 mg.

Younger than age 1, 0.1 to 0.2 mg/kg (0.75 to 2 mg) as I.V. bolus over 2 minutes. Dose may be repeated in 30 minutes if no response occurs.

Prevention of recurrent PSVT
• *Adult dosage:* 240 to 480 mg P.O. daily in three or four divided doses.

Control of ventricular rate in chronic atrial flutter or fibrillation
• *Adult dosage:* 240 to 320 mg P.O. daily in three to four divided doses.
• *Antiarrhythmic action:* Combined effects on SA and AV nodes help manage arrhythmias. Drug's primary effect is on AV node; slowed conduction reduces ventricular rate in atrial tachyarrhythmias and blocks reentry paths in PSVTs.

Hypertension
• *Adult dosage:* Usual starting dose is 80 mg P.O. t.i.d. Dosage may be increased at weekly intervals. Initiate therapy with extended-release tablets or capsules at 240 mg daily in a.m. or p.m. Adjust dosage based on clinical effectiveness 24 hours after dosing. Increase by 120 mg daily until maximum dose of 480 mg daily is given. Most patients respond to 240 mg daily. Extended-release capsules should be given only once daily. Extended-release tablets in daily dos-

ages greater than 240 mg should be given b.i.d. Elderly patients or those of small stature may do better with smaller doses (120 mg) P.O. b.i.d. Antihypertensive effects are usually seen within first week of therapy.
• *Antihypertensive action:* Reduces blood pressure mainly by dilating peripheral vessels.

Contraindications and cautions
• Don't use verapamil in patients with severe hypotension or cardiogenic shock because of the drug's antihypertensive effect.
• Don't use in patients with second- or third-degree AV block or SSS (unless a pacemaker is in place) because of the drug's effects on the cardiac conduction system.
• Use cautiously in patients with ventricular dysfunction or AV abnormalities who are receiving beta blockers because of the drug's negative inotropic effect and slowing of the cardiac conduction system.
• Use all forms with caution in left ventricular dysfunction or heart failure because the drug may precipitate or worsen these conditions.
• Use cautiously in patients with idiopathic hypertrophic cardiomyopathy, wide QRS complex, VT, SSS, or atrial fibrillation or flutter with an accessory bypass tract (such as WPW or Lown-Ganong-Levine syndrome) because the drug may cause serious and sometimes fatal adverse CV effects.
• Use with caution in patients with hepatic or renal impairment because the drug may accumulate.
• Use cautiously in patients receiving the drug I.V. because of possible adverse hemodynamic effects (hypoten-

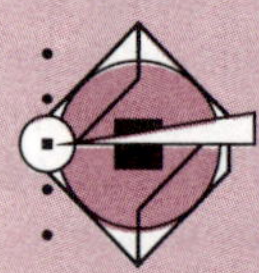

Life-threatening hazards of multidrug therapy with verapamil

Interacting drug	Effects
Beta blockers (such as propranolol and ophthalmic timolol)	May cause additive effects leading to CHF, conduction disturbances, arrhythmias, and hypotension
Carbamazepine (anticonvulsant agent)	Increases serum carbamazepine levels, posing risk of carbamazepine toxicity
Digoxin (digitalis glycoside)	Increases serum digoxin levels, posing risk of digitalis toxicity
Disopyramide (antiarrhythmic agent)	Combines negative inotropic effects, increasing the risk of CHF

sion) and adverse cardiac effects (such as bradycardia and heart block).
• Discontinue the drug if systolic pressure falls below 90 mm Hg, if heart failure worsens, or if arrhythmias, hemodynamically significant bradycardia, or second- or third-degree AV block occurs.
• Be aware that elderly patients may require lower dosages.
• Because the drug is excreted in breast milk, avoid use in breast-feeding women.
• Pregnancy risk category C

Life-threatening adverse reactions
• Ventricular asystole, CHF

Common adverse reactions
• Constipation

Infrequent adverse reactions
• Transient hypotension, heart failure, bradycardia, AV block, peripheral edema
• Pulmonary edema
• Dizziness, headache, fatigue
• Nausea (primarily with oral form), elevated liver enzyme levels
• Rash, flushing

Interactions
• *Antihypertensive agents, quinidine:* May cause hypotension. Monitor blood pressure daily.
• *Lithium:* Verapamil may decrease serum lithium levels. Monitor serum lithium levels closely.
• *Rifampin:* May decrease oral bioavailability of verapamil. Monitor patient for lack of effect.

For dangerous interactions, see *Life-threatening hazards of multidrug therapy with verapamil.* Also see *Verapamil combinations to avoid.*

Interventions
Preparation and administration
• Administer I.V. doses over at least 3 minutes to minimize the risk of adverse reactions.
• Know that giving extended-release tablets (but not capsules) with food may decrease the rate and extent of absorption but will result in smaller fluctuations of peak and trough blood levels.
• Be aware that generic extended-release verapamil tablets may be substituted only for Isoptin SR and Calan SR, but not for Verelan.
• Remember that the extended-release capsule formulation should be given only once daily.
• When using extended-release tablets, daily doses over 240 mg should be given b.i.d. (See *Taking verapamil at home,* page 320.)

Monitoring and supportive care
• If the patient is receiving I.V. verapamil, monitor his ECG and blood pressure continuously.

Safety tip. Administration of I.V. calcium may be useful in attenuating the antihypertensive effects of I.V. verapamil.
• Monitor blood pressure at the start of oral therapy and during dosage adjustments.

Safety tip. Help the patient walk because dizziness may occur.
• Be aware that if verapamil is being used to terminate supraventricular tachycardia, the doctor may have the

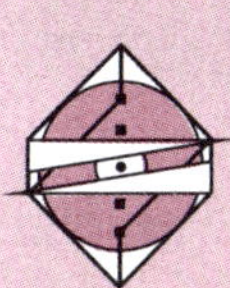

Be aware that verapamil is only compatible with parenteral solutions having a pH of 3 to 6. In solutions with a pH greater than 6, the drug will precipitate.

Verapamil is also incompatible with human albumin (cloudiness occurs), hydralazine hydrochloride (color changes to yellow), and amphotericin B or co-trimoxazole (precipitation occurs).

patient perform vagal maneuvers before or after receiving the drug.
• During long-term combination therapy with verapamil and digoxin, monitor the patient's ECG periodically to observe for AV block and bradycardia because of this drug's possible additive effects on the AV node.
• Know that patients with severely compromised cardiac function and those receiving beta blockers should receive lower verapamil doses. Monitor these patients closely.

Safety tip. Don't administer I.V. beta blockers at the same time as I.V. verapamil.
• The dosage in patients with renal or hepatic impairment should be reduced.
• Monitor liver function test results.
• Disopyramide should be discontinued 48 hours before starting verapamil therapy and reinstituted 24 hours after verapamil has been discontinued.

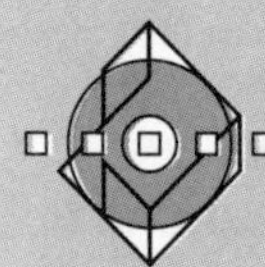

Patient-teaching checklist

Taking verapamil at home

In addition to explaining the drug's action and dosage, teach the patient who will continue verapamil therapy after discharge to follow these important guidelines.

Take your medication correctly

☐ Take short-acting verapamil on an empty stomach.

☐ Swallow the extended-release form of the drug whole (tablet or capsule). Don't crush or chew the extended-release form of the drug; however, you may break it. You may be instructed to take the tablet form with food to establish steadier drug levels in your blood.

☐ Take extended-release capsules only once daily (morning or evening). Extended-release tablets may be taken once or twice daily as prescribed.

☐ Keep in mind that you must not substitute a generic form of verapamil for Verelan capsules.

☐ Take verapamil as prescribed even when you're feeling well.

Consult with your doctor

☐ Continue taking the drug even if unpleasant adverse reactions occur because abrupt discontinuation may worsen angina or hypertension. But make sure you discuss any adverse reactions, especially swelling of your hands or feet or shortness of breath, with your doctor.

☐ If your doctor wants you to continue taking a prescribed nitrate at the beginning of verapamil therapy, it's important that you do so. Sublingual nitroglycerin, especially, may be taken as needed when anginal symptoms are acute.

Minimize adverse reactions

☐ Remember to change positions slowly (especially from lying flat to sitting upright) and to dangle your legs over the bedside for a few minutes before standing to minimize dizziness caused by the drug.

☐ Lie down immediately if dizziness or faintness occurs.

☐ Avoid driving or operating machinery until you've adjusted to the drug's effects.

☐ Restrict fluid and salt intake, if so instructed, to minimize fluid retention.

☐ Be aware that a headache may occur for a short time following each dose of verapamil. Take a mild analgesic such as acetaminophen as needed. The headache should become less noticeable after you've taken the drug for a while. If you continue experiencing headaches or they become severe, tell your doctor.

Other instructions

☐ Schedule daily activities to allow for adequate rest periods.

☐ Increase dietary fiber and fluid intake (if not contraindicated) to help prevent constipation.

☐ Check with your doctor or pharmacist before taking OTC medications.

• Assess for, report, and urge the patient to report signs of CHF, such as swelling of hands and feet or shortness of breath.
• Encourage the patient who is receiving nitrate therapy while his verapamil dosage is being titrated to comply with prescribed therapy.
• Encourage the patient to increase his intake of fiber (and fluids, if not contraindicated) to combat constipation. Administer a stool softener as prescribed.
• Know that preliminary studies show verapamil to be highly effective in preventing migraine headache.

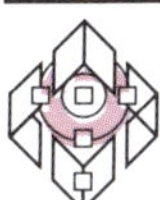 **MedTest**

1. When administering I.V. verapamil, give it:
  a. by continuous slow infusion.
  b. in a mini-bag over 20 to 30 minutes.
  c. using an infusion pump or controller.
  d. over at least 3 minutes.

2. Throughout administration of I.V. verapamil, you should continuously monitor the patient's:
  a. urine output.
  b. ECG and blood pressure.
  c. cardiac output.
  d. PAWP.

3. An ongoing common adverse effect of verapamil is:
  a. dizziness.
  b. nausea.
  c. constipation.
  d. pruritus.

Warfarin sodium

Also known by the brand names Coumadin, Panwarfin, Sofarin, and (in Canada) Warfilone Sodium, warfarin is a coumarin derivative that's classified therapeutically as an anticoagulant. It's available in 1-, 2-, 2.5-, 5-, 7.5-, and 10-mg tablets.

Pharmacokinetics
• *Absorption:* Rapidly and completely absorbed from GI tract.
• *Distribution:* Highly bound to plasma protein, especially albumin; drug crosses placenta but doesn't appear to accumulate in breast milk.
• *Metabolism:* Hydroxylated by the liver into inactive metabolites.
• *Excretion:* Metabolites reabsorbed from bile and excreted in urine. Half-life of parent drug is 1 to 3 days. Because therapeutic effect is more dependent on clotting factor depletion, PT will not peak for $1\frac{1}{2}$ to 3 days. Loading doses won't shorten onset of effect. Duration of action is 2 to 5 days, more closely reflecting drug's half-life.

Indications, dosage, and action
Prevention and treatment of pulmonary emboli and emboli associated with deep vein thrombosis, MI, rheumatic heart disease with valve damage, prosthetic heart valves, and atrial arrhythmias
• *Adult dosage:* 5 to 10 mg P.O. for 3 days; then dosage is based on daily

PT or international normalized ratio (INR). Usual maintenance dosage is 2 to 10 mg P.O. daily. Alternative regimen is to start on dose most likely to be used for maintenance (such as 5 mg/day), check PT in 4 days, and readjust accordingly.

• *Action:* Inhibits vitamin K–dependent activation of clotting factors II, VII, IX, and X, which are formed in the liver.

Contraindication and cautions

• Don't use in patients with bleeding or hemorrhagic tendencies, open wounds, visceral cancer, GI ulcers, severe hepatic or renal disease, severe uncontrolled hypertension, subacute bacterial endocarditis, polycythemia vera, or vitamin K deficiency or in those who've recently undergone surgery of the eye, brain, or spinal cord because excessive bleeding can occur.

• Use cautiously in patients with diverticulitis, colitis, mild or moderate hypertension, or mild or moderate hepatic or renal disease; with drainage tubes in any orifice; with regional or lumbar block anesthesia; or with any condition that increases the risk of hemorrhage.

• Know that elderly patients are more susceptible to the effects of anticoagulants and are at an increased risk for hemorrhage.

• Use cautiously in breast-feeding women.

• Be aware that infants, especially neonates, may be more susceptible to anticoagulants because of vitamin K deficiency. Observe breast-feeding infants of mothers taking this drug for unexpected bleeding.

• Pregnancy risk category D

Life-threatening adverse reactions

• Hemorrhage

Common adverse reactions

• Rash
• Fever

Infrequent adverse reactions

• Paralytic ileus, intestinal obstruction (both resulting from hemorrhage), diarrhea, vomiting, cramps, nausea, hepatitis, jaundice
• Excessive uterine bleeding, priapism
• Eosinophilia, leukopenia
• Dermatitis, urticaria, necrosis, gangrene, alopecia

Interactions

• *Amiodarone, anabolic steroids, broad-spectrum antibiotics, chloramphenicol, cimetidine, ciprofloxacin, clofibrate, diflunisal, disulfiram, ethacrynic acid, glucagon, heparin, methimazole, metronidazole, NSAIDs, propylthiouracil, salicylates, sulfinpyrazone, sulfonamides, sulindac, thyroid drugs, vitamin E:* Increased PT. Monitor patient carefully for bleeding. Warfarin dosage may need to be reduced.

• *Barbiturates:* Inhibition of hypoprothrombinemic effect of anticoagulants. If barbiturates are withdrawn, anticoagulant dose should be reduced; inhibition may last weeks after barbiturate is withdrawn, but fatal hemorrhage can occur when inhibition disappears.

• *Carbamazepine, ethchlorvynol, griseofulvin, paraldehyde, rifampin:* Decreased PT with reduced anti-

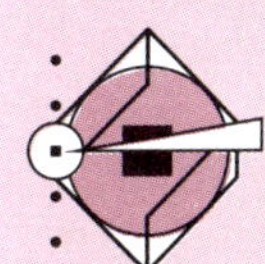

Interactions alert

Life-threatening hazards of multidrug therapy with warfarin

Interacting drug	Effects
Any agent that can cause bleeding (such as NSAIDs, ticlopidine, heparin)	May cause excessive bleeding
Barbiturates (such as phenobarbital)	Increase risk of excessive bleeding

coagulant effect. Monitor patient closely.

• *Chloral hydrate, glutethimide*: Increased or decreased PT. Avoid use, if possible, or monitor patient carefully.

• *Cholestyramine:* Decreased response when taken too close together. Administer 6 hours after oral anticoagulants.

• *Hydantoins:* Increased serum levels of hydantoins. Monitor serum levels closely.

• *Sulfonylureas (oral antidiabetic agents):* Increased hypoglycemic response. Monitor blood glucose levels.

For dangerous interactions, see *Life-threatening hazards of multidrug therapy with warfarin.*

Interventions
Preparation and administration

• Give at the same time daily (usually late afternoon) to allow time to obtain PT or INR. Dosage may be adjusted accordingly. (See *Taking warfarin at home,* pages 324 and 325.)

Monitoring and supportive care

• Use PT determinations for proper control. Know that there's a high incidence of bleeding when PT exceeds 3 times control values. The therapeutic goal is usually to maintain PT at $1\frac{1}{2}$ to 2 times normal, but the range may be higher for patients with mechanical heart valves.

• Know that INR is the more current standard for maintaining control. Desired INR levels for anticoagulation are 2 to 3; however, when mechanical valve implants are present, INR should be 2.5 to 3.5.

• Because the onset of action is delayed, heparin sodium is often given during the first few days of treatment. When heparin is being given simultaneously, don't draw blood for PT within 5 hours of intermittent I.V. heparin administration. However, you can draw blood for PT at any time during continuous heparin infusion.

• The half-life of warfarin's anticoagulant effect is 36 to 44 hours. You can neutralize this effect with phytonadione (5 to 25 mg, rarely up to 50 mg). In emergency situations (severe hemorrhage), return clotting factors to

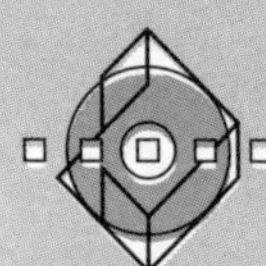

Taking warfarin at home

In addition to explaining the drug's action and dosage, teach the patient who will continue warfarin therapy after discharge to follow these important guidelines.

Take your medication correctly

☐ Take warfarin at the same time every day (usually in the late afternoon). You may take it with or without food.

☐ If you miss a dose of warfarin, take it as soon as possible. However, if it's almost time for your next dose, don't take the missed dose at all and don't double the next one. Doubling the dose may cause bleeding. Instead, go back to your regular dosing schedule. To avoid mistakes, keep a record of each dose as you use it.

☐ Take warfarin exactly as prescribed even when you're feeling well. Be aware that the drug will take up to 3 days to produce optimal effects.

Know when to call your doctor

☐ Continue taking the drug even if unpleasant adverse reactions occur. But make sure you discuss any adverse reactions with your doctor.

☐ Notify your doctor immediately if you experience signs of bleeding, such as bleeding gums, bruises on your arms or legs, small purplish spots on your skin, nosebleeds, black tarry stools, or blood in your urine or vomitus.

Modify your diet

☐ Don't drink alcoholic beverages on a daily basis or take more than one or two drinks at any one time because drinking too much alcohol may change the way warfarin affects blood clotting.

☐ Try to limit the amount of leafy green vegetables that you eat. However, if you eat them regularly, make sure you eat the same amount every day because leafy green vegetables contain vitamin K, which may alter anticoagulant effects. Avoid green tea, which greatly increases vitamin K levels.

☐ Don't go on a weight-loss diet, make other changes in your eating habits, start taking vitamins, or begin using other nutritional supplements until you have first checked with your doctor.

Guard against injuries

☐ Avoid contact sports and other activities that may cause you to be injured. Also report any falls, blows to the body or head, or other injuries because serious bleeding inside your body may occur without your knowing about it.

☐ Take special care in brushing your teeth and shaving. Use a soft toothbrush and floss gently. Also, use an

Taking warfarin at home *(continued)*

electric shaver rather than a razor blade if possible.

Other instructions
☐ Avoid OTC medications containing aspirin or other salicylates because they may cause excess bleeding. Also check with your doctor or pharmacist before taking other OTC medications because serious interactions may occur.

☐ Tell all doctors and dentists you visit that you're taking warfarin.
☐ Notify your doctor if you're scheduled for surgery, tooth extraction, or an angiogram. You may need to discontinue warfarin 2 to 4 days prior to the procedure.
☐ Carry medical identification stating that you're taking warfarin.

---

normal by administering fresh frozen plasma or factor IX complex.
• Regularly inspect the patient for bleeding gums, bruises on his arms or legs, petechiae, nosebleeds, melena, black tarry stools, hematuria, and hematemesis.
• Fever and rash signal severe adverse reactions. If these signs occur, withhold the drug and call the doctor immediately.
• Assess female patients for and report heavier-than-usual menstrual flow. This tendency may require dosage adjustment.
• Supply the patient with an electric razor to use when shaving to avoid scratching his skin and a soft toothbrush or sponge-stick for oral hygiene.
• Be aware that warfarin prolongs both PT and PTT; it also may enhance uric acid excretion, elevate serum transaminase levels, increase LD activity, and cause false-negative serum theophylline levels.

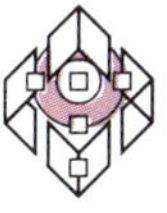 **MedTest**

1. Warfarin should be administered:
   a. without food.
   b. with food.
   c. at the same time each day.
   d. in the morning or evening.

2. A high incidence of serious bleeding is related to a PT exceeding:
   a. 1 to $1\frac{1}{2}$ times the control value.
   b. 2 times the control value.
   c. $2\frac{1}{2}$ times the control value.
   d. 3 times the control value.

3. Warfarin's effect can be neutralized using:
   a. protamine sulfate.
   b. phytonadione.
   c. naloxone hydrochloride.
   d. potassium chloride.

Comparing beta blockers

DRUG AND ROUTE	CV INDICATIONS	ONSET, PEAK, AND DURATION
Acebutolol (Oral) cardioselective	• Hypertension • Ventricular arrhythmias • Angina	*Onset:* Unknown *Peak:* 2½ to 3½ hours *Duration:* 12 to 24 hours
Atenolol (Oral, I.V.) cardioselective	• Hypertension • Chronic stable angina pectoris • To reduce risk of CV mortality in acute MI	**Oral** *Onset:* 1 hour *Peak:* 2 to 4 hours *Duration:* 24 hours **I.V.** *Onset:* 0 to 5 minutes *Peak:* 5 minutes *Duration:* 12 hours
Betaxolol (Oral) noncardioselective	• Hypertension	*Onset:* 3 to 6 hours *Peak:* 3 to 6 hours *Duration:* 24 hours
Carteolol (Oral) noncardioselective	• Hypertension	*Onset:* 1 to 3 hours *Peak:* 1 to 3 hours *Duration:* 24 hours
Esmolol (I.V.) noncardioselective	• Supraventricular tachycardia	*Onset:* Immediate *Peak:* 5 minutes *Duration:* 20 to 30 minutes
Labetalol (Oral, I.V.) noncardioselective; also blocks alpha-receptors	• Hypertension • Severe hypertension and hypertensive emergencies	**Oral** *Onset:* 20 minutes to 2 hours *Peak:* 1 to 2 hours *Duration:* 8 to 10 hours **I.V.** *Onset:* Immediate *Peak:* 5 minutes *Duration:* 2 to 4 hours
Metoprolol (Oral, I.V.) cardioselective	• Hypertension • Early intervention in acute MI • Angina	**Oral** *Onset:* 10 minutes *Peak:* 1½ hours *Duration:* Up to 6 hours **I.V.** *Onset:* Immediate Peak: 20 minutes *Duration:* 5 to 8 hours

SPECIAL CONSIDERATIONS

• May alter blood glucose levels in diabetics and masks tachycardia associated with a hypoglycemic reaction.

• May alter blood glucose levels in diabetics and masks tachycardia associated with hypoglycemia, but doesn't potentiate insulin-induced hypoglycemia or delay recovery of serum glucose to normal levels.

• May also be used as eyedrops to treat chronic, open-angle glaucoma and ocular hypertension.
• Masks tachycardia associated with hypoglycemic reactions in diabetics.

• May be used alone or in combination with other antihypertensive agents, especially thiazide diuretics.
• May inhibit glycogenolysis and attenuate insulin release.

• Requires a loading dose followed by a continuous infusion.
• Masks tachycardia associated with hypoglycemia in diabetic patients.

• Unlabeled clinical use includes treatment of hypertension associated with pheochromocytoma and clonidine-withdrawal hypertension.
• Investigational uses include managing chronic stable angina pectoris, excessive sympathetic activity associated with tetanus, and uncontrolled hypertension before and during anesthesia.
• Masks tachycardia associated with hypoglycemia or hyperthyroidism.

• Most patients with asthma or bronchitis can safely use this drug in low doses (daily doses less than 100 mg) without fear of worsening their condition.
• Masks tachycardia associated with hypoglycemic reactions in diabetics.

(continued)

Comparing beta blockers *(continued)*

DRUG AND ROUTE	CV INDICATIONS	ONSET, PEAK, AND DURATION
Nadolol (Oral) noncardioselective	• Hypertension • Long-term prophylactic management of chronic stable angina pectoris	*Onset:* Unknown *Peak:* 2 to 4 hours *Duration:* 24 hours
Penbutolol (Oral) noncardioselective	• Hypertension	*Onset:* Unknown *Peak:* 2 to 3 hours *Duration:* 12 to 24 hours
Pindolol (Oral) noncardioselective	• Hypertension • Angina pectoris	*Onset:* 1 to 2 hours *Peak:* 1 to 2 hours *Duration:* 24 hours
Propranolol (Oral, I.V.) noncardioselective	• Hypertension • Angina pectoris • Supraventricular and ventricular arrhythmias; tachyarrhythmias caused by excessive catecholamine stimulation • To reduce mortality after MI	**Oral** *Onset:* 30 minutes *Peak:* 1 to 1½ hours *Duration:* 6 hours **I.V.** *Onset:* 2 minutes *Peak:* 15 minutes *Duration:* 3 to 6 hours
Sotalol (Oral) noncardioselective	• Documentated life-threatening ventricular arrhythmias	*Onset:* Unknown *Peak:* 2½ to 4 hours *Duration:* About 12 hours
Timolol (Oral) noncardioselective	• Hypertension • To reduce risk of CV mortality and reinfarction after MI • Angina	*Onset:* 30 minutes *Peak:* 1 to 2 hours *Duration:* 4 to 6 hours

SPECIAL CONSIDERATIONS

• Unlabeled clinical use includes use as an antiarrhythmic agent and as a prophylactic agent for migraine headaches.
• Masks tachycardia associated with hypoglycemia and hyperthyroidism.

• Usually given with other antihypertensive agents such as thiazide diuretics.
• May alter hypoglycemic response to insulin or oral hypoglycemic agents.
• Masks tachycardia associated with hypoglycemia.

• Drug should be discontinued if signs of cardiac failure develop.
• Masks tachycardia associated with hypoglycemia or hyperthyroidism.

• Used to prevent frequent, severe, uncontrollable, or disabling migraine or vascular headache.
• Unlabeled clinical use includes adjunctive treatment of anxiety; treatment of essential, familial, or senile movement tremors; and adjunctive treatment of thyrotoxicosis.
• Masks tachycardia associated with hypoglycemia or hyperthyroidism.

• Used in Canada to treat hypertension and angina.
• Masks tachycardia associated with hypoglycemia in diabetic patients.

• May be used (as eyedrops) to treat glaucoma.
• Masks tachycardia associated with hypoglycemia in diabetic patients.

Comparing ACE inhibitors

DRUG AND ROUTE	CV INDICATIONS	ONSET, PEAK, AND DURATION
Benazepril (Oral)	• Hypertension	*Onset:* 1 hour *Peak:* 30 minutes to 2 hours *Duration:* 24 hours
Captopril (Oral)	• Hypertension • CHF	*Onset:* 15 minutes *Peak:* 1 to 2 hours *Duration:* 2 to 6 hours usually, but may be as long as 12 hours
Enalapril (Oral)	• Hypertension • CHF	*Onset:* 1 hour *Peak:* 4 to 6 hours *Duration:* 24 hours
Enalaprilat (I.V.)	• Hypertension • CHF	*Onset:* 15 minutes *Peak:* 1 to 4 hours *Duration:* 6 hours
Fosinopril (Oral)	• Hypertension	*Onset:* 1 hour *Peak:* 3 hours *Duration:* 24 hours
Lisinopril (Oral)	• Hypertension	*Onset:* 1 hour *Peak:* 6 hours *Duration:* 24 hours
Quinapril (Oral)	• Hypertension	*Onset:* 1 hour *Peak:* 2 to 6 hours *Duration:* 24 hours
Ramipril (Oral)	• Hypertension	*Onset:* 1 to 2 hours *Peak:* 4 hours *Duration:* 24 hours

SPECIAL CONSIDERATIONS

• Blood pressure measurements should be made when drug levels are at peak (2 to 6 hours after dosing) and at trough (just before a dose) to verify adequate blood pressure control.

• May cause false-positive results for urinary acetone levels.

• Symptomatic hypotension may occur after first dose in patients taking diuretics. Discontinue diuretic therapy 2 to 3 days before starting enalapril therapy.

• Drug should be discontinued if neutropenia or renal failure occurs.

• Effectiveness of fosinopril is unaffected by age, sex, or weight.
• False-low measurements of digoxin levels may result with the DIGI-TAB radioimmunoassay kit for digoxin; other kits may be used.

• Beneficial effects may require several weeks of therapy.

• Blood pressure measurements should be made when drug levels are at peak (2 to 6 hours) after dosing and at trough (just before a dose) to verify adequate blood pressure control.

• Effectiveness of ramipril is unaffected by age, sex, or weight.

Comparing antilipemics

DRUG AND ROUTE	CV INDICATIONS	ONSET, PEAK, AND DURATION
Cholestyramine (Oral)	• Hyperlipidemia • Hypercholesterolemia	*Onset:* Not applicable *Peak:* Not applicable *Duration:* Not applicable
Clofibrate (Oral)	• Hyperlipidemia	*Onset:* 2 to 5 days *Peak:* 3 weeks with continued use *Duration:* Return to pretreatment VLDL concentrations within 3 weeks after drug is withdrawn
Colestipol (Oral)	• Primary hypercholesterolemia	*Onset:* Not applicable *Peak:* Not applicable *Duration:* Not applicable
Gemfibrozil (Oral)	• Type IV hyperlipidemia • Severe hypercholesterolemia unresponsive to diet and other drugs	*Onset:* 2 to 5 days *Peak:* 4 weeks *Duration:* Unknown
Lovastatin (Oral)	• Primary hypercholesterolemia (types IIa and IIb)	*Onset:* 3 days *Peak:* 4 to 6 weeks *Duration:* Probably a few weeks

SPECIAL CONSIDERATIONS

• Not absorbed from the GI tract.
• Reduction of plasma cholesterol occurs generally within 24 to 48 hours after initiation of therapy but may continue to fall for up to 1 year.
• After withdrawal of drug, cholesterol levels return to baseline in about 2 to 4 weeks.
• May also be used to treat pruritus associated with partial biliary obstruction.
• Unlabeled indications include treatment of diarrhea due to bile acids, treatment of hyperoxaluria, and treatment of digitalis glycoside overdose.

• Studies suggest clofibrate may increase risk of death from cancer, postcholecystectomy complications, and pancreatitis.
• May also be used to treat xanthoma tuberosum.

• Not absorbed from the GI tract.
• Plasma cholesterol levels generally reduced within 24 to 48 hours after therapy begins.
• Reaches its peak effectiveness in 1 month.
• After withdrawal of colestipol, cholesterol levels return to baseline in about 1 month.
• May also be used to treat xanthomas.
• Unlabeled indications include treatment of diarrhea due to bile acids, treatment of pruritus associated with partial biliary obstruction, and treatment of digitalis glycoside overdose.

• Because gemfibrozil is pharmacologically related to clofibrate, hazards of clofibrate therapy, such as increased risk of death from cancer, postcholecystecomy complications, and pancreatitis, should be kept in mind even though these hazards haven't been studied in gemfibrozil.

• Drug should be temporarily discontinued in any patient with an acute condition that suggests a developing myopathy or in patients having risk factors that may predispose them to development of renal failure secondary to rhabdomyolysis (including severe acute infection; severe endocrine, metabolic, or electrolyte disorders; hypotension; major surgery; or uncontrolled seizures).
• Drug should be discontinued if liver function studies show signs of hepatotoxicity or if patient develops myositis or renal failure secondary to rhabdomyolysis.

(continued)

Comparing antilipemics *(continued)*

DRUG AND ROUTE	CV INDICATIONS	ONSET, PEAK, AND DURATION
Pravastatin (Oral)	• Primary hypercholesterolemia (types IIa and IIb)	*Onset:* 3 days *Peak:* 4 to 6 weeks *Duration:* Probably a few weeks
Probucol (Oral)	• Primary hypercholesterolemia (types IIa and IIb)	*Onset:* 1 to 3 months *Peak:* Unknown *Duration:* Unknown
Simvastatin (Oral)	• Primary hypercholesterolemia (types IIa and IIb)	*Onset:* 3 days *Peak:* 4 to 6 weeks *Duration:* Probably a few weeks

SPECIAL CONSIDERATIONS

• Drug should be temporarily discontinued in any patient with an acute condition that suggests a developing myopathy or in patients having risk factors that may predispose them to development of renal failure secondary to rhabdomyolysis (including severe acute infection; severe endocrine, metabolic, or electrolyte disorders; hypotension; major surgery; or uncontrolled seizures).
• Drug should be discontinued if liver function studies show signs of hepatotoxicity or if patient develops myositis or renal failure secondary to rhabdomyolysis.

• Drug should be discontinued if cardiac arrhythmia or prolonged QT interval occurs.
• Dosage should not exceed 1 g daily.
• ECG should be done before and during drug therapy.

• Drug should be temporarily discontinued in any patient with an acute condition that suggests a developing myopathy or in patients having risk factors that may predispose them to development of renal failure secondary to rhabdomyolysis (including severe acute infection; severe endocrine, metabolic, or electrolyte disorders; hypotension; major surgery; or uncontrolled seizures).
• Drug should be discontinued if liver function studies show signs of hepatotoxicity or if patient develops myositis or renal failure secondary to rhabdomyolysis.

Comparing calcium channel blockers

DRUG AND ROUTE	CV INDICATIONS	ONSET, PEAK, AND DURATION
Amlodipine (Oral)	• Prinzmetal's, variant, or chronic stable angina pectoris • Hypertension	*Onset:* Unknown *Peak:* 6 to 12 hours *Duration:* 24 hours
Bepridil (Oral)	• Chronic stable angina pectoris	*Onset:* 1 hour *Peak:* 2 to 3 hours *Duration:* 24 hours
Diltiazem (Oral, I.V.)	• Prinzmetal's, variant, or chronic stable angina pectoris • Hypertension • Atrial fibrillation or flutter	**Oral** *Onset:* 30 to 60 minutes (extended-release: 2 to 3 hours) *Peak:* 2 to 3 hours (extended-release: 6 to 11 hours) *Duration:* 4 to 8 hours (extended-release: 12 hours) **I.V.** *Onset:* Immediate *Peak:* Immediate *Duration:* 3 to 5 hours
Felodipine (Oral)	• Hypertension	*Onset:* 30 minutes to $1\frac{1}{2}$ hours *Peak:* $2\frac{1}{2}$ to 5 hours *Duration:* 24 hours
Isradipine (Oral)	• Hypertension	*Onset:* 30 minutes to $1\frac{1}{2}$ hours *Peak:* $1\frac{1}{2}$ hours *Duration:* 12 hours
Nicardipine (Oral)	• Hypertension • Chronic stable angina	*Onset:* 20 minutes *Peak:* 30 minutes to 2 hours *Duration:* 8 hours
Nifedipine (Oral)	• Hypertension • Prinzmetal's, variant, or chronic stable angina pectoris	*Onset:* 20 minutes *Peak:* 30 minutes *Duration:* 6 to 8 hours

SPECIAL CONSIDERATIONS

- May be taken without regard to meals.
- Once-daily dosing may improve compliance.
- Has little, if any, direct effects on the heart.

- Drug has been associated with serious arrhythmias (such as torsades de pointes) and agranulocytosis.
- Reserved for use in patients who can't tolerate or don't respond to other antianginal agents.

- Has been used investigationally to prevent reinfarction after non – Q wave MI, as an adjunct in the treatment of peripheral vascular disorders, and in the treatment of a variety of spastic smooth muscle disorders, including esophageal spasm.

- The adverse reaction peripheral edema appears to be both dose- and age-dependent. It's more common in patients taking higher doses, especially those who are ages 60 and over.
- Has little or no direct effect on the heart.

- Administration with food increases the time to reach peak concentrations by about 1 hour, but has no effect on total bioavailability of the drug.
- Elevated liver function test results have been reported in some patients.
- Has little or no direct effect on the heart.

- When treating hypertension, blood pressure measurements should be made at trough plasma levels (approximately 8 hours after a dose, or immediately before subsequent doses). Because of the prominent effects that may occur at peak plasma levels, additional blood pressure measurements should be made 1 to 2 hours after a dose.

- Although rebound effect hasn't been observed when drug is stopped, be aware that the dosage should be reduced slowly under medical supervision.

(continued)

Comparing calcium channel blockers *(continued)*

DRUG AND ROUTE	CV INDICATIONS	ONSET, PEAK, AND DURATION
Verapamil (Oral, I.V.)	• Hypertension • Prinzmetal's, variant, or chronic stable angina pectoris • Supraventricular tachyarrhythmias • Prevention of recurrent PSVT • Control of ventricular rate in digitalized patients with chronic atrial flutter or fibrillation	**Oral** *Onset:* 30 to 60 minutes *Peak:* 2 hours *Duration:* 6 to 8 hours **I.V.** *Onset:* Immediate *Peak:* Immediate to 5 minutes *Duration:* 30 to 60 minutes

SPECIAL CONSIDERATIONS

• Drug should be discontinued if systolic blood pressure falls below 90 mm Hg, if heart failure worsens, or if arrhythmias, hemodynamically significant bradycardia, or second- or third-degree heart block occurs.
• Be aware that generic sustained-release verapamil tablets may be substituted only for Isoptin SR and Calan SR, not Verelan capsules. The capsule formulation should be given only once daily. When using sustained-release tablets, doses over 240 mg should be given b.i.d.

Comparing adrenergics

DRUG AND ROUTE	CV INDICATIONS	ONSET, PEAK, AND DURATION
Dobutamine (I.V.)	• To increase cardiac output in short-term treatment of cardiac decompensation caused by depressed contractility	*Onset:* 1 to 3 minutes *Peak:* 10 minutes or less *Duration:* 10 minutes or less
Dopamine (I.V.)	• Adjunct in shock to increase cardiac output, blood pressure, and urine flow • Short-term treatment of severe, refractory, chronic CHF	*Onset:* 2 to 5 minutes *Peak:* Up to 10 minutes *Duration:* 5 to 10 minutes
Epinephrine (S.C., I.V., intratracheal, intracardiac)	• To restore cardiac rhythm in cardiac arrest	**S.C.** *Onset:* 3 to 5 minutes *Peak:* 20 minutes *Duration:* Unknown **I.V., intratracheal, and intracardiac use** *Onset:* 5 to 10 minutes *Peak:* Immediate *Duration:* 8 to 10 hours
Isoproterenol (Sublingual, I.V.)	• To treat or prevent AV heart block • Emergency treatment of cardiac arrhythmias including atropine-resistant bradycardia • Adjunct treatment of shock	**Sublingual** *Onset:* Immediate to 10 minutes *Peak:* Immediate upon absorption *Duration:* 1 to 2 hours **I.V.** *Onset:* Immediate *Peak:* Immediate *Duration:* Less than 1 hour

SPECIAL CONSIDERATIONS

• Drug should be discontinued if hypersensitivity reaction to drug or sulfites or if cardiac arrhythmia occurs.
• Before administration of drug, hypovolemia should be corrected with appropriate plasma volume expanders.
• Pink discoloration of solution indicates slight oxidation but no significant loss of potency.
• Concentration of infusion solution shouldn't exceed 5,000 mcg/ml; solution should be used within 24 hours. Rate and duration of infusion depend on patient's response.

• Drug should be discontinued if patient develops signs of hypersensitivity reaction to drug or sulfite preservative, cardiac arrhythmia, or tachyphylaxis.
• Before administration of drug, hypovolemia should be corrected with appropriate plasma volume expanders
• Severe hypotension may result with abrupt withdrawal of infusion; therefore, dose should be reduced gradually.
• If extravasation occurs, stop infusion and infiltrate site promptly with 10 to 15 ml of 0.9% NaCl injection containing 5 to 10 mg of phentolamine as prescribed. Use syringe with a fine needle, and infiltrate area liberally with phentolamine solution.

• Epinephrine may also be prescribed to treat severe anaphylaxis or asthma, bronchospasms, or open-angle glaucoma; to prolong local anesthetic effect; and to function as a hemostatic agent.
• Monitor diabetic patient's blood glucose level closely because drug may raise blood glucose levels.

• Isoproterenol may also be prescribed to treat bronchospasms that may occur during asthma attacks, in COPD, and during anesthesia.
• Drug should be discontinued if precordial distress, angina, ventricular arrhythmias, or swelling of parotids occurs or airway resistance develops.
• Be aware that hypotension must be corrected before isoproterenol is administered.

(continued)

Comparing adrenergics *(continued)*

DRUG AND ROUTE	CV INDICATIONS	ONSET, PEAK, AND DURATION
Metaraminol (S.C., I.M., I.V.)	• Hypotension	**S.C.** *Onset:* 5 to 20 minutes *Peak:* Unknown *Duration:* 20 to 60 minutes **I.M.** *Onset:* 10 minutes *Peak:* Unknown *Duration:* 20 to 60 minutes **I.V.** *Onset:* 1 to 2 minutes *Peak:* 5 to 10 minutes *Duration:* 20 to 60 minutes
Norepinephrine (I.V.)	• To maintain blood pressure in acute hypotensive states	*Onset:* Immediate *Peak:* Immediate *Duration:* 1 to 2 minutes
Phenylephrine (S.C., I.M., I.V.)	• To treat or prevent hypotension • To prevent PSVT • Adjunct treatment in shock	**S.C.** *Onset:* 1 to 15 minutes *Peak:* Unknown *Duration:* 30 to 50 minutes **I.M.** *Onset:* 1 to 5 minutes *Peak:* Unknown *Duration:* 30 to 50 minutes **I.V.** *Onset:* Immediate *Peak:* Immediate *Duration:* 15 to 20 minutes

---

SPECIAL CONSIDERATIONS

• Metaraminol should be discontinued if patient develops a hypersensitivity to drug or sulfite preservative, or if infiltration or thrombosis occurs during I.V. administration.
• Treat extravasation promptly with 10 to 15 ml 0.9% NaCl solution containing 5 to 10 mg phentolamine infiltrated into site with a fine needle as prescribed.
• Allow at least 10 minutes to elapse before administering additional doses because maximum effect isn't immediately apparent.
• Monitor diabetic patient's blood glucose levels closely because insulin adjustments may be needed.

• Norepinephrine has also been used to control upper GI bleeding.
• Norepinephrine should be discontinued if patient develops hypersensitivity reaction, infiltration, or thrombosis.
• Treat extravasation promptly with 10 to 15 ml 0.9% NaCl solution containing 5 to 10 mg phentolamine infiltrated into site with a fine needle as prescribed.

• Phenylephrine may also be used to treat mydriasis, posterior synechia, postoperative malignant glaucoma, conjunctival congestion, and nasal, sinus, or eustachian tube congestion. Sometimes it's added to local anesthetics to prolong their duration of action.
• Drug should be discontinued if patient develops a hypersensitivity reaction or cardiac arrhythmias.
• Treat extravasation promptly with 10 to 15 ml 0.9% NaCl solution containing 5 to 10 mg phentolamine infiltrated into site with a fine needle as prescribed.

Comparing commonly used antiarrhythmics

DRUG AND ROUTE	CV INDICATIONS	ONSET, PEAK, AND DURATION
Adenosine (I.V.)	• Conversion of PSVT to sinus rhythm	*Onset:* Immediate *Peak:* Immediate *Duration:* Less than 2 minutes
Amiodarone (Oral)	• Ventricular and supraventricular arrhythmias	*Onset:* 2 to 3 days to 2 to 3 months, even with loading doses *Peak:* 3 to 7 hours *Duration:* Weeks to months
Bretylium (I.M., I.V.)	• Ventricular fibrillation • Unstable VT and other ventricular arrhythmias	**I.M.** *Onset:* 20 to 60 minutes *Peak:* 1 hour *Duration:* 6 to 24 hours **I.V.** *Onset:* 5 to 10 minutes *Peak:* Immediate *Duration:* 6 to 24 hours
Disopyramide (Oral)	• PVCs • VT not severe enough to require electrocardio-version	*Onset:* 30 minutes *Peak:* 2 to 5 hours *Duration:* 6 to 7 hours
Flecainide (Oral)	• Life-threatening VT • Paroxysmal atrial flutter and PSVT in the absence of structural heart defects	*Onset:* 1 to 2 hours (blood level); 1 to 4 days (clinical effects) *Peak:* Up to 4 days *Duration:* Approximately 12 hours
Lidocaine (I.V.)	• Ventricular arrhythmias	*Onset:* Immediate *Peak:* Immediate *Duration:* 10 to 20 minutes
Mexiletine (Oral)	• Refractory ventricular arrhythmias	*Onset:* 30 minutes *Peak:* 2 to 3 hours *Duration:* 8 to 12 hours

SPECIAL CONSIDERATIONS

- Be aware that adenosine may produce a transient first-, second-, or third-degree heart block because it decreases conduction through AV node. Because drug has short half-life, these effects are usually transient. However, patients who develop significant block after a dose of adenosine shouldn't receive additional doses.

- Amiodarone should be discontinued if signs or symptoms of pulmonary toxicity, liver disease, or epididymitis occur.
- Adverse effects are more prevalent with high doses but usually resolve within about 4 months after drug therapy stops.

- Be aware that bretylium isn't a first-line agent, according to ACLS guidelines. With ventricular fibrillation, drug should follow lidocaine; with VT, drug should follow lidocaine or procainamide.
- Drug may cause hypotension.

- Drug should be discontinued if hypotension, progressive heart failure, or heart block occurs; if QRS complex widens by 25% to 50% over baseline; or if QT interval lengthens.

- Drug should be discontinued if CHF worsens despite optimum therapy and reduced dosage; if second- or third-degree AV block or bifascicular block occurs (unless an artificial pacemaker is in place); or if unexplained jaundice, signs of hepatic dysfunction, or blood dyscrasias develop.
- Drug is not recommended for chronic atrial fibrillation.

- Know that lidocaine may also be used as local anesthetic to relieve pain and as topical agent in symptomatic relief of sunburn or skin irritation.
- Be aware that infusion rate of drug that's greater than 4 mg/minute isn't recommended because it greatly increases risk of toxicity.

- Know that therapeutic serum drug levels range from 0.75 to 2 mcg/ml.

(continued)

Comparing commonly used antiarrhythmics *(continued)*

DRUG AND ROUTE	CV INDICATIONS	ONSET, PEAK, AND DURATION
Procainamide (Oral, I.M., I.V.)	• PVCs • VT • Atrial fibrillation and flutter unresponsive to quinidine • PAT	**Oral** *Onset:* 30 to 60 minutes *Peak:* 60 to 90 minutes *Duration:* 4 to 6 hours **I.M.** *Onset:* 10 to 30 minutes *Peak:* 1 hour *Duration:* 2 to 4 hours **I.V.** *Onset:* Immediate *Peak:* Immediate *Duration:* 2 to 4 hours
Propafenone (Oral)	• Life-threatening ventricular arrhythmias	*Onset:* 1 to 2 hours (blood levels); 1 to 3 days (clinical effects) *Peak:* 3½ hours (blood levels); 1 to 3 days (clinical effects) *Duration:* 8 to 12 hours
Quinidine (Oral, I.M.)	• Atrial fibrillation or flutter • PSVT • PATs and PVCs • AV junctional rhythm or atrial tachycardia and VT, maintenance of cardio-version	**Oral** *Onset:* 30 minutes to 1 hour *Peak:* 1 to 1½ hours (quinidine sulfate); 3 to 4 hours (quinidine gluconate); 6 hours (quinidine polygalacturonate) *Duration:* 6 to 12 hours **I.M.** *Onset:* 15 to 30 minutes *Peak:* 1 hour *Duration:* 4 to 6 hours
Tocainide (Oral)	• Ventricular arrhythmias	*Onset:* 30 minutes *Peak:* 30 minutes to 2 hours *Duration:* 8 to 12 hours

SPECIAL CONSIDERATIONS

• Drug should be discontinued if granulocytopenia or lupus-like syndrome occurs, unless drug's benefits outweigh risks.
• Be aware that I.V. drug form is more likely to cause adverse cardiac effects, possibly resulting in severe hypotension.

• Know that maximum daily dosage is **900 mg**.

• Drug should be discontinued if the following problems develop: blood dyscrasias; hepatic dysfunction; renal dysfunction; syncope; cardiotoxicity, including conduction defects (25% widening of QRS complex); VT or ventricular flutter; frequent PVCs; or complete AV block
• An unlabeled use of quinidine gluconate is treatment of malaria when quinine is unavailable.

• Drug should be discontinued if signs or symptoms of adverse hematologic, pulmonary, or cardiac effects (including worsening CHF or cardiac conductivity, despite adequate therapy or without external pacing) occur.
• Know that drug is considered an oral lidocaine and may be used to ease transition from I.V. lidocaine to oral antiarrhythmic therapy.

Comparing diuretics

DRUG AND ROUTE	CV INDICATIONS	ONSET, PEAK, AND DURATION
Amiloride (Oral)	• Hypertension • Edema associated with CHF	*Onset:* Within 2 hours *Peak:* 6 to 10 hours *Duration:* 24 hours
Bumetanide (Oral, I.M., I.V.)	• Edema associated with CHF or hepatic or renal disease	**Oral** *Onset:* 30 to 60 minutes *Peak:* 1 to 2 hours *Duration:* 4 to 6 hours **I.M.** *Onset:* 40 minutes *Peak:* 1 to 2 hours *Duration:* 4 hours **I.V.** *Onset:* Immediate *Peak:* 15 to 30 minutes *Duration:* $3\frac{1}{2}$ to 4 hours
Ethacrynate sodium, ethacrynic acid (Oral, I.V.)	• Acute pulmonary edema • Edema	**Oral** *Onset:* 30 minutes *Peak:* 2 hours *Duration:* 6 to 8 hours **I.V.** *Onset:* 5 minutes *Peak:* 15 to 30 minutes *Duration:* 2 hours
Furosemide (Oral, I.M., I.V.)	• Acute pulmonary edema • Edema • Hypertension • Hypertensive crisis	**Oral** *Onset:* 20 to 60 minutes *Peak:* 1 to 2 hours *Duration:* 6 to 8 hours **I.M.** *Onset:* 15 to 30 minutes *Peak:* 30 to 45 minutes *Duration:* 2 to 3 hours **I.V.** *Onset:* 5 minutes *Peak:* Within 30 minutes *Duration:* 2 hours
Hydrochlorothiazide (Oral)	• Hypertension • Edema	*Onset:* 2 hours *Peak:* 4 hours *Duration:* 6 to 12 hours

SPECIAL CONSIDERATIONS

• Drug should be discontinued if hyperkalemia occurs.

• Drug should be discontinued if dehydration or hypotension occurs.
• Report rising BUN and serum creatinine levels, and use cautiously.

• Know that ethacrynate sodium has been used to treat hypercalcemia and to manage ethylene glycol poisoning and bromide intoxication.
• Drug should be discontinued if excessive diuresis, electrolyte abnormalities, increasing azotemia, oliguria, hematuria, bloody stools, or severe or watery diarrhea occurs.
• Don't give ethacrynate sodium I.M. or S.C. because it may cause severe local pain and irritation.

• Drug may also be used to treat acute and chronic renal failure as well as hypercalcemia.
• Drug should be discontinued if dehydration or hypotension occurs.
• Report rising BUN and creatinine levels, and use cautiously.

• Drug should be discontinued if rising BUN and serum creatinine levels indicate renal impairment or if patient shows signs of impending coma.
• Elderly and debilitated patients are more sensitive to developing excess diuresis because of age-related changes in CV and renal function.

(continued)

Comparing diuretics *(continued)*

DRUG AND ROUTE	CV INDICATIONS	ONSET, PEAK, AND DURATION
Indapamide (Oral)	• Hypertension • Edema	*Onset:* 1 hour *Peak:* 2 hours *Duration:* 8 to 12 hours
Spironolactone (Oral)	• Hypertension • Edema	*Onset:* 1 to 2 days *Peak:* 2 to 3 days *Duration:* 2 to 3 days
Torsemide (Oral, I.V.)	• Hypertension • Edema associated with CHF and cirrhosis	**Oral** *Onset:* Less than 1 hour *Peak:* drug, 1 hour; active metabolites, 1 to 2 hours; clinical activity, 4 hours *Duration:* 8 to 12 hours **I.V.** *Onset:* Immediate *Peak:* Less than 4 hours *Duration:* 6 hours

SPECIAL CONSIDERATIONS

• Drug should be discontinued if rising BUN and serum creatinine levels indicate renal impairment or if patient shows signs of impending coma.
• Elderly and debilitated patients are more sensitive to developing excess diuresis because of age-related changes in CV and renal function.

• Drug is also used to treat diuretic-induced hypokalemia. Unlabeled uses include detection of primary hyperaldosteronism and treatment of hirsutism.

• Drug has longer duration of action than furosemide and isn't associated with rebound antidiuretic effect observed with shorter-acting loop diuretics. In addition, it may produce less excretion of potassium and calcium than furosemide.
• Torsemide is newest loop diuretic to be approved by FDA.

Comparing vasodilators

DRUG AND ROUTE	CV INDICATIONS	ONSET, PEAK, AND DURATION
Amrinone (I.V.)	• Short-term management of CHF	*Onset:* Immediate *Peak:* 10 minutes *Duration:* 30 minutes (750 mcg/kg); 2 hours (3 mg/kg)
Diazoxide (I.V.)	• Hypertensive crisis	*Onset:* 1 to 3 minutes *Peak:* 2 to 5 minutes *Duration:* Usually 3 to 12 hours, but ranges from 1 to 72 hours
Hydralazine (Oral, I.M., I.V.)	• Hypertension • Short-term management of severe CHF	**Oral** *Onset:* 20 to 30 minutes *Peak:* 2 hours *Duration:* 2 to 8 hours **I.M.** *Onset:* 10 to 30 minutes *Peak:* 1 hour *Duration:* 2 to 6 hours **I.V.** *Onset:* 5 to 20 minutes *Peak:* 10 to 80 minutes *Duration:* 2 to 6 hours
Milrinone (I.V.)	• Short-term management of CHF	*Onset:* Immediate *Peak:* 5 to 15 minutes *Duration:* Variable; mean elimination half-life about 2½ hours
Minoxidil (Oral)	• Severe hypertension	*Onset:* 30 minutes *Peak:* 2 to 8 hours *Duration:* 2 to 5 days
Nitroprusside (I.V.)	• Hypertensive emergencies	*Onset:* Immediate *Peak:* Immediate *Duration:* 1 to 10 minutes after infusion stops

SPECIAL CONSIDERATIONS

• Know that amrinone is prescribed primarily for those patients who have not responded to therapy with digitalis glycosides, diuretics, and other vasodilators.
• Drug should be discontinued if thrombocytopenia becomes clinically significant.

• Oral form of drug may also be used to treat hypoglycemia resulting from hyperinsulinism; it's not used to treat functional hypoglycemia. It may be used temporarily to control preoperative or postoperative hypoglycemia in patients with hyperinsulinism.
• Be aware that using oral form of drug to treat hypoglycemia doesn't cause significant hypotension.

• Drug should be discontinued if patient develops lupus-like syndrome, blood dyscrasias, a positive ANA titer, or positive LE cell preparation.
• Know that incidence of hydralazine-induced lupus-like syndrome is greatest in patients receiving more than 200 mg/day for prolonged periods.

• Milrinone is often used in patients receiving digitalis glycosides.
• Duration of drug therapy depends on the patient's responsiveness.

• Minoxidil has been used in 2% topical solutions to promote hair growth.
• Drug should be discontinued if pericardial effusion develops.

• Nitroprusside has been used in patients with acute MI, refractory heart failure, and severe mitral insufficiency.
• Drug should be discontinued if metabolic acidosis occurs; it may indicate cyanogen toxicity.

Answers to MedTests

Acebutolol (pp. 62 and 63)
1. (c) Acebutolol may mask signs of hypoglycemia, such as tachycardia.

2. (d) Acebutolol is contraindicated in patients with persistent bradycardia.

3. (c) If your patient is scheduled for surgery, you should notify the anesthesiologist that he's receiving acebutolol.

Adenosine (p. 65)
1. (a) Adenosine is especially useful in treating WPW syndrome.

2. (d) If when preparing adenosine for injection you note the presence of crystals in the solution, you should slowly warm the solution to room temperature.

3. (c) Because it may produce a transient first-, second-, or third-degree AV block, adenosine is contraindicated in SSS.

Alteplase (p. 68)
1. (c) After the onset of MI symptoms, alteplase should be given within 6 hours.

2. (b) You should prepare the alteplase solution using sterile water for injection.

3. (c) Because of the high risk of bleeding from an alteplase infusion, you should avoid I.M. injections and venipunctures.

Amiloride hydrochloride (pp. 70 to 72)
1. (d) Monitor the serum potassium level in a patient receiving amiloride.

2. (a) Amiloride exerts its diuretic effects by acting on the distal renal tubule to inhibit sodium reabsorption.

3. (b) Dietary guidelines for the patient taking amiloride include moderation in the use of potassium-rich foods.

Amiodarone hydrochloride (p. 75)
1. (c) Amiodarone is excreted mainly through the biliary tree.

2. (a) To assess for visual disturbances, recommend weekly, then monthly, eye examinations.

3. (a) To assess for the most significant adverse reaction to amiodarone, monitor your patient for exertional dyspnea, nonproductive cough, and pleuritic pain.

Amlodipine besylate (pp. 77 and 78)
1. (c) Amlodipine is classified pharmacologically as a calcium channel blocker.

2. (d) Dosage reductions of amlodipine may be required for patients with hepatic failure.

3. (d) Administer amlodipine once daily, without regard to meals.

Amrinone lactate (p. 80)
1. (c) Amrinone produces its vasodilating effect by direct effect on vascular smooth muscle.

2. (b) Amrinone's main use is for short-term management of CHF.

3. (a) While monitoring your patient's blood pressure during amrinone infusion, you note a gradual, asymptomatic decrease. You then slow the administration rate and continue careful monitoring.

Atenolol (p. 82)
1. (d) Before giving each dose of atenolol, you should check the patient's apical pulse.

2. (b) Atenolol's negative inotropic and chronotropic action, which decreases myocardial contractility and heart rate to reduce myocardial oxygen consumption, makes it useful in treating chronic stable angina.

3. (b) Dizziness is the most common adverse reaction in patients taking atenolol.

Atropine sulfate (pp. 84 and 85)
1. (c) For symptomatic bradycardia, give I.V. doses of atropine into a large vein or I.V. tubing over 1 to 2 minutes.

2. (b) The antidote for atropine overdose is physostigmine salicylate.

3. (d) If an I.V. line isn't in place and atropine is required for immediate treatment of symptomatic bradycardia, the next best route for rapid absorption is endotracheal insufflation.

Benazepril hydrochloride (p. 88)
1. (c) Benazepril is effective in treating CHF because it reduces afterload and pulmonary vascular resistance.

2. (d) To verify adequate blood pressure control in the patient receiving benazepril, check the patient's blood pressure at peak and trough drug level times.

3. (b) A clinically insignificant adverse effect that benazepril, like other ACE inhibitors, causes is a dry, persistent, tickling, nonproductive cough.

Bepridil hydrochloride (p. 90)
1. (c) Bepridil is pharmacologically classified as a calcium channel blocker.

2. (d) Bepridil's main use is in the treatment of angina.

3. (d) When initiating bepridil therapy, closely monitor the patient's QT interval.

Betaxolol hydrochloride (p. 93)
1. (b) The cardioselective beta$_1$-adrenergic blocking action of betaxolol is helpful in managing hypertension because it slows heart rate and decreases cardiac output.

2. (a) Bronchospasm is a life-threatening adverse reaction to betaxolol.

3. (d) When discontinuing betaxolol, the patient should be told to reduce dosage gradually over at least 2 weeks.

Bretylium tosylate (p. 96)
1. (b) Following I.V. administration of bretylium, suppression of VT and

other ventricular arrhythmias usually occurs within 20 minutes to 2 hours.

2. (a) When administering bretylium, monitor the patient's heart rate and rhythm and blood pressure continuously throughout therapy.

3. (a) Bretylium should be avoided if the patient is already receiving a digitalis glycoside.

Bumetanide (p. 99)
1. (d) Bumetanide should be used with caution in patients allergic to sulfonamides.

2. (a) The doctor has indicated a change in dosage from once a day to b.i.d. The patient's second dose should be given in the early afternoon.

3. (a) Assess (and include in your patient teaching) symptoms of hypokalemia, such as muscle weakness and cramps.

Captopril (pp. 101 and 102)
1. (a) Patients taking captopril should have the serum electrolyte potassium monitored because captopril can cause hyperkalemia.

2. (d) Captopril's antihypertensive action occurs in part because the drug reduces sodium and water retention.

3. (a) A possible life-threatening adverse effect of captopril is agranulocytosis.

Cholestyramine (pp. 104 and 105)
1. (b) Administer cholestyramine powder in a fluid volume of at least 90 ml.

2. (d) Constipation is the adverse reaction that the patient is most likely to experience and that would require assessment and intervention.

3. (a) Cholestyramine therapy puts the patient at risk for deficiencies of vitamins A, D, E, and K.

Clofibrate (pp. 107 and 108)
1. (a) Clofibrate is contraindicated in patients with hepatic or renal dysfunction because of potential drug accumulation, thus increasing the incidence of adverse reactions.

2. (c) Administer clofibrate with meals to minimize GI discomfort.

3. (b) Serum amylase, cholesterol, and triglyceride levels should be monitored frequently during clofibrate therapy.

Clonidine hydrochloride (p. 112)
1. (c) When clonidine is prescribed in a transdermal patch, it should be applied weekly.

2. (c) Patients taking clonidine should report any weight gain in excess of 5 lb (2.3 kg) per week.

3. (d) If your patient is taking oral clonidine b.i.d., the last dose should be taken h.s.

Colestipol hydrochloride (p. 115)
1. (d) To ensure that your patient receives his entire dose of colestipol, follow the dose with additional liquid swirled in the same glass.

2. (d) Peak decreases in cholesterol levels occur in 1 month.

3. (c) If constipation worsens after dosage reduction, stop the colestipol.

Diazoxide (p. 118)
1. (b) Following administration of I.V. diazoxide, the maximum hypotensive effect should occur within 5 minutes.

2. (a) Keep the patient in a supine position for 1 hour following administration of diazoxide.

3. (d) In addition to closely monitoring your patient's blood pressure during and following administration of diazoxide, your follow-up care includes close monitoring of intake, output, and body weight.

Digoxin (p. 124)
1. (d) Capsules are the most completely absorbed of all the oral and parenteral administration forms of digoxin.

2. (c) It customarily takes 7 days or more to achieve steady-state levels of digoxin.

3. (d) When taking the patient's apical pulse for a full minute before administering the dose, monitor carefully for significant changes.

Digoxin immune FAB (p. 127)
1. (c) While the dosage of digoxin immune FAB varies according to the amount of drug to be neutralized, the average dose is about 400 mg or 10 vials. This will bind approximately 6 mg of digoxin or digitoxin.

2. (a) The toxicity will begin to subside within 30 minutes after the 15-

to 30-minute infusion of digoxin immune FAB.

3. (d) Use digoxin immune FAB for life-threatening overdoses only.

Diltiazem hydrochloride (p. 130)
1. (b) Instruct patients to take sustained- and extended-release forms of diltiazem q 12 hours or daily.

2. (c) If a patient develops headaches during initial use of extended-release diltiazem, he should take the drug with aspirin or acetaminophen, if not contraindicated.

3. (a) If a patient experiences increased fatigue when taking diltiazem with nitrates, he should space administration of the two drug doses.

Dipyridamole (p. 133)
1. (d) The only FDA-approved use for oral dipyridamole is as a platelet adhesion inhibitor.

2. (b) Given I.V. as part of a thallium scan in place of exercise, dipyridamole should be diluted to 40 ml and administered over 10 minutes.

3. (c) When administering I.V. dipyridamole, monitor the patient closely for hypotension.

Disopyramide phosphate (p. 136)
1. (d) Disopyramide is used to treat PVCs because it suppresses automaticity.

2. (c) Because of its anticholinergic effect, disopyramide must be used with caution or not at all in patients

with urine retention related to benign prostatic hyperplasia.

3. (b) The most common adverse reaction to disopyramide is dry mouth.

Dobutamine hydrochloride (p. 139)
1. (b) Peak concentrations of I.V. dobutamine occur within 10 minutes.

2. (b) Dobutamine increases myocardial contractility and stroke volume by stimulating beta$_1$-adrenergic receptors.

3. (a) Most patients respond to dobutamine with an increase in systolic blood pressure of 10 to 20 mm Hg.

Dopamine hydrochloride (p. 143)
1. (b) Administer dopamine through a large vein to prevent extravasation and local necrosis and tissue sloughing.

2. (c) If extravasation does occur, you should infiltrate the site with a phentolamine solution.

3. (b) Unless alpha-receptor stimulation and vasoconstriction is the desired response, decrease the infusion rate if the patient demonstrates a marked decrease in pulse pressure.

Enalaprilat and enalapril maleate (p. 146)
1. (b) The peak antihypertensive effect of enalapril given P.O. occurs within 4 to 6 hours.

2. (d) Enalapril should be administered without regard to meals.

3. (c) Enalapril may have to be discontinued if the patient experiences loss of taste.

Epinephrine hydrochloride (pp. 149 and 150)
1. (d) In cardiac arrest, if an I.V. site is not available, the next best administration route for epinephrine is intratracheal.

2. (a) While administering epinephrine I.V., you should monitor cardiac status continually and the patient's blood pressure repeatedly during the first 5 minutes and then q 3 to 5 minutes until stable.

3. (b) If epinephrine is administered by intracardiac injection, it will require external cardiac massage to move the drug into coronary circulation.

Esmolol (p. 153)
1. (d) To achieve an antiarrhythmic effect, administer esmolol I.V.

2. (b) During treatment with esmolol, monitor the patient's ECG and blood pressure.

3. (a) Following the initial loading dose and maintenance therapy, tachycardia should subside within 5 minutes.

Ethacrynate sodium and ethacrynic acid (pp. 156 and 157)
1. (c) Ethacrynic acid's diuretic action in the proximal part of the ascending loop of Henle promotes excretion of sodium, water, chloride, and potassium.

2. (d) When assessing patients taking ethacrynic acid, be particularly alert for hearing loss.

3. (a) The proper diluent for reconstituting ethacrynic acid is D_5W or 0.9% NaCl solution.

Flecainide acetate (pp. 159 and 160)
1. (a) When initiating therapy with flecainide, closely monitor the patient's heart rate and rhythm.

2. (d) Dosage increases of 50 mg should occur q 4 days.

3. (c) While awaiting full therapeutic effect, the patient may be maintained on I.V. lidocaine.

Fosinopril sodium (p. 162)
1. (c) Administration of an antacid should be separated by 2 hours from fosinopril.

2. (c) The antihypertensive effect of fosinopril usually lasts 24 hours.

3. (b) Adjust the dosage of fosinopril based on peak and trough blood pressures.

Furosemide (p. 166)
1. (b) Following oral administration of furosemide, expect diuresis to begin within 30 to 60 minutes.

2. (b) Furosemide is contraindicated in patients with oliguria or anuria.

3. (d) With rapid I.V. administration of furosemide, a possible adverse reaction is transient or permanent deafness.

Gemfibrozil (pp. 167 and 168)
1. (a) For optimal absorption, the patient should take gemfibrozil 30 minutes before breakfast and dinner.

2. (d) Advise the patient taking gemfibrozil to examine his bowel movements and to report changes, especially bulky, fatty stools.

3. (d) Because of the special risks that gemfibrozil poses, CBC and liver function tests should be monitored periodically during the first 12 months of therapy.

Heparin calcium, heparin sodium (p. 174)
1. (b) When administering heparin S.C. inject slowly, deep into S.C. fat.

2. (d) You should monitor the platelet count every 3 days to avoid "white clot" syndrome.

3. (a) If severe hemorrhaging occurs, treat the patient, as prescribed, with protamine sulfate.

Hydralazine hydrochloride (p. 177)
1. (c) Hydralazine's antihypertensive action occurs primarily because of its direct vasodilating action on arteries and arterioles.

2. (d) A common adverse effect of hydralazine is headache.

3. (c) You should teach patients to take their hydralazine with food to enhance absorption and minimize gastric irritation.

Hydrochlorothiazide (pp. 179 and 181)
1. (a) You should discuss with the doctor discontinuing hydrochlorothiazide if the patient develops signs of renal failure.

2. (d) Hydrochlorothiazide is most effective and causes the patient less lifestyle disruption when administered first thing in the morning.

3. (b) Hydrochlorothiazide shouldn't be used for patients with known hypersensitivity to sulfoanamides.

Isoproterenol (pp. 184 and 185)
1. (d) If the patient's heart rate exceeds 110 beats/minute while receiving I.V. isoproterenol, you should decrease the infusion rate.

2. (a) A common CNS adverse effect of isoproterenol that you would warn the patient about is headache.

3. (c) The primary cardiac use of isoproterenol is management of AV block.

Isosorbide dinitrate, isosorbide mononitrate (pp. 187 and 189)
1. (a) The onset of action of chewable isosorbide dinitrate is less than 5 minutes.

2. (d) Isosorbide's vasodilator action occurs primarily in capacitance vessels (veins and venules).

3. (b) You should advise your patient that he may initially experience headache when taking isosorbide.

Labetalol hydrochloride (p. 192)
1. (d) When labetalol is first administered I.V., you should monitor blood pressure closely (q 5 minutes for 30 minutes).

2. (a) The most troublesome adverse effect of labetalol is dizziness.

3. (b) Tachycardia is a sign of hypoglycemia that would not be evident in the diabetic patient taking labetalol.

Lidocaine hydrochloride (p. 196)
1. (c) Your 165-lb (75-kg) male patient is in ventricular fibrillation. According to current ACLS criteria, you would administer a lidocaine bolus of 112.5 mg.

2. (b) You would administer this bolus at the rate of 25 to 50 mg/minute.

3. (d) Your patient has been receiving lidocaine by continuous infusion at a rate of 2 mg/minute, and it's to be discontinued. You should shut off the lidocaine infusion.

Lisinopril (p. 199)
1. (a) Diuretics should be discontinued before starting lisinopril therapy.

2. (d) Common adverse effects of lisinopril include headache or dizziness.

3. (c) Quinapril produces the greatest decrease in peripheral vascular resistance.

Lovastatin (pp. 201 and 202)
1. (b) Lovastatin produces its anti-lipemic effect by inhibiting an enzyme that's an early step in synthesizing cholesterol.

2. (c) A life-threatening adverse effect of lovastatin is rhabdomyolysis.

3. (c) The patient should take lovastatin once daily with dinner.

Metaraminol bitartrate (p. 206)
1. (d) Before administering metaraminol, you should ask the patient if he's allergic to sulfites.

2. (b) While administering metaraminol, you should closely monitor the patient's blood pressure and watch for extravasation at the infusion site.

3. (c) A symptom that would alert you to an excessive metaraminol response (hypertension) is headache.

Methyldopa (p. 210)
1. (d) Administer I.V. methyldopa over a period of 30 to 60 minutes.

2. (d) A common distressing reaction for the patient taking methyldopa is impotence.

3. (c) Involuntary choreoathetoid movements might signal the need to discontinue I.V. methyldopa.

Metolazone (p. 213)
1. (b) Metolazone is contraindicated in patients with known sensitivity to sulfonamides.

2. (a) Metolazone should be administered in the morning to prevent nocturia.

3. (a) While taking metolazone, the patient may need to consume potassium-rich foods, such as tomatoes, dates, and apricots.

Metoprolol tartrate (p. 216)
1. (b) The maintenance dosage for oral metoprolol in hypertension is 100 to 450 mg daily.

2. (d) To enhance absorption of oral metoprolol, you would give the drug with meals.

3. (c) Your diabetic patient receiving metoprolol is at risk for insulin-induced hypoglycemia, so you teach her to watch for dizziness, headache, and mental status changes.

Mexiletine hydrochloride (p. 218)
1. (b) Mexiletine is structurally similar to lidocaine.

2. (c) Mexiletine should be administered with food or an antacid to limit nausea.

3. (a) An early sign of mexiletine toxicity is a fine hand tremor.

Milrinone lactate (pp. 220 and 221)
1. (c) A common adverse reaction to assess for when administering milrinone is ventricular ectopic activity.

2. (b) Milrinone is classified pharmacologically as an inotropic and vasodilating agent.

3. (c) Milrinone is administered I.V. as a bolus followed by a continuous infusion.

Moricizine hydrochloride (p. 223)
1. (d) Moricizine is classified pharmacologically as a sodium channel blocker.

2. (a.) A common adverse effect of moricizine is dizziness.

3. (d) Moricizine should be used to treat only life-threatening ventricular arrhythmias.

Morphine sulfate (p. 225)
1. (d) Morphine proves effective in treating pain from acute MI because it produces analgesia and reduces afterload.

2. (c) A common adverse reaction to assess for when administering morphine is hypotension.

3. (d) Morphine achieves its peak analgesic effect 30 to 60 minutes after administration.

Nadolol (pp. 227 and 228)
1. (b) Bronchospasm is a life-threatening adverse reaction to nadolol.

2. (d) Reduced dosage of nadolol may be required in patients with renal impairment.

3. (d) Nadolol should be administered with or without food.

Nicardipine hydrochloride (p. 230)
1. (c) Nicardipine is classified pharmacologically as a calcium channel blocker.

2. (d) Nicardipine dosage should be reduced in patients with hepatic or renal impairment.

3. (a) When using the immediate-release form of nicardipine, the maximum blood pressure effect will occur in about 1 hour.

Nifedipine (pp. 232 and 233)
1. (d) If a patient develops angina during titration of his nifedipine dosage, the appropriate response should be to administer sublingual nitroglycerin.

2. (c) One of the common adverse reactions to nifedipine is dizziness.

3. (a) When nifedipine is given sublingually, 20% or less of it reaches systemic circulation.

Nitroglycerin (p. 239)
1. (c) If your patient develops tolerance to his nitroglycerin, manage it best by allowing an 8-hour nitrate-free interval daily.

2. (a) When taking the transmucosal form of nitroglycerin, the patient should place the tablet under his upper lip or in the buccal pouch and allow it to dissolve.

3. (b) If your patient is using nitroglycerin aerosol spray, you would teach him to release the spray onto his tongue.

Nitroprusside sodium (pp. 242 and 243)

1. (b) When preparing nitroprusside, you should protect the I.V. container from light with foil wrap.

2. (a) While administering nitroprusside, you should monitor the patient's blood pressure q 5 minutes at the start of the infusion and then q 15 minutes for the duration.

3. (c) Concerned that your patient receiving nitroprusside may develop cyanide toxicity, you assess for dyspnea, ataxia, and vomiting.

Norepinephrine bitartrate (p. 246)

1. (c) The recommended dilution for norepinephrine is 4 mg to 1,000 ml of D_5W to equal 4 mcg/ml.

2. (d) To check for extravasation of norepinephrine, you would assess the site for blanching along the course of the infused vein.

3. (c) When administering norepinephrine, you monitor blood pressure q 2 minutes until stabilized and then q 5 minutes.

Pentoxifylline (pp. 247 and 248)

1. (b) Pentoxifylline increases capillary blood flow by increasing erythrocyte flexibility.

2. (c) Pentoxifylline should be taken with meals to reduce GI distress.

3. (d) If GI or CNS adverse reactions occur in a patient taking pentoxifylline, change the frequency to b.i.d.

Phenoxybenzamine hydrochloride (p. 251)

1. (a) Phenoxybenzamine is pharmacologically classified as an alpha-adrenergic blocker.

2. (c) Common adverse effects of phenoxybenzamine includes impotence and ejaculation inhibition.

3. (d) If your patient experiences nasal stuffiness while taking phenoxybenzamine, you would tell him it will probably subside as he continues therapy.

Phentolamine mesylate (p. 254)

1. (d) Phentolamine is classified pharmacologically as an alpha-adrenergic blocking agent.

2. (b) The plasma half-life of phentolamine after I.V. injection is 19 minutes.

3. (c) To prevent extravasation sloughing from I.V. norepinephrine, phentolamine may be added to the norepinephrine infusion (10 mg/liter).

Phenylephrine hydrochloride (pp. 257 and 258)

1. (a) When administering phenylephrine I.V., you should monitor the patient's blood pressure, pulse rate, and CVP q 2 to 5 minutes.

2. (a) In a previously normotensive patient receiving phenylephrine, you aim to maintain systolic blood pressure at 80 to 100 mm Hg.

3. (d) When discontinuing a phenyl-ephrine infusion, you should withdraw the drug gradually, monitoring blood pressure and patient response.

Phenytoin (pp. 261 and 262)
1. (c) Your patient has a peripheral I.V. of D_5W. To administer I.V. phenytoin, you should first clear the line with 0.9% NaCl solution.

2. (d) Warn the patient that phenytoin may turn his urine pink, red, or reddish brown.

3. (a) Phenytoin's CV use is to treat ventricular arrhythmias unresponsive to lidocaine or procainamide.

Pravastatin sodium (p. 265)
1. (c) Pravastatin is therapeutically classified as an antilipemic.

2. (d) The patient should take pravastatin h.s.

3. (d) You should advise the patient receiving pravastatin to restrict his intake of alcoholic beverages.

Prazosin hydrochloride (p. 269)
1. (b) Prazosin is excreted primarily in feces.

2. (a) A common adverse reaction to prazosin is dizziness.

3. (d) Prazosin should be administered h.s.

Probucol (pp. 271 and 272)
1. (c) You should administer probucol with meals to enhance drug absorption.

2. (b) A common adverse reaction to probucol is hyperhidrosis.

3. (b) Because of persistent drug levels, six months should elapse between discontinuation of probucol therapy and attempts to become pregnant.

Procainamide hydrochloride (p. 276)
1. (b) For life-threatening arrhythmias, the initial dose of procainamide should be administered by slow I.V. push, no more than 50 mg/minute.

2. (b) When giving the extended-release tablet form, be aware and warn the patient that a wax-matrix capsule may appear in his stools; however, the drug has been absorbed.

3. (a) An extremely common adverse reaction to procainamide is an increased ANA titer.

Propafenone hydrochloride (p. 279)
1. (c) Propafenone is pharmacologically classified as a sodium channel blocker.

2. (a) Common adverse reactions to propafenone include nausea and vomiting.

3. (b) Propafenone should be administered with food to minimize adverse GI reactions.

Propranolol (p. 283)
1. (c) Elderly patients require lower dosing with propranolol.

2. (c) You administer propranolol with meals to enhance absorption.

3. (d) Your diabetic patient is taking propranolol, which can mask beta-adrenergic signs of hypoglycemia. Rapid heart rate is a hypoglycemic indicator, which may not be present as a clue for the patient.

Quinidine (p. 288)
1. (c) Quinidine is used to treat atrial and ventricular tachyarrhythmias.

2. (b) Oral quinidine preparations should generally be administered with meals to reduce GI symptoms.

3. (d) Check serum quinidine levels for possible toxicity if your patient develops diarrhea.

Reserpine (p. 291)
1. (b) Reserpine is an antihypertensive agent that's classified pharmacologically as an anti-adrenergic agent.

2. (d) Common adverse reactions to reserpine include dry mouth and nasal stuffiness.

3. (b) Drowsiness and dizziness are common adverse reactions in early reserpine therapy.

Simvastatin (pp. 293 and 294)
1. (d) Administer simvastatin in the evening.

2. (c) Laboratory findings in simvastatin toxicity include marked, persistent serum transaminase level elevations.

3. (b) Patients taking simvastatin should be cautioned to avoid alcohol intake.

Sotalol (pp. 297 and 298)
1. (d) A common adverse reaction to sotalol is dyspnea.

2. (b) Administer sotalol consistently, either with or without food.

3. (c) Upon initiation and dosage adjustment of sotalol, you would closely monitor ECG waveforms (QT interval).

Spironolactone (p. 301)
1. (c) Spironolactone is a diuretic that's further classified as potassium sparing.

2. (b) Gynecomastia is the adverse reaction to spironolactone that may not disappear after the drug is withdrawn.

3. (c) The maximum antihypertensive response to spironolactone can be expected to occur within 3 to 4 days.

Streptokinase (p. 305)
1. (a) Before initiating streptokinase therapy, you should determine APTT, PT, and thrombin time.

2. (d) If your patient receiving streptokinase develops a fever above 104° F (40° C), you should treat it with acetaminophen.

3. (a) If major bleeding occurs while the patient is receiving streptokinase, you should discontinue therapy.

Timolol maleate (p. 307)
1. (d) Patients with hepatic or renal impairment may require adjustment of timolol dosage.

2. (d) Because timolol masks beta-adrenergic signs of hypoglycemia in the diabetic patient, you should monitor for restlessness.

3. (c) If your patient's timolol therapy is to be discontinued, the drug should be withdrawn over a period of 1 to 2 weeks.

Tocainide hydrochloride (p. 310)
1. (b) Tocainide is an amide antiarrhythmic and may be used to ease transition from lidocaine to oral antiarrhythmic therapy.

2. (c) Tremors are an early sign of tocainide toxicity.

3. (c) A patient who is given tocainide at the same time he is receiving lidocaine may experience CNS toxicity.

Torsemide (p. 313)
1. (d) Torsemide is pharmacologically classified as a loop diuretic.

2. (a) Torsemide's advantage over other drugs in its class may be that it is less potassium wasting.

3. (b) You watch for ototoxicity when giving torsemide at high doses or with rapid I.V. administration.

Triamterene (pp. 314 to 316)
1. (c) Triamterene should be administered p.c. to prevent nausea.

2. (a) When initiating triamterene therapy, while adjusting dosage, and periodically throughout therapy, you should monitor blood pressure and BUN and serum electrolyte levels.

3. (d) If the patient's folic acid level falls, he is at risk for megaloblastic anemia.

Verapamil hydrochloride (p. 321)
1. (d) When administering I.V. verapamil, give it over at least 3 minutes.

2. (b) Throughout administration of I.V. verapamil, you should continuously monitor the ECG.

3. (c) An ongoing common adverse reaction of verapamil is constipation.

Warfarin sodium (p. 325)
1. (c) Warfarin should be administered at the same time each day.

2. (d) A high incidence of serious bleeding is related to a PT exceeding 3 times the control value.

3. (b) Warfarin's effect can be neutralized by using phytonadione.

Index

G
gemfibrozil, 166-168
    patient teaching for, 168

H
Heart failure, 21-22
Hepalean, 169
Heparin, 169-174
    administration guidelines for, 171
    combinations to avoid with, 172
    patient teaching for, 173
Hydopa, 206
hydralazine hydrochloride, 174-177
    patient teaching for, 176
hydrochlorothiazide, 177-181
    patient teaching for, 180
HydroDIURIL, 177
Hyperetic, 177
Hyperlipidemia, 22-23
Hyperstat I.V., 116
Hypertension, 23-24
Hypertensive crisis, 24-25
Hypertrophic cardiomyopathy, 25-26
Hypovolemic shock, 26-27
Hytrin, 266

I
Idiopathic hypertrophic subaortic stenosis, 25-26
Idioventricular rhythm, 27
Inderal, 280
Inderal LA, 280
Inocor, 78
Inocor Lactate Injection 78
Intra-aortic balloon pump, 17
Intrinsic sympathomimetic activity, 61
Intropin, 139
Ipran, 280
Ismo, 185
Iso-Bid, 185
Isonate, 185
isoproterenol, 181-185
    multidrug therapy hazards with, 183t
    patient teaching for, 184
Isoptin, 316
Isoptin SR, 316
Isorbid, 185
Isordil, 185
isosorbide dinitrate, 185-189
    multidrug therapy hazards with, 187t
    patient teaching for, 188
isosorbide mononitrate, 185-189
    multidrug therapy hazards with, 187t
    patient teaching for, 188
isradipine, 231
Isuprel, 181

J
Junctional rhythm, 27-28
Junctional tachycardia, 28

K
Kabikinase, 301
Kerlone, 91
Kinidin Durules, 284

L
labetalol hydrochloride, 189-192
    changing dos
    combinations
    patient teach
Lanoxicaps, 118
Lanoxin, 118
Laser surgery,
Lasix, 162
Lasix Special,
L-caine, 192
Levatol, 61
Levophed, 243
lidocaine hydrochloride
    I.V. adminis
    multidrug therapy hazards with, 195t
Lidoject, 192
Lido Pen Auto-Injector, 192
Liquaemin Sodium, 169
lisinopril, 196-199
    multidrug therapy hazards with, 199t
Loop diuretics, patient teaching for, 98
Lopid, 166
Lopresor, 213
Lopresor SR, 213
Lopressor, 213
Lorelco, 269
Lotensin, 85
lovastatin, 199-202
    multidrug therapy hazards with, 201t
    patient teaching for, 202
Lown-Ganong-Levine syndrome, 29
Lumbar sympathectomy, 6
Lurselle, 269

M
metaraminol bitartrate, 202-206
    combinations to avoid with, 205
    multidrug therapy hazards with, 204t
methyldopa, 206-210
    patient teaching for, 209
metolazone, 210-213
    patient teaching for, 212
metoprolol tartrate, 213-216
Mevacor, 199
mexiletine hydrochloride, 216-218
Mexitil, 216